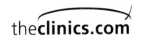

ANESTHESIOLOGY CLINICS

Obstetric Anesthesia

GUEST EDITOR
Gurinder M. Vasdev, MD

CONSULTING EDITOR
Lee A. Fleisher, MD

March 2008 • Volume 26 • Number 1

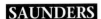

An Imprint of Elsevier, Inc.
PHILADELPHIA   LONDON   TORONTO   MONTREAL   SYDNEY   TOKYO

W.B. SAUNDERS COMPANY
A Division of Elsevier Inc.

1600 John F. Kennedy Boulevard, Suite 1800 • Philadelphia, Pennsylvania 19103-2899

http://www.theclinics.com

ANESTHESIOLOGY CLINICS　　　　　　　　　　　　　Volume 26, Number 1
March 2008　　　　　　　　　　　　　　　　　　　　　　　ISSN 1932-2275
Editor: Rachel Glover　　　　　　　　　　　　　ISBN-13: 978-1-4160-6062-8
　　　　　　　　　　　　　　　　　　　　　　　　　　ISBN-10: 1-4160-6062-6

The ideas and opinions expressed in *Anesthesiology Clinics* do not necessarily reflect those of the Publisher. The Publisher does not assume any responsibility for any injury and/or damage to persons or property arising out of or related to any use of the material contained in this periodical. The reader is advised to check the appropriate medical literature and the product information currently provided by the manufacturer of each drug to be administered to verify the dosage, the method and duration of administration, or contraindications. It is the responsibility of the treating physician or other health care professional, relying on independent experience and knowledge of the patient, to determine drug dosages and the best treatment for the patient. Mention of any product in this issue should not be construed as endorsement by the contributors, editors, or the Publisher of the product or manufacturers' claims.

Anesthesiology Clinics (ISSN 1932-2275) is published quarterly by Elsevier Inc., 360 Park Avenue South, New York, NY 10010-1710. Months of issue are March, June, September, and December. Business and Editorial Offices: 1600 John F. Kennedy Blvd., Suite 1800, Philadelphia, PA 19103-2899. Customer Service Office: 6277 Sea Harbor Drive, Orlando, FL 32887-4800. Periodicals postage paid at New York, NY and additional mailing offices. Subscription prices are $111.00 per year (US student/resident), $222.00 per year (US individuals), $271.00 per year (Canadian individuals), $332.00 per year (US institutions), $403.00 per year (Canadian institutions), $147.00 per year (Canadian and foreign student/resident), $289.00 per year (foreign individuals), and $403.00 per year (foreign institutions). To receive student and resident rate, orders must be accompanied by name of affiliated institution, date of term, and the *signature* of program/residency coordinator on institutions letterhead. Orders will be billed at individual rate until proof of status is received. Foreign air speed delivery is included in all *Clinics'* subscription prices. All prices are subject to change without notice. POSTMASTER: Send address changes to *Anesthesiology Clinics*, Elsevier Periodicals Customer Service, 6277 Sea Harbor Drive, Orlando, FL 32887-4800. Customer Service: 1-800-654-2452 (US). From outside the United States, call 1-407-563-6020. Fax: 1-407-363-9661. E-mail: JournalsCustomerService-usa@elsevier.com.

Anesthesiology Clinics, is also published in Spanish by McGraw-Hill Inter-americana Editores S. A., P.O. Box 5-237, 06500 Mexico D. F., Mexico.

Anesthesiology Clinics, is covered in *Index Medicus, Current Contents/Clinical Medicine, Excerpta Medica, ISI/BIOMED*, and *Chemical Abstracts*.

Printed in the United States of America.

CONSULTING EDITOR

LEE A. FLEISHER, MD, Robert D. Dripps Professor of Medicine; Chair, Anesthesiology and Critical Care, University of Pennsylvania School of Medicine, Philadelphia, Pennsylvania

GUEST EDITOR

GURINDER M. VASDEV, MD, President, Society of Obstetric Anesthesia and Perinatology; Assistant Professor of Anesthesiology, Department of Anesthesiology, Mayo Clinic College of Medicine, Rochester, Minnesota

CONTRIBUTORS

DOUGLAS R. BACON, MD, MA, Professor of Anesthesiology and History of Medicine, Department of Anesthesiology, College of Medicine, Mayo Clinic, Rochester, Minnesota

DAVID J. BIRNBACH, MD, MPH, Professor; Director, University of Miami-Jackson Memorial Hospital Center for Patient Safety, Miller School of Medicine, University of Miami, Miami, Florida

JOSE CARLOS ALMEIDA CARVALHO, MD, PhD, FANZCA, FRCPC, Associate Professor of Anesthesia and Obstetrics and Gynecology, University of Toronto; Director of Obstetric Anesthesia, Mount Sinai Hospital, Toronto, Ontario, Canada

PAULA A. CRAIGO, MD, Department of Anesthesiology, Mayo Clinic, Rochester, Minnesota

JOANNE DOUGLAS, MD, FRCPC, Clinical Professor, Department of Anesthesiology, Pharmacology and Therapeutics, University of British Columbia; BC Women's Hospital and Health Centre, Vancouver, BC, Canada

ROSHAN FERNANDO, MB BCh, FRCA, Consultant Anaesthetist; Honorary Senior Lecturer, University College Hospital, London, United Kingdom

ERIC GOLDSZMIDT, MD, FRCPC, Assistant Professor of Anesthesia, University of Toronto; Staff Anesthesiologist, Department of Anesthesia and Pain Management, Mount Sinai Hospital, Toronto, Ontario, Canada

RACHEL HIGNETT, MA, MB BChir, MRCP, FRCA, Consultant Anaesthetist, The Royal Infirmary of Edinburgh, Little France Crescent, Edinburgh, United Kingdom

DAVID HILL, MD, FCARCSI, Dip Pain Med RCSI, Honorary Senior Lecturer, Queen's University, Department of Anaesthesia, Ulster Hospital, Belfast, United Kingdom

TERESE T. HORLOCKER, MD, Professor of Anesthesiology and Orthopedics, Department of Anesthesiology, Mayo Graduate School of Medicine, Rochester, Minnesota

SANDRA L. KOPP, MD, Assistant Professor of Anesthesiology, Department of Anesthesiology, Mayo Graduate School of Medicine, Rochester, Minnesota

RUTH LANDAU, MD, PD, Service d'Anesthésiologie, Département APSI, Hôpitaux Universitaires de Genève, Switzerland

FREDERIC J. MERCIER, MD, PhD, Department of Anesthesia and Intensive Care, Hopital Antoine Beclere—APHP and Universite Paris-Sud, Clamart Cedex, France

JASON REIDY, MBBS, FRCA, Fellow, Department of Anesthesiology, Pharmacology and Therapeutics, University of British Columbia; BC Women's Hospital and Health Centre, Vancouver, BC, Canada

FELICITY REYNOLDS, MB BS, MD, FRCA, FRCOG ad eudem, Emeritus Professor of Obstetric Anaesthesia, St Thomas's Hospital, London, United Kingdom

EDUARDO SALAS, PhD, Professor; Trustee Chair, Department of Psychology, and Institute for Simulation and Training, University of Central Florida, Orlando, Florida

MAYA S. SURESH, MD, Professor of Anesthesiology; Interim Chairman, Department of Anesthesiology, Baylor College of Medicine, Faculty Center, Houston, Texas

LAURENCE C. TORSHER, MD, FRCPC, Department of Anesthesiology, Mayo Clinic, Rochester, Minnesota

MARC VAN DE VELDE, MD, PhD, Department of Anaesthesiology, University Hospitals Gasthuisberg, Katholieke Universiteit Leuven, Leuven, Belgium

ASHUTOSH WALI, MD, FFARCSI, Associate Professor, Department of Anesthesiology, Baylor College of Medicine, Faculty Center, Houston, Texas

CONTENTS

Foreword   xi
Lee A. Fleisher

Preface   xiii
Gurinder M. Vasdev

Anticoagulation in Pregnancy and Neuraxial Blocks   1
Sandra L. Kopp and Terese T. Horlocker

> The peripartum management of the anticoagulated parturient
> represents a significant clinical challenge to both the obstetrician
> and the anesthesiologist. This review discusses the causes of
> thrombosis in the pregnant population, the anticoagulants used for
> prophylaxis, and treatment of these disorders, along with
> recommendations for neuraxial blockade in parturients who
> receive peripartum anticoagulation.

Neurological Infections After Neuraxial Anesthesia   23
Felicity Reynolds

> Infection is the commonest cause of serious neurologic sequelae of
> neuraxial anesthesia. The incidence depends on operator skill and
> patient population. Meningitis, a complication of dural puncture, is
> usually caused by viridans streptococci. The risk factors are dural
> puncture during labor, no mask and poor aseptic technique,
> vaginal infection and bacteremia. Epidural abscess is a complica-
> tion of epidural catheterization, route of entry the catheter track
> and the organism usually the staphylococcus. Principal risk factors
> are prolonged catheterization, poor aseptic technique and trau-
> matic insertion. Prevention includes wearing a mask, using a full
> sterile technique, avoiding prolonged catheterization and prescrib-
> ing antibiotics in a high-risk situation.

Major Obstetric Hemorrhage

53

Frederic J. Mercier and Marc Van de Velde

Major obstetric hemorrhage remains the leading cause of maternal mortality and morbidity worldwide, and is associated with a high rate of substandard care. A well-defined and multidisciplinary approach that aims to act quickly and avoid omissions or conflicting strategies is key. The most common etiologies of hemorrhage are abruptio placenta, placenta previa/accreta, uterine rupture in the antepartum period and retained placenta, uterine atony, and genital-tract trauma in the postpartum period. Basic treatment of postpartum hemorrhage relies on manual removal of the placenta or manual exploration of the uterus plus bladder emptying and oxytocin administration. If this does not arrest bleeding, or if there is any suspicion of genital-tract trauma, examination of the vagina and cervix with appropriate valves and analgesia/anesthesia must follow quickly. Postpartum uterine atony resistant to oxytocin must be treated with prostaglandin within 15 to 30 minutes; uterine balloon tamponade can be also useful at this stage. Aggressive transfusion therapy and resuscitation are mandatory in major obstetric hemorrhage. Specific invasive treatment must be considered within no more than 30 to 60 minutes, if previous measures have failed—and even earlier in some particular etiologies. The two main options are radiologic embolization and surgical artery ligations. Recombinant factor VIIa may also be considered, but should not delay the performance of a life-saving procedure such as embolization or surgery. Hysterectomy must be implemented when all other interventions have failed.

The Historical Narrative: Tales of Professionalism?

67

Douglas R. Bacon

The historical narrative is a story told to illustrate a point, however subconsciously. The "giants" of obstetric anesthesia—Simpson, Snow, Apgar—and countless other less well-known physicians all contributed to the history of obstetric anesthesia. We remember them by retelling this history to illustrate elements of professionalism and how we as a profession wish to act. The Physician Charter is an excellent first approximation of a workable definition of this quality, which can and does change over time. By using the three principles and 10 professional responsibilities as a template, the past comes alive as a teaching method to each and every obstetric anesthesiologist.

Vasopressors in Obstetrics

75

Jason Reidy and Joanne Douglas

Hypotension is a common, treatable side effect of neuraxial anesthesia, which has significant side effects for the mother and demonstrable biochemical effects in the fetus. It is clear that a shift in management of hypotension in the obstetric population is in order, but we can only speculate on the benefits for the compromised fetus due to the lack of available information in that patient population.

Obstetric Anesthesia: Outside the Labor and Delivery Unit

89

Paula A. Craigo and Laurence C. Torsher

The maternal mortality rate in the United States has stagnated for the past 2 decades. To further lower morbidity and mortality, we must take a broader perspective. When a pregnant woman is treated in a nonobstetric part of the hospital, care must adapt quickly to her special needs. Excessive concern as to medication, radiation, and litigation may render her care neither safe, timely, efficient, effective, nor patient-centered. Anesthesiologists can significantly improve the care of the pregnant patient by applying their uniquely broad-based skills, experience, and knowledge outside the labor unit.

Principles and Practices of Obstetric Airway Management

109

Eric Goldszmidt

Although maternal mortality resulting from anesthesia is declining, airway causes predominate. Although there are many physiologic and nonphysiologic factors that contribute to potential difficulties when intubating parturients, whether or not the maternal airway is more difficult anatomically continues to be debatable. What is more certain, however, is that the situation is more complex than other settings. Vigilance, avoidance, and preparation continue to be key to management. In cases of unexpected difficulty, which likely are unavoidable, several rescue devices may be helpful.

Anesthesia for the Pregnant HIV Patient

127

Rachel Hignett and Roshan Fernando

Numbers of HIV-infected individuals across the globe are increasing, as is the proportion of women infected with HIV. However, better understanding of the HIV virus, and rapidly evolving treatments has provided hope for millions of people world-wide. In the pregnant population, recent understanding of factors influencing vertical transmission has enabled dramatic reductions in mother-to-child transmission. The anesthesiologist is likely to encounter HIV-infected parturients in the delivery suite as part of routine practice, and should be aware of the current trends in obstetric—as well as anesthetic—best practice and management.

Ultrasound-Facilitated Epidurals and Spinals in Obstetrics

145

Jose Carlos Almeida Carvalho

Regional anesthesia is currently the gold standard of practice for pain control in obstetrics. Failures and complications of regional anesthesia can be related to many causes, one of the most important being the blind nature of such techniques. The practice of epidurals and spinals relies primarily on the palpation of anatomic landmarks that are not always easy to find. Ultrasound has recently been introduced into clinical anesthesia to facilitate lumbar spinals and epidurals. The use of preprocedure ultrasound imaging or, eventually, real-time ultrasound guidance should improve not only clinical practice, but also teaching. This article describes the techniques, challenges, and benefits related to the use of ultrasound in guiding lumbar spinals and epidurals.

Can Medical Simulation and Team Training Reduce Errors in Labor and Delivery? 159
David J. Birnbach and Eduardo Salas

Patient safety is one of the most pressing challenges in health care today, and there is no question that medical errors occur and that patients are worried about them. Currently, there is a belief that the availability of medical simulations and the knowledge gained from the science of team training may improve patient outcomes, and there is a paradigm shift occurring in many universities and training programs. This article discusses two strategies that, when combined, may reduce medical error in the labor and delivery suite: team training and medical simulation.

The Use of Remifentanil in Obstetrics 169
David Hill

Remifentanil has been proposed as the most suitable systemic opioid for use in obstetrics. Although the onset and offset are rapid, it cannot achieve maximum effect within the time period of a single uterine contraction. Nevertheless, it provides worthwhile analgesia mainly for the first stage of labor with consistently high maternal satisfaction. Maternal oxygen desaturation limits the dose and suitable monitoring during use is advised. As an adjunct to general anesthesia, it is successful in blunting responses to airway manipulation and providing hemodynamic stability in high-risk women. Neonatal effects when used in labor are minimal, but when combined with general anesthesia neonatal depression is unpredictable and more likely with an infusion dose greater than 0.1 µg/kg/min.

Pharmacogenetics and Obstetric Anesthesia 183
Ruth Landau

The ultimate goal of pharmacogenetics research is to help doctors tailor doses of medicines to a person's unique genetic make-up, making medicines safer and more effective for everyone. Although there still are no guidelines and immediate clinical implications for practitioners providing analgesia or anesthesia, it is essential to realize that trial-and-error pharmacotherapy and one-size-fits-all dogmas are bound to die. This review briefly outlines the genetic variability of pharmacokinetics and pharmacodynamics and discusses selected fields relevant to obstetric anesthesiologists for whom the challenges of translating pharmacogenetics to clinical practice hopefully are on their way.

Maternal Morbidity, Mortality, and Risk Assessment 197
Ashutosh Wali and Maya S. Suresh

Maternal deaths in developed countries continue to decline and are rare. Maternal mortality statistics are essentially similar in the United States and United Kingdom. However, the situation is completely different in developing countries, where maternal mortality exceeds 0.5 million every year. This article not only assesses morbidity risks in some of the leading causes of maternal death but also highlights strategies to minimize the risks and to prevent maternal morbidity and mortality.

Index 231

FORTHCOMING ISSUES

June 2008
  Thoracic Anesthesia
  Peter D. Slinger, MD, *Guest Editor*

September 2008
  Cardiac Anesthesia: Today and Tomorrow
  Davy Cheng, MD, *Guest Editor*

December 2008
  Value-Based Anesthesia
  Alex Macario, MD, MBA, *Guest Editor*

RECENT ISSUES

December 2007
  Pain Management
  Howard S. Smith, MD, *Guest Editor*

September 2007
  Neurosurgical Anesthesia and Critical Care
  Ansgar M Brambrink, MD, PhD,
  and Jeffrey R. Kirsch, MD, *Guest Editors*

June 2007
  New Vistas in Patient Safety and Simulation
  W. Andrew Kofke, MD, MBA, FCCM, and
  Vinay M. Nadkarni, MD, *Guest Editors*

ELSEVIER
SAUNDERS

Anesthesiology Clin
26 (2008) xi

ANESTHESIOLOGY
CLINICS

Foreword

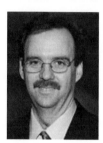

Lee A. Fleisher, MD
Consulting Editor

It is hard to imagine an area of anesthesia that has been a mainstay of practice like that of obstetric anesthesia. Many practiced as they were trained in their residency, focusing on the provision of labor analgesia and anesthesia for cesarean sections. Yet in trying to continue the tradition of looking forward and providing state-of-the-art reviews, this issue of obstetrical anesthesia has addressed modern treatment of many difficult anesthesia problems, as well as new areas including pharmacogenetics and the use of medical simulation and remifentanil.

In trying to choose a consulting editor for this issue of *Anesthesiology Clinics*, Gurinder Vasdev quickly came to mind. He is currently assistant professor of Anesthesiology at the College of Medicine at the Mayo Clinic and a consultant in the department. Having been educated in the United Kingdom, he completed his fellowship in obstetric anesthesia at the Mayo Clinic. Importantly, he has been an active member of the Society of Obstetric Anesthesia and Perinatology and is currently president of that subspecialty society. He has assembled an outstanding group of authors, and I hope you will learn as much as I did about the changing face of obstetric anesthesia.

Lee. A. Fleisher, MD
Anesthesiology and Critical Care
University of Pennsylvania
6 Dulles, 3400 Spruce Street
Philadelphia, PA 19104, USA

E-mail address: fleishel@uphs.upenn.edu

1932-2275/08/$ - see front matter © 2008 Elsevier Inc. All rights reserved.
doi:10.1016/j.anclin.2008.02.001

ELSEVIER
SAUNDERS

Anesthesiology Clin
26 (2008) xiii

ANESTHESIOLOGY
CLINICS

Preface

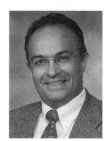

Gurinder M. Vasdev, MD
Guest Editor

The roots of modern anesthesia practice can be traced to the pioneering work of John Snow and his administration of chloroform to Queen Victoria as she gave birth to Prince Leopold in 1853. Thus, obstetrical anesthesia has been at the forefront of innovation since the beginnings of our specialty. In keeping with this forward-looking tradition, obstetric anesthesia continues to evolve and serve as a leader in scientific investigation, patient safety, and clinical excellence. It is no longer "just about epidurals." Today, obstetric anesthesiologists are involved in a large variety of activities which epitomize the best in our profession. These range from cutting-edge genomics research to extending our clinical duties beyond the labor floor. This professionalism has been exemplified in this issue of *Anesthesiology Clinics.*

I hope you enjoy these articles and agree that we are, indeed, a very broad-based specialty.

My sincere thanks to all the contributing authors; Rachel Glover; Janet Henderson; and my family, Billie, Amrit, Ranveer, and Tanveer, for their timely support and endurance during this project.

Gurinder M. Vasdev, MD
Department of Anesthesiology
Mayo Clinic College of Medicine
200 First Street SW
Rochester, MN 55905, USA

E-mail address: vasdev.gurinder@mayo.edu

ANESTHESIOLOGY
CLINICS

Anesthesiology Clin
26 (2008) 1–22

Anticoagulation in Pregnancy and Neuraxial Blocks

Sandra L. Kopp, MD*, Terese T. Horlocker, MD

*Department of Anesthesiology, Mayo Graduate School of Medicine,
200 First Street SW, Rochester, MN 55905, USA*

The peripartum management of the anticoagulated parturient represents a significant clinical challenge to both the obstetrician and the anesthesiologist. This review discusses the causes of thrombosis in the pregnant population, the anticoagulants used for prophylaxis, and treatment of these disorders, along with recommendations for neuraxial blockade in parturients who receive peripartum anticoagulation.

Normal pregnancy is a well-established risk factor for venous thromboembolism (VTE), which includes superficial and deep thrombophlebitis, pulmonary embolus, septic pelvic thrombophlebitis, and thrombosis. All three components of Virchow's triad (venous stasis, endothelial damage, and a hypercoagulable state) are present during normal pregnancy. "Venous stasis" results from decreased venous tone, obstruction of venous outflow by the enlarged uterus, and possibly decreased mobility. "Endothelial damage" of the pelvic veins can occur from venous hypertension or as a result of delivery. The "hypercoagulable state" is caused by increased levels of procoagulant factors VII, VIII, X, von Willebrand factor, and a pronounced increase in fibrinogen. There also is an acquired resistance to activated protein C, a decrease in protein S levels, and impaired fibrinolysis during pregnancy. These changes in the coagulation system begin with conception, do not return to baseline until approximately 8 weeks postpartum [1], and most likely evolved as a mechanism to protect women from hemorrhage during childbirth or miscarriage.

Incidence and timing of thrombosis

Despite decreased maternal mortality over the last 70 years, pulmonary embolism (PE) continues to be one of the most common causes of maternal

---

* Corresponding author.
E-mail address: kopp.sandra@mayo.edu (S.L. Kopp).

doi:10.1016/j.anclin.2007.12.002   *anesthesiology.theclinics.com*

death in both the United States and the United Kingdom [2]. The age-adjusted incidence of VTE ranges from 5 to 50 times higher in pregnant versus nonpregnant women [3]. Interestingly, in pregnant women, 90% of deep venous thrombosis (DVT) presents on the left side, compared with only 55% in the nonpregnant patient. This is likely caused by increased venous stasis in the left leg caused by compression of the left iliac vein by the right iliac artery as well as compression of the inferior vena cava by the gravid uterus [4]. More than 70% of gestational DVT develops in the ileo-femoral area compared with only 9% in the nonpregnant woman, where DVT in the calf is more common. This puts the pregnant patient at much higher risk, because ileo-femoral DVT is more likely to embolize and cause a pulmonary embolus [4].

Common risk factors that increase the incidence of thrombosis in pregnant women include increasing age, prolonged immobilization, obesity, thrombophilia, previous thromboembolism, and cesarean delivery. The puerperium, defined as the 6-week period after delivery, is associated with a higher rate of thrombosis than that associated with pregnancy itself [4]. A recent review found the relative risk for VTE among pregnant or postpartum women to be 4.29 (95% CI, 3.49 to 5.22; $P < .001$), and the overall incidence of VTE (absolute risk) was 199.7 per 100,000 woman-years in this patient population. The annual incidence was 5 times higher among postpartum women than pregnant women (511.2 versus 95.8 per 100,000). PE was also much more common in the postpartum period than during pregnancy (159.7 versus 10.6 per 100,000), and the overall incidence of VTE and PE was highest in the first postpartum week and steadily declined until returning to baseline at approximately 8 weeks postpartum [2].

Thrombophilias

"Thrombophilia" is the propensity of thrombosis (blood clots) to develop because of an abnormality in the system of coagulation. Inherited and acquired thrombophilias are a varied group of conditions that have been implicated in multiple pregnancy-related complications. There is evidence that thrombophilias may play a role in recurrent miscarriages, late fetal loss, abruptio placentae, preeclampsia, and intrauterine growth restriction (IUGR) as well as increased incidence of VTE [5,6]. The first manifestation of a woman's underlying thrombophilia may be a VTE during pregnancy. In at least 50% of the cases of VTE during pregnancy, one or more acquired or inherited thrombophilias are identified [4]. The two most common inherited thrombophilias are Factor V Leiden and the prothrombin gene mutation G20210A, and when these two defects are present in the same patient, the incidence of VTE is increased significantly with an odds ratio of 107 [4]. Other more rare inherited disorders include deficiencies of protein C, protein S, and antithrombin (Table 1). Because of the multigenic nature of these disorders, more than one inherited or acquired

Table 1
Inherited thrombophilias in pregnancy

Thrombophilia	Prevalence % (healthy subjects)	Risk of thrombosis
AT-III deficiency	0.02–0.10	• Most common congenital clotting disorder in women • 70%–90% lifetime risk of thrombosis [7] • 60% chance of thrombosis during pregnancy and 33% during the puerperium [6]
Factor V Leiden		• 10%–15% during pregnancy and 20% during puerperium in heterozygous [8]
Heterozygous	3.6–6.0	• Risk of thrombosis increased more than 100 fold if homozygous [8]
Homozygous	0.1–0.2	• Mutation rate varies among ethnic groups
Protein C deficiency	0.2–0.5	• 5% during pregnancy and 20% during puerperium [8]
Protein S deficiency	0.03–1.3	• 5% during pregnancy and 20% puerperium [8] • Protein S declines during normal pregnancy
Prothrombin G2010A	1–4	• Risk of thrombosis in asymptomatic pregnant carrier is 0.5% [9] • Homozygosity carries a significant risk of thrombosis [7]

thrombophilia may be present in a pregnant patient presenting with a VTE or coagulation disorder.

Inherited thrombophilias

Activated protein C resistance (Factor V Leiden)

Activated protein C resistance, usually referred to as Factor V Leiden mutation, is the most common inherited coagulopathy, primarily inherited in an autosomal dominant fashion, and carries a 30% lifetime risk of thromboembolism [8]. The point mutation in the Factor V gene prevents protein C from inactivating active factor V. The usual decreases in Protein S levels seen in normal pregnancies can further increase the prothrombotic effects of the factor V Leiden mutation. Therefore, heterozygote patients, who typically have up to a 10-fold increased risk of VTE, may actually have a 50-fold increase during pregnancy. The risk of VTE can approach greater than 100-fold in the rare pregnant patient who is homozygous for the factor V Leiden mutation [8].

Antithrombin III deficiency

Antithrombin is a serine protease inhibitor that naturally acts as an anticoagulant by inhibiting thrombin as well as factors Xa, IXa, VIIIa, and plasmin. Antithrombin III deficiency is the most thrombogenic of the inherited coagulopathies, usually inherited in an autosomal dominant fashion, and without thromboprophylaxis carries a greater than 70% to 90% lifetime risk of thromboembolism [7]. The prevalence of antithrombin III deficiency is very low, although the risk of thrombosis among pregnant patients is up to 60% during pregnancy and 33% during the puerperium [6].

Protein C and S deficiencies

Protein C and protein S are vitamin K–dependent glycoproteins with several anticoagulant functions, which basically act to maintain blood fluidity by dampening the coagulation cascade [8]. The lifetime risk of thromboembolism in all patients with protein C or protein S deficiencies is approximately 50%. The risk of VTE in pregnant patients with protein C and protein S deficiency is approximately 3% to 10% during pregnancy and 7% to 19% during the puerperium and 0% to 6% during pregnancy and 7% to 22% during the puerperium, respectively [8].

Prothrombin gene mutation G2010A

The prothrombin gene mutation G2010A (PGM) is a mutation in the prothrombin gene and is associated with increased plasma prothrombin levels leading to an increased risk of pregnancy complications as well as thrombosis [9]. Heterozygosity of the PGM mutation is present in 2% to 3% of healthy controls and leads to increased levels of prothrombin (150%–200%). Carriers of PGM have an approximately 3-fold increased risk of thrombosis, and the much more rare homozygous mutation carries a significantly higher risk of VTE, similar to that of homozygosity of Factor V Leiden [7].

Acquired thrombophilias

In addition to pregnancy itself, there are several acquired disease states and patient characteristics that can cause a hypercoagulable state (Box 1). The most common cause of acquired thrombophilia in pregnancy is

---

Box 1. Common acquired hypercoagulable syndromes encountered in pregnancy

Antiphospholipid syndrome
    Anticardiolipin antibodies (aCL)
    Lupus anticoagulant (LA)
Autoimmune disease
    Systemic lupus erythematosus
    Ulcerative colitis
Pre-eclampsia
Thrombocythemia
Heparin-induced thrombocytopenia
Immobility
Estrogen use
Smoking obesity

antiphospholipid syndrome (APS), which is a multisystem disorder associated with various medical and obstetric complications. Although the prevalence of obstetric complications in women with APS is around 15% to 20%, it is regarded as one of the few treatable causes of recurrent pregnancy loss [9]. APS predominantly affects young women and is associated with recurrent pregnancy loss, pre-eclampsia, intrauterine growth restriction, and thrombosis. Patients may present with a wide range of clinical features including arterial or venous thrombosis, and nearly any organ system can be affected. There are several proposed hypotheses to explain the mechanisms by which APS induce thrombosis: (1) activation of endothelial cells, (2) oxidant-mediated injury of the vascular endothelium, and (3) interference or modulation of the function of phospholipid-binding proteins involved in the regulation of coagulation [10]. The most common manifestation is DVT of the legs, which tends to be recurrent. The already increased risk of thrombosis in patients with APS is augmented by the hypercoagulable state of pregnancy.

Anticardiolipin antibodies and lupus anticoagulant are the two antiphospholipid antibodies that are associated most commonly with recurrent pregnancy loss and thromboembolism [10]. The name "lupus anticoagulant" is a misnomer for two reasons. Although these antibodies were initially discovered in patients with systemic lupus erythematosus, not all patients with lupus anticoagulant will have systemic lupus erythematosus. Secondly, the name appears to be based on the in vitro finding of bleeding from anticoagulation, rather than the in vivo association with thrombosis.

Indications for thromboprophylaxis during pregnancy, delivery, and the postpartum period

Although there is an increased risk of thrombosis during normal pregnancy, in the majority of women, the benefits of thromboprophylaxis do not outweigh the maternal and fetal risks. The exception is the pregnant woman with an acquired or inherited thrombophilia. A recent randomized trial found improved outcomes in women with a history of a single fetal loss at >10 weeks' gestation and an inherited thrombophilia. Sixty-nine of 80 women taking enoxaparin 40 mg per day had a healthy, live birth compared with 23 of 80 women taking low-dose aspirin (placebo) [11]. Likewise, thromboprophylaxis with unfractionated heparin (UFH) or low-molecular-weight heparin (LMWH), either alone or in combination with aspirin, has been recommended in women with antiphospholipid syndrome. A systematic review of 13 trials (849 participants) evaluating the effects of aspirin and/or heparin to improve pregnancy outcome concluded combined UFH and aspirin reduced pregnancy loss by 54% [12].

The American College of Chest Physicians (ACCP) guidelines on the use of antithrombotic agents during pregnancy have not recommended anticoagulation in pregnant women without thrombophilia or women with thrombophilia in the absence of a history of thromboembolism or poor pregnancy outcome. Because of the high risk of thrombosis, the exceptions to this recommendation are women with (1) antithrombin deficiency, (2) homozygosity for the Factor V Leiden mutation, (3) homozygosity for the prothrombin gene G20210A mutation, or (4) heterozygosity for both mutations [13]. Although there are no large clinical trials showing maternal or fetal benefits of anticoagulation during pregnancy, the current guidelines established during the Seventh ACCP Conference on Antithrombotic and Thrombolytic Therapy [13] are summarized in Table 2. There are several physiologic changes unique to pregnancy that will influence the dosing of anticoagulants, such as the increased volume of distribution, the increased glomerular filtration rate and resultant increased renal excretion, and the increase in protein binding of heparin [14]. Additionally, the potential maternal and fetal complications of anticoagulants will need to be considered, especially the teratogenic effects during the period of organogenesis (fourth to eighth week after conception).

Delivery and postpartum anticoagulation

Whenever possible, the delivery should be scheduled for the pregnant woman who is at high risk for VTE/PE. A consultation with anesthesiology before the onset of labor is essential to establish an appropriate plan for labor and delivery. It is important that the patient be informed and understand her options for analgesia during labor and delivery. Vaginal delivery is safe in most cases, and cesarean delivery should be considered if there are other obstetric concerns. To minimize the risk of maternal and fetal hemorrhage during delivery the following should be considered: (1) at no later than 36 weeks, oral anticoagulants should be switched to LMWH or UFH with similar administration and monitoring as when used for anticoagulation throughout pregnancy; (2) at least 36 hours before induction of labor or cesarean section, use of LMWH should be discontinued and the patient's drug should be converted to intravenous (IV) or subcutaneous (SC) UFH if needed; (3) use of IV UFH should be discontinued 4 to 6 hours before anticipated delivery [14]. Adherence to these guidelines facilitates the performance of neuraxial techniques for labor and delivery.

The plan for reinitiating anticoagulation postpartum must also be considered when planning the anesthetic management and often is the limiting factor when determining the safety of a neuraxial technique. Typically, anticoagulation should be held until at least 12 hours after vaginal delivery or epidural removal (which ever is later). After cesarean delivery, thromboprophylaxis should be held for at least 24 hours [14]. Warfarin does not enter the breast milk; therefore, the American Academy of Pediatrics Committee on Drugs supports the use of warfarin in women who choose to breast feed [15]. However, most women on chronic warfarin therapy will be bridged with UFH or LMWH until a therapeutic international normalized ratio (INR) is obtained with warfarin. Women who had a thrombotic event during pregnancy should be anticoagulated for at least 3 to 6 months. A high proportion of both postpartum DVT and PE manifest after discharge from the hospital; therefore, continued surveillance in the puerperium is extremely important in at-risk women.

Management of pregnant women with prosthetic heart valves

Due to the maternal and fetal complications, the anticoagulation regimen for the pregnant woman with a prosthetic heart valve is particularly difficult to manage and requires special consideration. The management of these patients is challenging because there are no available controlled clinical trials to provide guidelines for effective and safe antithrombotic therapy. The current recommendations are largely based on data from nonpregnant patients, case series of pregnant patients, and case reports. The choice of anticoagulation regimens should be made by balancing the two main risks: maternal morbidity and mortality from thromboembolism or hemorrhage and fetal embryopathy or loss. There are several common anticoagulation regimens used, each with their own risks and benefits to the fetus and the mother. The American College of Cardiology (ACC) and the American Heart Association (AHA) concluded that it is reasonable to use one of the following three regimens: (1) LMWH or UFH between 6 and 12 weeks and close to term only, with warfarin anticoagulation at other times; (2) aggressive dose-adjusted UFH throughout pregnancy; or (3) aggressive adjusted-dose LMWH throughout pregnancy [16]. The incidence of major bleeding complications, independent of the regimen used, is approximately 2.5%, with the majority (80%) occurring during delivery [17].

Subcutaneous UFH has been used as an alternative to warfarin during the first 6 to 12 weeks and the last 2 weeks of pregnancy. However, there are several case series and reports revealing a high incidence of thromboembolic complications (12%–24%), including fatal valve thrombosis, especially in high-risk parturients [16]. In several studies, when heparin is substituted for warfarin during the first trimester, the risks of maternal thromboembolism and maternal death are more than doubled [18,19]. Although these studies have been criticized because of the inclusion of a large percentage of women with older, more thrombogenic prostheses and inadequate heparin administration, it is clear that the efficacy of subcutaneous heparin has not been established. The ACC/AHA practice guidelines state that women who choose to use UFH up to 36 weeks should be informed that although the fetal risk is lower, the maternal risks of prosthetic valve thrombosis, systemic embolization, infection, osteoporosis, and heparin-induced thrombocytopenia are relatively higher. It is also recommended that pregnant women with prosthetic valves receiving dose-adjusted UFH should have an activated partial thromboplastin time (aPTT) at least twice control [16].

Although LMWHs have been used successfully to treat pregnant women with deep venous thrombosis, the use of LMWH in pregnant women with prosthetic valves remains controversial. The controversy started with

Table 2
Anticoagulation during pregnancy

Thrombotic disorder	Anticoagulant
Treatment of VTE during pregnancy	Adjusted dose LMWH *or* Adjusted dose UFH
History of thrombophilia *without* prior VTE	Surveillance Prophylactic LMWH *or* Mini-dose UFH
Thrombophilia *with* history of single episode of VTE	Prophylactic or intermediate-dose LMWH or Mini-dose or moderate-dose UFH
No history of VTE *and* • Antithrombin deficiency • Prothrombin G20210A *and* factor V Leiden • Homozygotes for the above disorders	Prophylactic LMWH or Mini-dose UFH
History of VTE *and* • Antithrombin deficiency • Prothrombin G20210A *and* factor V Leiden • Homozygotes for the above disorders	Prophylactic intermediate-dose LMWH or Moderate-dose UFH
Multiple (2 or more) episodes of VTE *and/or* Receiving long-term anticoagulants before pregnancy	Adjusted-dose UFH or Adjusted-dose LMWH
Congenital thrombophilic deficit *and* History of pregnancy complication	Low dose aspirin *plus* Mini-dose UFH or Prophylactic LMWH
Antiphospholipid antibodies *without* history of VTE or pregnancy complication	Surveillance *or* Mini-dose heparin *or* Prophylactic LMWH *and/or* Low-dose aspirin
Antiphospholipid antibodies *and* History of multiple pregnancy complications[a]	Low dose aspirin *plus* Mini-dose or moderated dose UFH or Prophylactic LMWH
Antiphospholipid antibodies *and* history of VTE	Adjusted-dose LMWH or UFH therapy *plus* low-dose aspirin

Mini-dose UFH: 5000 U subcutaneously (SC) every (q) 12 hour (h).

Moderate-dose UFH: UFH SC q 12h in doses adjusted to target and anti-Xa level of 0.1-0.3U/mL.

Adjusted dose UFH: UFH SC q 12h in doses adjusted to target a mid-interval aPTT into the therapeutic range.

Prophylactic LMWH: dalteparin 5,000 U SC q24h, or enoxaparin 40 mg SC q24h (extremes of weight may require dose modification).

Intermediate-dose LMWH: dalteparin 5,000 U SC q12h, or enoxaparin 40 mg SC q12h.

Adjusted dose LMWH: weight-adjusted, full-treatment doses of LMWH administered once or twice daily (dalteparin 200 U/kg dq, or 100 U/kg q12h, or enoxaparin 1 mg/kg q12h).

Postpartum anticoagulants: warfarin for 4 to 6 weeks with a target INR of 2.0 to 3.0, with initial UFH or LMWH overlap until INR is ≥2.0.

[a] Pregnancy complications include multiple early pregnancy losses, one or more late pregnancy loss, pre-eclampsia, abruption, IUGR.

Data from Bates SM, Greer IA, Hirsh J, Ginsberg JS. Use of antithrombotic agents during pregnancy: the Seventh ACCP Conference on Antithrombotic and Thrombolytic Therapy. Chest 2004;126(3 Suppl):627S–44S.

a warning issued by the US Food and Drug Administration (FDA) and a manufacturer of LMWH in 2001 describing case reports of deadly valve thrombosis in pregnant women anticoagulated with LMWH. After further review, in 2004 the FDA approved labeling that specifically stated that the use of LMWH for thromboprophylaxis in pregnant women with prosthetic heart valves had not been adequately studied [16]. Although there are several case reports of valve thrombosis in pregnant women receiving LMWH anticoagulation, it appears that this occurs most often when factor Xa levels are not monitored [20]. The ACC/AHA guidelines recommend that if pregnant women with prosthetic valves are receiving dose-adjusted LMWH it should be administered twice daily to maintain an anti-Xa level between 0.7 and 1.2 U/mL 4 hours after administration. In addition, they specifically state that LMWH should not be administered to this population without measuring anti-Xa levels 4 to 6 hours after administration [16].

Chan and colleagues [17] performed a systematic review of the literature surrounding fetal and maternal outcomes of pregnant women with heart valves. Unfortunately, the review consisted solely of prospective and retrospective cohort trials. This review suggested that warfarin is more efficacious than UFH for thromboprophylaxis in pregnant women with prosthetic heart valves, although there was an increased incidence of embryopathy. The use of low-dose UFH was found to be inadequate, and the use of adjusted-dose UFH requires aggressive monitoring and appropriate dose adjustment to maintain a minimum aPTT ratio of at least twice control. In the case of urgent delivery, the risk of hemorrhage must be balanced against the potentially catastrophic risk of valve thrombosis if anticoagulation is reversed.

Assuming adequate hemostasis is achieved, UFH or LMWH should be resumed within 4 to 6 hours after delivery with concomitant resumption of warfarin. Heparin (UFH or LMWH) should be used in combination with warfarin until a therapeutic INR is obtained.

Spinal hematoma

Spinal hematoma is a rare but potentially serious neurologic disorder that can lead to permanent neurologic deficit or death without the appropriate treatment. Although the incidence of such a rare event is difficult to accurately estimate, a meta-analysis concluded that the incidence of spinal hematoma after epidural and subarachnoid block was 1:150,000 and 1:200,000, respectively [21]. However, the presence of a coagulopathy dramatically increases the incidence of spinal hematoma formation [22,23].

Epidural hematomas are more common because of the prominent epidural venous plexus. Subarachnoid hematomas are the rarest of the intraspinal hematomas because of the diluting effect of the cerebral spinal fluid (CSF). Also, unlike the epidural space, the subarachnoid space does not contain major blood vessels. The source of subarachnoid bleeding is thought to be from the puncture of radicular vessels that run along the length of each nerve root [24]. There are several etiologies of spinal hematoma, such as spontaneous bleeding, trauma, coagulopathies, vascular malformations, and iatrogenic hemorrhage during lumbar puncture or neuraxial anesthesia.

Spinal hematoma in the obstetric patient

Although this review focuses on spinal hematomas after neuraxial procedures, it is well documented that spinal hematomas can occur in the obstetric population in the absence of a neuraxial bock. In a case report of a spontaneous thoracic epidural hematoma in a preeclamptic woman, Doblar and Schumacher [25] present an additional six cases of spontaneous epidural hematoma in *healthy* parturients. The etiology of these spontaneous hematomas is not currently understood, although if not treated appropriately and expeditiously, the outcome can be devastating for these young mothers.

The incidence of spinal hematoma after neuraxial blockade is very difficult to determine, although, it is widely reported that obstetric patients have a significantly lower incidence of complications than their elderly counterparts [26–28]. It is important to note that neurologic complications associated with pregnancy and delivery, are much more common than complications directly related to neuraxial blockade [27]. Moen and colleagues [26] recently reviewed complications after 1,260,000 spinal blocks and 450,000 epidural blocks, including 200,000 epidural blocks for pain relief in labor. There were two spinal hematomas in the obstetric population studied; one after a subarachnoid block and one after the removal of an epidural catheter. Interestingly, signs of severe coagulopathy were present in both patients. The investigators reported the incidence of spinal hematoma after obstetric epidural blockade was 1:200,000, which was significantly lower than the incidence of 1:3,600 elderly women undergoing total knee arthroplasty. Among the published case reports of parturients who have experienced a spinal hematoma after neuraxial blockade, a significant proportion of patients had altered coagulation at the time of block placement or epidural catheter removal (Table 3).

Anticoagulants commonly used in pregnancy and recommendations for neuraxial blockade

In response to the patient safety issues surrounding neuraxial blockade in the setting of potent antithrombotic drugs, the American Society of Regional Anesthesia and Pain Medicine (ASRA) convened its Second Consensus Conference on Neuraxial Anesthesia and Anticoagulation [39]. Although the consensus statements are based on a thorough evaluation of the available information, in many cases the data are few, specifically when considering the obstetric population. The consensus statements are designed to help guide the anesthesiologist toward safe options for neuraxial blockade in the anticoagulated patient, including the parturient.

Table 3
Spinal hematomas in obstetric patients

Author	Technique	Coagulopathy	Outcome	Miscellaneous
Nguyen et al, [29]	Epidural	Postpartum hemorrhage Thrombocytopenia Elevated thrombin time	Recovered	• Epidural catheter inadvertently removed while coagulopathic
Moen et al, [26]	Epidural	HELLP	Unknown	• Epidural catheter removed in setting of coagulopathy
Moen et al, [26]	Subarachnoid	HELLP	Unknown	• Evidence of coagulopathy
Esler et al, [30]	Epidural	None	Recovered	• Neurofibromatosis • Presented on second postpartum day
Yuen et al, [31]	Epidural	Severe pre-eclampsia Thrombocytopenia	Recovered	• Presented within hours • Surgical laminectomy
Yarnell and D'Alton [32]	Epidural	Elevated aPTT Elevated PT	Mild weakness of right leg	• Presented 12 hours after epidural • Surgical treatment
Lao et al, [33]	Epidural	Preeclampsia & Lupus anticoagulant Abnormal aPTT	Residual urinary and bowel dysfunction	• Presented 1 day postpartum • Surgical treatment
Scott and Hibbard [34]	Epidural	Not reported	Improving	• Surgical treatment
Sibai et al, [35]	Epidural	Thrombocytopenia	Unknown	• No information
Crawford [28]	Epidural	Unknown	Recovered	• Presented several weeks postpartum
Roscoe and Barrington [36]	Epidural	None	Residual leg weakness	• Epidural ependymoma • Presented 3 days postpartum • Surgical treatment
Newman [37]	Epidural	None	Minimal weakness and paresthesia	• Presented 2 hours after delivery
Ballin [38]	Epidural	None	Recovered	• Spinal stenosis

HELLP, syndrome of hemolysis, elevated liver enzymes, and low platelets.

Table 4
Anticoagulants commonly used in pregnancy

Agent	Pregnancy category[a]	Half-life	Peak effect	Time to normal hemostasis after discontinuation	Monitoring	Placental transfer	Indication
Aspirin	D	15 min	30–40 min	5–8 days (the life of the platelet)	Platelet function analysis	Yes	Supplemental therapy in women with mechanical heart valves or antiphospholipid syndrome
Warfarin	X	36–42 hours	90 min	4–6 days	INR	Yes	Mechanical heart valves
Unfractionated heparin	C	1–2 hours	2 hours	4–6 hours	aPTT	None	Treatment or prophylaxis
Low-molecular-weight heparin	B	3–5 hours	3–4 hours	12–24 hours	Antifactor Xa levels	None	Treatment or prophylaxis

[a] Category B, Animal studies show no risks or human data are reassuring; Category C, Human data are lacking, animal studies positive or not done; Category D, Human data show risk, benefit may outweigh; Category X, Animal or human data positive, no benefit.

Aspirin

Aspirin is an antiplatelet drug that permanently inactivates cyclooxyge-nase, leading to platelet dysfunction for the life of the platelet (Table 4). Large, randomized trials have found no increased risk of miscarriage, con-genital anomalies, fetal hemorrhage, or placental abruption [40]. The use of low-dose aspirin also does not appear to be associated with premature clo-sure of the fetal ductus arteriosus or excessive surgical bleeding. Although aspirin appears to be safe during pregnancy, rarely is it sufficient to prevent thrombosis in most cases. In women with a mechanical heart valve or a his-tory of antiphospholipid syndrome, low-dose aspirin may be used in combi-nation with UFH or LMWH [13].

Neuraxial anesthesia and aspirin

Several studies involving a total of 4,714 patients have failed to demon-strate an increased risk of neuraxial blockade in patients treated with aspirin or nonsteroidal antiinflammatory drugs (NSAIDs) [41]. In the obstetric population, the Collaborative Low-dose Aspirin Study in Pregnancy (CLASP) group administered 60 mg of aspirin daily to high-risk parturients who subsequently underwent epidural anesthesia without any neurologic se-quelae [42]. Although, these findings are reassuring, it is impossible to con-clude the safety of aspirin use, especially in the obstetric population, until a much larger prospective study is performed. Because there is no widely ac-cepted test to determine a patient's risk of bleeding, a detailed history and good clinical examination with emphasis on signs of a bleeding tendency will help identify patients and parturients at risk (Box 2).

Warfarin

Warfarin is a vitamin K antagonist that interferes with the synthesis of vitamin K–dependent coagulation factors (II, VII, IX, X) with reduced

---

Box 2. Management of the pregnant patient receiving aspirin/NSAIDs

- Incidence of spinal hematoma is not significantly increased.
- No concerns regarding the timing of single-shot or catheter techniques in relationship to the administration of aspirin or NSAIDs, postoperative monitoring, or timing of catheter removal.

Data from Horlocker TT, Wedel DJ, Benzon H, et al. Regional anesthesia in the anticoagulated patient: defining the risks (the second ASRA Consensus Confer-ence on Neuraxial Anesthesia and Anticoagulation). Reg Anesth Pain Med 2003;28(3):172–97.

coagulant activity. Warfarin generally is contraindicated in pregnancy. When taken during the critical period of organogenesis, it carries up to a 30% risk of significant congenital anomalies. The effect of warfarin on calcium deposition and bone formation during embryologic ossification (6–9 weeks' gestation) may result in stippled calcification, shortened extremities, vertebral abnormalities, and nasal hypoplasia. The other adverse effects result from over–anticoagulation of the fetus, because warfarin easily crosses the placenta and may cause hemorrhage anytime during pregnancy and in any fetal organ [43]. Although the manufacturer considers the use of warfarin strictly contraindicated during pregnancy because of its association with embryopathy and central nervous system abnormalities, it often is used in high-risk patients, such as women with mechanical heart valves. The ACC/AHA 2006 guidelines recommend that women requiring long-term warfarin therapy who are contemplating pregnancy are encouraged to perform frequent pregnancy tests and consider substitution of UFH or LMWH for warfarin when pregnancy is first confirmed, until approximately 12 weeks of pregnancy [16]. In high-risk patients, warfarin occasionally is used during the second and third trimester of pregnancy, with an INR goal of 2.5 to 3.5, but because of the long half-life, the parturient should have their drug converted to UFH or LMWH several weeks before delivery.

Box 3. Management of the pregnant patient receiving warfarin

- Caution should be used when performing neuraxial techniques in patients who have recently discontinued chronic warfarin anticoagulation.
- Warfarin use should be discontinued for 4 to 5 days before delivery and a normal prothrombin time (PT)/INR documented before initiation of neuraxial blockade.
- Simultaneous use of other anticoagulant medications (NSAIDs, UFH, LMWH) can increase the bleeding risk without affecting the PT/INR.
- If an epidural catheter is left indwelling and oral anticoagulation is initiated
  - Monitor the patient's PT/INR daily before catheter removal.
  - Neuraxial catheters should be removed when the INR is <1.5.
  - Neurologic testing of sensory and motor function performed routinely during epidural analgesia and for at least 24 hours after catheter removal.

Data from Horlocker TT, Wedel DJ, Benzon H, et al. Regional anesthesia in the anticoagulated patient: defining the risks (the second ASRA Consensus Conference on Neuraxial Anesthesia and Anticoagulation). Reg Anesth Pain Med 2003;28(3):172–97.

Along with the maternal risks of being fully anticoagulated at the time of delivery, the placental transfer of warfarin can cause bleeding or cerebral hemorrhage in the fetus, especially if forceps are used during delivery [16].

Neuraxial anesthesia and warfarin

The relative safety of neuraxial anesthesia in patients receiving perioperative warfarin remains controversial. The ASRA consensus statements are based on warfarin pharmacology, series evaluating the risk of surgery in patients taking warfarin, and case reports of spinal hematomas in patients treated with warfarin for anticoagulation (Box 3).

Intravenous and subcutaneous unfractionated heparin

Unfractionated heparin is a heterogenous mixture of polysaccharide chains ranging in molecular weight from 3,000 to 30,000 Daltons and causes its anticoagulant effect by activating antithrombin. This interaction with antithrombin is mediated by a particular pentasaccharide sequence distributed along the heparin chains. Once binding occurs, a conformational change in antithrombin is initiated, which accelerates its interaction with thrombin and activated factor X (factor Xa) by about 1,000 times [44]. Because of the size of the pentasaccharide units, UFH has equivalent activity against factor Xa and thrombin, which is the main difference between UFH and LMWH. Intravenous injection of heparin results in immediate anticoagulation, whereas subcutaneous administration results in a 1- to 2-hour delay in anticoagulant activity. The side effects associated with prolonged use of UFH during pregnancy include the inconvenience of parenteral administration, a 2% risk of major bleeding, 2% incidence of osteoporotic fractures (17%–36% reduction in bone density), and the 1%–3% incidence of heparin-induced thrombocytopenia (HIT) [14,45]. Heparin-associated osteoporosis has been seen in patients who have been treated for at least 1 month and is likely related to a toxic effect of heparin on osteoblasts. The platelet count should be monitored for the first 2 weeks after initiating heparin because of the possibility of the development of HIT, which is a potentially serious complication that may lead to decreased platelet counts along with potentially deadly thromboses.

Neuraxial anesthesia and unfractionated heparin

Although there often is no detectable change in the coagulation parameters in parturients receiving prophylactic subcutaneous heparin doses of 5,000 U every 12 hours, there is a minority of patients in whom measurable changes in coagulation may develop and an even smaller subset who may become anticoagulated during subcutaneous heparin therapy [39]. A review of the literature by Schwander and Bachmann [46] found no spinal hematomas in more than 5,000 patients who underwent neuraxial anesthesia while receiving subcutaneous heparin. Although there are case reports of spinal hematomas in patients undergoing neuraxial anesthesia while receiving

---

Box 4. Management of the pregnant patient receiving unfractionated heparin

- Subcutaneous unfractionated heparin with twice-daily administration is not a strong contraindication to the performance of neuraxial anesthesia, providing the total daily dose is 10,000 units or less.
- Higher doses and more frequent administration may increase the risk, and neuraxial techniques are not recommended in these patients unless a normal aPTT has been documented.
  - Risk of hematoma may be reduced if the block is placed before the heparin injection.
  - Adequate platelet count should be confirmed if patient has been receiving heparin for longer than 4 days because of the risk of HIT.
  - The patient should not have confounding coagulopathies or anticoagulants.
  - Careful monitoring of neurologic status is recommended.
- Intravenous UFH should be stopped 4 to 6 hours before neuraxial blockade, and a normal aPTT should be confirmed before the placement of a neuraxial blockade.

Data from Horlocker TT, Wedel DJ, Benzon H, et al. Regional anesthesia in the anticoagulated patient: defining the risks (the second ASRA Consensus Conference on Neuraxial Anesthesia and Anticoagulation). Reg Anesth Pain Med 2003;28(3):172–97.

---

subcutaneous heparin, the majority of anesthesiologists believe that the subcutaneous heparin prophylaxis is not a strong contraindication to the performance of neuraxial anesthesia (Box 4) [39].

Low-molecular-weight heparin

Low-molecular-weight heparins are enzymatically or chemically depolymerized fragments of UFH yielding chains with a lower mean molecular weight of approximately 5,000 Daltons. Compared with UFH, LMWH has a greater activity against factor Xa and is less likely to bind to plasma proteins. It is this reduction in binding that leads to an increased bioavailability, half-life, and anticoagulant activity compared with UFH [44]. LMWH has greater than a 90% bioavailability after subcutaneous administration and a very predictable anticoagulant response when the dose is weight adjusted [22]. Peak anti-Xa activity occurs 3 to 4 hours after a subcutaneous LMWH injection. After a thromboprophylactic dose (see Table 2), significant anti-Xa activity is still present 12 hours after injection because of the long half-life (3–4 times that of standard heparin). With intermediate and treatment dosing, anticoagulant may persist 24 hours or longer. Unfortunately, there are no large comparative studies in pregnancy, although in nonpregnant patients, LMWHs have been associated with fewer side effects than UFH. Even though parenteral administration is still required, potential benefits compared with UFH include fewer daily injections, less bone loss, decreased incidence of HIT, more predictable anticoagulant response, and a longer half-life [13]. LMWH, like UFH does not cross the placenta and is safe during lactation.

Low-molecular-weight heparin and neuraxial anesthesia

There are several recommendations that have been devised to aid the anesthesiologist in reducing a patient's risk of spinal hematoma. Generally, the pregnant patient on LMWH should be advised to withhold her heparin injection if she believes she may be in labor until evaluated by her obstetrician. If it is determined that she is in labor, further doses usually are held until after delivery. When possible, an induction or elective cesarean section should be scheduled (Box 5).

Diagnosis and treatment of spinal hematoma

All patients receiving a neuraxial block should be monitored for the potential development of a spinal hematoma, especially those that are anticoagulated. It is important to remember that a continuous catheter technique with a local anesthetic infusion may hide the signs and symptoms of an early spinal hematoma. The symptoms of cord compression and ischemia include severe back pain, sensory or motor deficit outlasting the expected duration of the neuraxial block, and bowel and bladder dysfunction within the postoperative period. A review of 51 obstetric and nonobstetric spinal hematomas after epidural anesthesia from 1966 to 1995 found that the clinical symptoms were back pain (radicular), bladder dysfunction, and sensory and motor deficits [47].

The differential diagnosis of spinal hematoma includes spinal abscess, cauda equina syndrome, and anterior spinal artery syndrome. There are several distinguishing features of each of these disorders that will aid the physician in narrowing down the cause of a changing neurologic examination (Table 5). When spinal hematoma is suspected, it is imperative to get emergent imaging studies, including computed tomography (CT), magnetic resonance imaging (MRI), or myelography. The need for prompt diagnosis and intervention of a suspected spinal hematoma is supported in a review of the American Society of Anesthesiologists (ASA) Closed Claims database. In this review, Cheney and colleagues [48] noted that spinal cord injuries were the leading cause of claims in the 1990s, and spinal hematomas accounted for roughly half of the reported spinal cord injuries. Importantly, the significant increase in spinal cord injuries over time was attributed to neuraxial blocks in anticoagulated patients and blocks for chronic pain management. Medicolegally, patient care rarely met standards (1 of

---

Box 5. Management of the pregnant patient receiving low-molecular-weight heparin

- Patients receiving LMWH before surgery or delivery can be assumed to have altered coagulation.
  - In patients receiving prophylactic doses of LMWH, needle placement should occur at least 10 to12 hours after the last LMWH dose.
  - In patients receiving higher treatment doses of LMWH, needle placement should be delayed at least 24 hours.
- The anti-Xa level may be monitored to determine efficacy of therapy but is not predictive of the risk of neuraxial bleeding.
- Antiplatelet or oral anticoagulant medications given in combination with LMWH may increase the risk of spinal hematoma.
- If the needle or catheter placement is traumatic, initiation of postoperative LMWH should be delayed for at least 24 hours. Traumatic needle or catheter placement may increase the risk of spinal hematoma.
- Postoperative LMWH management is based on total daily dose, timing of the first postoperative dose, and dose schedule.
  - For single daily thromboprophylaxis dosing, the first postpartum dose should be administered 6 to 8 hours postoperatively/postpartum, and the second dose should not occur sooner than 24 hours after the initial dose. A neuraxial catheter should be removed a minimum of 10 to 12 hours after the last dose of LMWH, and a subsequent dose should occur a minimum of 2 hours after catheter removal (whichever is later).
  - Twice-daily intermediate or treatment dosing is associated with an increased risk of spinal hematoma. The first LMWH dose should be administered no earlier than 24 hours postoperatively/postpartum, in the presence of adequate hemostasis, and at least 2 hours after catheter removal (whichever is later).

Data from Horlocker TT, Wedel DJ, Benzon H, et al. Regional anesthesia in the anticoagulated patient: defining the risks (the second ASRA Consensus Conference on Neuraxial Anesthesia and Anticoagulation). Reg Anesth Pain Med 2003;28(3):172–97.

13 cases), in that the signs and symptoms of epidural hematoma were not readily appreciated by the caregivers. The presence of postoperative sensory or motor deficit was generally attributed to the effects of local anesthetic rather than to spinal cord compression or ischemia.

Table 5
Differential diagnosis of epidural abscess, epidural hemorrhage, and anterior spinal artery syndrome

Finding	Epidural abscess	Epidural hemorrhage	Anterior spinal artery syndrome
Age of patient	Any age	50% > 50 yr	Elderly
Previous history	Infection[a]	Anticoagulants	Arteriosclerosis, hypotension
Onset	1–3 days	Sudden	Sudden
Generalized symptoms	Fever, malaise, back pain	Sharp, transient back and leg pain	None
Sensory involvement	None of paresthesias	Variable, late	Minor, patchy
Motor involvement	Flaccid paralysis, later spastic	Flaccid paralysis	Flaccid paralysis
Segmental reflexes	Exacerbated[a], later obtunded	Abolished	Abolished
Myelogram/CT scan	Signs of extradural compression	Signs of extradural compression	Normal
Cerebrospinal fluid	Increased cell count	Normal	Normal
Blood data	Rise in sedimentation rate	Prolonged coagulation time[a]	Normal

[a] Infrequent findings.

From Wedel DJ, Horlocker TT: Risks of regional anesthesia—infectious, septic. Reg Anesth 1996;21:57–61; with permission.

The current practice recommends MRI as the diagnostic tool of choice because of its ability to define with a high degree of resolution the cranio-caudad spread of the hematoma and its effect on the spinal cord [49]. Also of note, the T1 and T2 signal intensity on the MRI can further delineate the age of the hematoma.

Because of the rare incidence, there are no clinical studies to date that have adequate power to definitively recommend a particular treatment modality in the patient with a documented spinal hematoma. In the setting of a progressive neurologic deficit, immediate decompressive laminectomy and hematoma evacuation is preferred; however, spontaneous recovery has been reported when severe deficits are present. Obviously, the operative risks must be weighed against the potential severity of the neurologic deficit; early consultation with a neurosurgeon is paramount. Overall, the less severe the preoperative neurologic deficit is, and the more quickly the hematoma evacuation is undertaken, the better a patient's chances are for a good neurologic recovery [50,51].

This review has highlighted the main causes of thrombosis in the pregnant population, the commonly used anticoagulants for prophylaxis and treatment of these disorders, as well as recommendations for neuraxial blockade in parturients who are currently or have recently been anticoagulated. It is estimated that greater than 50% of women in labor will request an epidural, and in some hospitals the rate of epidural usage is higher than 70% [52]. Also, the obstetric population is one of the few groups in which regional anesthesia has been shown to truly provide improved outcomes over general anesthesia, specifically for cesarean section delivery [53]. Therefore, it is essential that the anesthesiologist understand the implications of performing neuraxial blockade in the setting of anticoagulation. Unfortunately, the identification of patients at risk and establishment of guidelines will not eradicate the complication of spinal hematoma in the obstetric population. The importance of neurologic monitoring must be stressed, because early evaluation and treatment is the key to a favorable outcome. As the anticoagulant agents and the indications for those agents continue to evolve, it is crucial that the anesthesia care provider understand the pharmacologic properties as well as the individual risks and benefits of treatment. It is this knowledge that will allow for the appropriate balance of risk and benefit when managing the anticoagulated obstetric patient who desires neuraxial blockade. Understanding and respecting the recommendations to decrease the incidence of spinal hematoma will allow us to make neuraxial blockade safer, without withholding these techniques from women who not only desire them but who will most certainly benefit from them.

References

[1] Bremme KA. Haemostatic changes in pregnancy. Best Pract Res Clin Haematol 2003;16(2): 153–68.
[2] Heit JA, Kobbervig CE, James AH, et al. Trends in the incidence of venous thromboembolism during pregnancy or postpartum: a 30-year population-based study. Ann Intern Med 2005;143(10):697–706.
[3] Kujovich JL. Hormones and pregnancy: thromboembolic risks for women. Br J Haematol 2004;126(4):443–54.
[4] Greer IA. Prevention of venous thromboembolism in pregnancy. Best Pract Res Clin Haematol 2003;16(2):261–78.
[5] Alfirevic Z, Roberts D, Martlew V. How strong is the association between maternal thrombophilia and adverse pregnancy outcome? a systematic review. Eur J Obstet Gynecol Reprod Biol 2002;101(1):6–14.
[6] Lockwood CJ. Inherited thrombophilias in pregnant patients: detection and treatment paradigm. Obstet Gynecol 2002;99(2):333–41.
[7] Paidas MJ, Ku DH, Langhoff-Roos J, et al. Inherited thrombophilias and adverse pregnancy outcome: screening and management. Semin Perinatol 2005;29(3):150–63.
[8] Lockwood CJ. Heritable coagulopathies in pregnancy. Obstet Gynecol Surv 1999;54(12): 754–65.
[9] Gebhardt GS, Hall DR. Inherited and acquired thrombophilias and poor pregnancy outcome: should we be treating with heparin? Curr Opin Obstet Gynecol 2003;15(6): 501–6.
[10] Khare M, Nelson-Piercy C. Acquired thrombophilias and pregnancy. Best Pract Res Clin Obstet Gynaecol 2003;17(3):491–507.
[11] Gris JC, Mercier E, Quere I, et al. Low-molecular-weight heparin versus low-dose aspirin in women with one fetal loss and a constitutional thrombophilic disorder. Blood 2004;103(10): 3695–9.
[12] Empson M, Lassere M, Craig J, et al. Prevention of recurrent miscarriage for women with antiphospholipid antibody or lupus anticoagulant. Cochrane Database Syst Rev 2005;(2): CD002859.

[13] Bates SM, Greer IA, Hirsh J, et al. Use of antithrombotic agents during pregnancy: the Seventh ACCP Conference on Antithrombotic and Thrombolytic Therapy. Chest 2004; 126(Suppl 3):627S–44S.

[14] James AH, Abel DE, Brancazio LR. Anticoagulants in pregnancy. Obstet Gynecol Surv 2006;61(1):59–69 [quiz: 70–72].

[15] American Academy of Pediatrics Committee on Drugs. Transfer of drugs and other chemicals into human milk. Pediatrics 2001;108(3):776–89.

[16] Bonow RO, Carabello BA, Kanu C, et al. ACC/AHA 2006 guidelines for the management of patients with valvular heart disease: a report of the American College of Cardiology/American Heart Association Task Force on practice guidelines (writing committee to revise the 1998 guidelines for the management of patients with valvular heart disease): developed in collaboration with the society of cardiovascular anesthesiologists: endorsed by the society for cardiovascular angiography and interventions and the society of thoracic surgeons. Circulation 2006;114(5):e84–231.

[17] Chan WS, Anand S, Ginsberg JS. Anticoagulation of pregnant women with mechanical heart valves: a systematic review of the literature. Arch Intern Med 2000;160(2):191–6.

[18] Vitali E, Donatelli F, Quaini E, et al. Pregnancy in patients with mechanical prosthetic heart valves. Our experience regarding 98 pregnancies in 57 patients. J Cardiovasc Surg (Torino) 1986;27(2):221–7.

[19] Larrea JL, Nunez L, Reque JA, et al. Pregnancy and mechanical valve prostheses: a high-risk situation for the mother and the fetus. Ann Thorac Surg 1983;36(4):459–63.

[20] Oran B, Lee-Parritz A, Ansell J. Low molecular weight heparin for the prophylaxis of thromboembolism in women with prosthetic mechanical heart valves during pregnancy. Thromb Haemost 2004;92(4):747–51.

[21] Tryba M. [Epidural regional anesthesia and low molecular heparin: pro]. Anasthesiol Intensivmed Notfallmed Schmerzther 1993;28(3):179–81 [in German].

[22] Horlocker TT, Wedel DJ. Anticoagulation and neuraxial block: historical perspective, anesthetic implications, and risk management. Reg Anesth Pain Med 1998;23(6 Suppl 2): 129–34.

[23] Stafford-Smith M. Impaired haemostasis and regional anaesthesia. Can J Anaesth 1996; 43(5 Pt 2):R129–41.

[24] Evans RW. Complications of lumbar puncture. Neurol Clin 1998;16(1):83–105.

[25] Doblar DD, Schumacher SD. Spontaneous acute thoracic epidural hematoma causing paraplegia in a patient with severe preeclampsia in early labor. Int J Obstet Anesth 2005;14(3): 256–60.

[26] Moen V, Dahlgren N, Irestedt L. Severe neurological complications after central neuraxial blockades in Sweden 1990–1999. Anesthesiology 2004;101(4):950–9.

[27] Loo CC, Dahlgren G, Irestedt L. Neurological complications in obstetric regional anaesthesia. Int J Obstet Anesth 2000;9(2):99–124.

[28] Crawford JS. Some maternal complications of epidural analgesia for labour. Anaesthesia 1985;40(12):1219–25.

[29] Nguyen L, Riu B, Minville V, et al. [Epidural hematoma after hemorrhagic shock in a parturient]. Can J Anaesth 2006;53(3):252–7 [in French].

[30] Esler MD, Durbridge J, Kirby S. Epidural haematoma after dural puncture in a parturient with neurofibromatosis. Br J Anaesth 2001;87(6):932–4.

[31] Yuen TS, Kua JS, Tan IK. Spinal haematoma following epidural anaesthesia in a patient with eclampsia. Anaesthesia 1999;54(4):350–4.

[32] Yarnell RW, D'Alton ME. Epidural hematoma complicating cholestasis of pregnancy. Curr Opin Obstet Gynecol 1996;8(3):239–42.

[33] Lao TT, Halpern SH, MacDonald D, et al. Spinal subdural haematoma in a parturient after attempted epidural anaesthesia. Can J Anaesth 1993;40(4):340–5.

[34] Scott DB, Hibbard BM. Serious non-fatal complications associated with extradural block in obstetric practice. Br J Anaesth 1990;64(5):537–41.

[35] Sibai BM, Taslimi MM, el-Nazer A, et al. Maternal-perinatal outcome associated with the syndrome of hemolysis, elevated liver enzymes, and low platelets in severe preeclampsia-eclampsia. Am J Obstet Gynecol 1986;155(3):501–9.

[36] Roscoe MW, Barrington TW. Acute spinal subdural hematoma. A case report and review of literature. Spine 1984;9(7):672–5.

[37] Newman B. Postnatal paraparesis following epidural analgesia and forceps delivery. Anaesthesia 1983;38(4):350–1.

[38] Ballin NC. Paraplegia following epidural analgesia. Anaesthesia 1981;36(10):952–3.

[39] Horlocker TT, Wedel DJ, Benzon H, et al. Regional anesthesia in the anticoagulated patient: defining the risks (the second ASRA Consensus Conference on Neuraxial Anesthesia and Anticoagulation). Reg Anesth Pain Med 2003;28(3):172–97.

[40] Duley L, Henderson-Smart D, Knight M, et al. Antiplatelet drugs for prevention of pre-eclampsia and its consequences: systematic review. BMJ 2001;322(7282):329–33.

[41] Urmey WF, Rowlingson J. Do antiplatelet agents contribute to the development of perioperative spinal hematoma? Reg Anesth Pain Med 1998;23(6 Suppl 2):146–51.

[42] CLASP: a randomised trial of low-dose aspirin for the prevention and treatment of pre-eclampsia among 9364 pregnant women. CLASP (Collaborative Low-dose Aspirin Study in Pregnancy) collaborative group. Lancet 1994;343(8898):619–29.

[43] Blickstein D, Blickstein I. The risk of fetal loss associated with Warfarin anticoagulation. Int J Gynaecol Obstet 2002;78(3):221–5.

[44] Weitz JI. Low-molecular-weight heparins. N Engl J Med 1997;337(10):688–98.

[45] Greer IA. Anticoagulants in pregnancy. J Thromb Thrombolysis 2006;21(1):57–65.

[46] Schwander D, Bachmann F. [Heparin and spinal or epidural anesthesia: decision analysis]. Ann Fr Anesth Reanim 1991;10(3):284–96 [in French].

[47] Wulf H. Epidural anaesthesia and spinal haematoma. Can J Anaesth 1996;43(12):1260–71.

[48] Cheney FW, Domino KB, Caplan RA, et al. Nerve injury associated with anesthesia: a closed claims analysis. Anesthesiology 1999;90(4):1062–9.

[49] Binder DK, Sonne DC, Lawton MT. Spinal epidural hematoma. Neurosurgery Quarterly 2004;14(1):51–9.

[50] Lawton MT, Porter RW, Heiserman JE, et al. Surgical management of spinal epidural hematoma: relationship between surgical timing and neurological outcome. J Neurosurg 1995;83(1):1–7.

[51] Kreppel D, Antoniadis G, Seeling W. Spinal hematoma: a literature survey with meta-analysis of 613 patients. Neurosurg Rev 2003;26(1):1–49.

[52] Bucklin BA, Hawkins JL, Anderson JR, et al. Obstetric anesthesia workforce survey: twenty-year update. Anesthesiology 2005;103(3):645–53.

[53] Hawkins JL, Koonin LM, Palmer SK, et al. Anesthesia-related deaths during obstetric delivery in the United States, 1979–1990. Anesthesiology 1997;86(2):277–84.

ELSEVIER
SAUNDERS

Anesthesiology Clin
26 (2008) 23–52

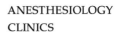

ANESTHESIOLOGY
CLINICS

Neurological Infections After Neuraxial Anesthesia

Felicity Reynolds, MB BS, MD, FRCA, FRCOG ad eudem

Department of Anaesthetics, St Thomas's Hospital, London, SE1 7EH, UK

Nowadays various forms of neuraxial analgesia and anesthesia are widely used in obstetrics. Just over a century ago spinal analgesia was first applied in late labor [1]; it continued to be used by enthusiasts until the practice of continuous lumbar epidural analgesia and then the local anesthetic bupivacaine took the stage in the 1960s and 1970s. The reemergence of atraumatic spinal needles in the latter part of the twentieth century then opened the way for the wider use of spinal and combined spinal-epidural blockade. Over the years the complications associated with the various techniques have emerged and been tackled, so that currently serious complications of neuraxial blockade are extremely rare, particularly among the obstetric population, who are usually young and fit. Among these serious complications, however, neuraxial infection, comprising meningitis and epidural and para-epidural infection, is probably the most important, for two reasons. First, infection is the now commonest cause of neuraxial injury claims among obstetric patients in the United States [2]. Second, by our own actions we may affect its occurrence. Every case of infection following neuraxial blockade therefore deserves our close attention.

Although both epidural abscess and meningitis are complications of neuraxial anesthesia, their causation and risk factors are disparate. While epidural abscess is primarily a complication of epidural catheter use, the route of infection via the catheter entry point and the causative organism, the *Staphylococcus*, nosocomial meningitis is a complication of dural puncture (for whatever purpose) and is usually caused by streptococci of the viridans type, commonly found in the upper air passages and the vagina.

The rarity of both types of complication makes incidence, relative risk, and efficacy of preventive measures impossible to establish using high-quality

E-mail address: felicity.reynolds@btinternet.com

1932-2275/08/$ - see front matter © 2008 Elsevier Inc. All rights reserved.
doi:10.1016/j.anclin.2007.11.006   *anesthesiology.theclinics.com*

evidence. Reliance therefore has to be placed on case reports, indirect evidence, and common sense.

Incidence

Expectant mothers often ask about the incidence of complications of neuraxial anesthesia, but there is, in truth, no such thing as "an incidence" of meningitis or epidural abscess, accurate or otherwise. The incidence of problems varies widely, depending on the skill and training of the practitioners concerned, as well as on the risk factors in the population. The frequent occurrence of case clusters gives the lie to any attempt to measure a true incidence. Anesthesiologists, nevertheless, have a duty to inform patients of the complications associated with a proposed procedure and are expected to give some figure for the level of risk, however futile such estimates may be.

A number of surveys have been published that attempted to establish the frequency of serious complications of neuraxial blockade, but the findings vary widely, for many reasons. Some old surveys, although they may be based on accurate local records, relate to a time when practices and preparation of equipment and drugs were less safe than they are today. Local audit is likely to be more accurate than any multicenter survey, but now, with the incidence of complications so much reduced, small numbers lack the power to estimate it. Moreover, level of skill can still have a major impact. For example, a Danish national survey of the incidence of epidural abscess after epidural analgesia demonstrated an incidence of 1:5661 in university hospitals and of 1:796 in community hospitals [3]. The problems associated with all such surveys are summarized in Box 1.

Surveys of regional block complications that include both surgical and obstetric patients indicate that complications arise less frequently among the latter. Moen and colleagues [4] detected 29 cases of meningitis (albeit clustered) in a Swedish national survey involving 1,260,000 spinal anesthetics for surgical patients, but none among a possible 55,000 spinals for cesarean section, and 12 epidural abscesses among 450,000 surgical epidurals and one among 200,000 for labor. A French national survey also found fewer complications among obstetric than surgical patients [5]. The sterility of the delivery suite may not be so scrupulously controlled as that of the operating room (OR), but the parturient, being usually young and fit, seems to come off relatively lightly.

The numbers of infectious complications found in surveys of neuraxial blocks in obstetric patients are given in Table 1 [6–13]. Surveys that were not designed to detect such complications, or those that were prompted by the occurrence of a case or case series, as reflecting an inevitable bias, are excluded. The included surveys, given in chronologic order, initially focused on epidural analgesia, but with increased use of spinal and combined spinal-epidural (CSE) blocks, such limitations became appropriate. Little

---

Box 1. Reasons for inaccuracy in surveys of infective complications of neuraxial blockade in obstetric patients

1. Many questionnaire surveys suffer from a poor response rate, and potentially, therefore, a reporting bias.
2. Clinical practice has changed radically since the older surveys were conducted.
3. Small local audit may be more precise than larger multicenter surveys, but with improvement in practice, smaller studies lack power to assess incidence of rare disorders with accuracy.
4. Level of skill and training vary from place to place.
5. Denominator data are inaccurate, while numerators may lack diagnostic precision.
6. Cases arising late, in the community, may be missed.
7. Surveys that are prompted by the occurrence of a case or cluster of cases have a built-in positive reporting bias.
8. Infectious complications usually arise for a specific reason; they are not natural events with "an incidence" as such.

---

reliance should be placed on a recent attempt to collate the findings of surveys of epidural complications in obstetric patients [14], as it overlooked the wide use of spinal and hybrid techniques and used faulty denominators. The studies included in Table 1 provide denominators of 116,987 spinals and CSEs and 908,270 epidurals. There were only 629 spinals in the regional survey by Holdcroft and colleagues, [10] too few for inclusion. The prospective multicenter study by Scott and Tunstall [9] mentioned two unconfirmed cases of meningitis. If these are included and presumed to fall among the spinal anesthetics, this gives an aggregated incidence of meningitis among the spinals in all these surveys of 1:39,000 or 25.6 per million (95% confidence interval [CI]: 5.3 to 74.9 per million) and of epidural abscesses among the epidurals of 1:303,000 or 3.3 per million (95% CI: 0.7 to 9.7 per million). I would not vouch for either the accuracy or the validity of these figures nor rely on their confidence intervals!

Information from surveys involving surgical patients emphasizes the idiosyncratic nature of infectious complications. In a US retrospective review of 4767 spinal anesthetics from a single institution, there were no infective complications [15]; similarly in a Swedish follow-up study of 8501 spinals and 9232 epidurals, there were no instances of meningitis or abscess [16], whereas in a Danish survey of 17,372 epidural anesthetics, there were nine epidural abscesses, admittedly all in elderly people, eight of whom were immunocompromised [3]. In a Brazilian survey there were three cases of meningitis following 38,128 spinal anesthetics, and none in 12,822

Table 1
Incidence of infectious complications of neuraxial anesthesia in obstetric patients, derived from published surveys

Author	Type of study	Denominator	Numbers of cases	
			Meningitis	Epidural abscess
Crawford 1985 [6]	Local audit	27,000 epidurals		1
Ong et al [7]	Chart review	9403 epidurals		0
Scott and Hibbard [8]	Retrospective multicenter review	505,000 epidurals		1
Scott and Tunstall [9]	Prospective multicenter survey	108,133 epidurals 14,856 spinals	0 2?	0 0
Holdcroft et al [10]	Regionwide audit	13,007 epidurals	0	0
Paech [11]	Prospective local audit	10,995 epidurals	0	0
Albright and Foster [12]	Local audit	4164 CSEs	0	0
Holloway et al [13]	Retrospective multicenter review	29,698 spinals 12,254 CSEs	0 1	0 0
Auroy et al [5]	Prospective multicenter survey	29,732 epidurals 5640 spinals	0 0	0 0
Moen et al [4]	Postal survey and search of administrative files	205,000 epidurals 55,000 spinals for CS	0 0	1 0

Abbreviations: CS, cesarean section; CSE, combined spinal-epidural.

patients who received other types of anesthesia [17]. Interestingly, because there were too few cases to attain statistical significance, the authors stated "The incidence of meningitis was similar in patients subjected to spinal anesthesia and in those subjected to another anesthetic technique." Oh the mockery of statistics!

It is sometimes supposed that neuraxial infection may be a chance event in relation to neuraxial anesthesia. Indeed, in an excellent review of neurologic complications of neuraxial anesthesia in obstetrics, Loo and colleagues [18] highlight the numbers of case reports of epidural abscess in obstetric patients that occurred in the absence of anesthesia. In the case of meningitis, the causative agents in nosocomial infection are quite different from those in community-acquired disease [18], so the two are readily distinguished.

Meningitis

Meningitis may follow diagnostic lumbar puncture and myelography as well as neuraxial anesthesia. Despite the paucity of cases that are detected in surveys of neuraxial anesthesia, case reports abound. Thirty-eight concerning obstetric patients are summarized in Table 2 [19–46]. There is one case of viral meningitis (case 8 [24]) and one of community-acquired disease (case 29 [43]) but neuraxial anesthesia is implicated in the rest. The first seven cases listed followed saddle-block spinal anesthesia using nondisposable equipment and tetracaine, a practice then popular in the United States for the second stage of labor. Cases 1 to 3 were from a US army hospital in Germany where spinals were given by obstetricians, and all occurred within 3 weeks [21]. They were ascribed to chemical meningitis attributed to detergent used to wash equipment. This poses the question: why the low cerebrospinal fluid (CSF) glucose? This is, of course, a diagnostic feature of bacterial meningitis. In these cases, as in case 4 [22], undetected bacterial infection would seem more likely. Cases 5 to 7, another case cluster, resulted from extraordinary practice by a single anesthesia provider [23]. Thereafter, causation is more subtle. Two cases that were *reported* as meningitis (cases 11 and 28) [24,40] rather resembled epidural infection or abscess.

Clinical features and management

Among the patients listed in Table 2, symptoms appeared hours or a few days after anesthesia, the exception being among the cases of *Aspergillus* meningitis, in whom the onset time was up to 1 month [45,46].

The initial clinical picture is of headache and fever, often with backache and emetic symptoms, classical signs of meningism, drowsiness, and lethargy. Some cases have been confused initially with dural puncture headache, one receiving two blood patches [23]. The condition is usually benign when treated promptly. In severe and untreated cases, the patient may become unrousable, with diabetes insipidus and other signs of cerebral edema [44–46]. Among the 38 cases in Table 2, there were six deaths, three due to the *Aspergillus* (see below under "Causative organisms"). There can be no cause for complaisance in this condition, particularly as resistant organisms are emerging even among the meek viridans *Streptococcus* [47].

The CSF is often cloudy and shows a raised white cell count, predominantly neutrophils, raised protein, and low glucose concentrations. CSF culture may yield no growth, as in cases 1 to 4, 12 to 15, 19, 21, 24, and 27 (see Table 2), even when bacteria are visible on microscopy. Such cases are sometimes diagnosed as chemical meningitis, but previous antibiotic treatment may contribute to this finding, while the white cell count and still more the low CSF glucose suggest a bacterial origin.

Lumbar puncture aids diagnosis, but it should be remembered that it is risky in the presence of raised intracranial pressure [44] and, indeed, epidural abscess. Imaging may therefore take precedence in doubtful cases. It is clearly important to give appropriate antibiotics early, which will usually be before the causative organism or its sensitivity is established, recognizing that antibiotics may impede its culture. Vancomycin, with third-generation cephalosporins,

Table 2
Case reports of meningitis in obstetric patients

Author	Procedure	Onset	Organism and findings	Treatment	Comments and outcome
Gibbons [19] US Army in Germany	1. Spinal for labor, forceps delivery	2 h	In all cases, CSF typical for bacterial meningitis, including low glucose, but no growth. Ascribed to "chemical meningitis" due to detergent	Ampicillin	Recovered
	2. Spinal for labor, forceps delivery	6 h		Penicillin, chloramphenicol	Recovered
	3. Spinal for labor, forceps delivery	3 h		Penicillin, chloramphenicol	Recovered
Phillips [20] USA	4. Spinal for labor	2 h	2nd LP consistent with bacterial meningitis	Colistin, cefalotin, hydrocortisone	Recovered
Corbett and Rosenstein [21] USA	5. Spinal for labor	36 h	Case cluster: *Pseudomonas aeruginosa* in all cases, also grown from multiuse bottle of saline used to rinse stylet before insertion	Colistin, polymyxin B	Recovered
	6. Spinal for labor	3 days		Colistin, polymyxin B	Recovered
	7. Spinal for labor	4 days		Colistin, polymyxin B	Recovered
Neumark et al [22] Austria	8. Uncomplicated epidural for labor	8 days	Coxsackie B (unrelated)	Intensive care, no mention of antibiotics	h/o TB; stormy passage, recovered
Berga and Trierweiler [23] USA	9. Accidental dural puncture in labor Epidural blood patch × 2	?1 day	*Streptococcus sanguis*	Oxacillin, cefotaxime	Recovered
Ready and Helfer [24] USA	10. Uncomplicated epidural for labor PI to skin	1 day	*Streptococcus uberis* (α-hemolytic)	Ceftriaxone, vancomycin, then ampicillin	Recovered

Reference	Case	Onset	Findings	Antibiotics	Outcome
Roberts and Petts [25] UK	11. Uncomplicated epidural for CS. PCEA hydromorphone for 48 h	5 days	Streptococcus faecalis; epidural inflammation; not drowsy	Gentamycin, ceftazidime, vancomycin, penicillin G	Recovered
	12. Spinal for retained placenta	18 h	CSF typical for bacterial meningitis but no growth	Ceftazidime, flucloxacillin	Recovered
Sansome et al [26] UK	13. Accidental dural puncture; chlorhexidine; epidural replaced	3 days	CSF typical for bacterial meningitis but glucose near normal and no growth	Rifampicin, cefotaxime	Recovered
Bugedo [27] Chile	14. Spinal for CS	5 h	Signs of bacterial meningitis		Recovered
Lee and Parry [28] UK	15. Early labor, cesarean for genital herpes, spinal chlorhexidine, spinal three attempts. Mask not worn as of doubtful value (sic)	16 h	CSF typical for bacterial meningitis but no growth	Benzyl-penicillin, cefotaxime, flucloxacillin, gentamycin	Recovered
Davis et al [29] UK	16. Uncomplicated epidural for labor "full aseptic technique" no mask!	2 days	Group B Streptococcus from blood and vagina	Amoxicillin, vancomycin, metronidazole	Recovered
Newton et al [30] USA	17. Spinal for labor; mask worn, PI to skin; vaginal delivery	12 h	Streptococcus salivarius	Ampicillin, vancomycin, ceftriaxone	Recovered
Lurie et al [31] Israel	18. Spinal for labor; chlorhexidine	12 h	Streptococcus viridans	Broad-spectrum antibiotics	Recovered
Harding et al [32] UK	19. CSE for labor, sterile gown and gloves, no mask assumed; chlorhexidine; forceps delivery	3 days	Bacterial meningitis picture except normal glucose, no growth	Chloramphenicol, benzyl penicillin, ampicillin, flucloxacillin, metronidazole	Recovered

(continued on next page)

Table 2 (continued)

Author	Procedure	Onset	Organism and findings	Treatment	Comments and outcome
	20. CSE, early labor, chlorhexidine, epidural re-sited, spinal for emergency CS: blood patch	21 h	Staphloccus epidermidis	Vancomycin, cefotaxime	Recovered
Stallard and Barry [33] UK	21. Epidural × 2 for labor; mask and chlorhexidine; spinal for cesarean same space	18 h	Bacterial (no growth)	IV antibiotics	Recovered but had PDPH
Goldstein et al [34] USA	22. Epidural for labor and CS	6 days	Group B Streptococcus		Cortical blindness 2° to meningitis Recovered
Cascio and Heath [35] USA	23. CSE for labor	16 h	S salivarius (dismissed as contaminant)	Vancomycin, ceftriaxone	Recovered
Donnelly et al [36] UK	24. Membranes ruptured; spinal for CS; chlorhexidine; no mask	4 days	CSF no growth, glucose not measured; bacterial meningitis diagnosed	Ampicillin, cefotaxime	Recovered
Bouhemad et al [37] France	25. CSE for labor; wore a mask, iodine skin prep, vaginal delivery	14 h	S salivarius	Amoxicillin, cefotaxime, fosfomycin	Recovered
Duflo et al [38] France	26. CSE for labor ("all hygienic measures taken" but sufentanil ampoule shared), vaginal delivery	8 days	S viridans	Ceftriaxone	Recovered
Choy [39] Singapore	27. Epidural for labor; first attempt failed; mask worn; PI skin prep	3 days	Delayed diagnosis of meningitis, no growth but low CSF glucose	Ceftriaxone, metronidazole then ceftazidime, isoniazid, rifampicin, acyclovir	Died

Study	Procedure	Onset	Organism/notes	Treatment	Outcome
Trautman et al [40] Germany	28. Epidural for twin delivery	2 days	Staphylococcus aureus from anesthesiologist's nose; called meningitis but actually abscess	Ceftriaxone, netilmicin	Recovered
Pinder and Dresner [41] UK	29. CSE for labor	1 day	Neisseria meningitidis (ie, chance event)	Cefotaxime, amoxicillin	Recovered
Vermis et al [42] France	30. CSE for labor		One case of meningitis in the course of a randomized trial		Recovered
Thomas and Cooper [43] UK	31. Spinal for CS in preeclampsia; no mention of mask or antibiotic cover		CSF findings not mentioned		Died
Baer [44] USA	32. Accidental dural puncture, epidural replaced, delivered vaginally	<1 day	Staphylococcus simulans from CSF, S salivarius from blood	Ceftriaxone, vancomycin, meropenem, dexamethasone	Died
Rodrigo et al [45] Sri Lanka	33. Spinal for elective CS	7 days	Aspergillus fumigatus	Broad-spectrum antibiotics, fluconazole	Died
	34. Spinal for emergency CS	10 days	A fumigatus	Antibiotics, amphotericin	Died
	35. Spinal for elective CS	1 month	A fumigatus	Amphotericin, voriconazole	Survived
	36. Spinal for elective CS	23 days	A fumigatus	Itraconazole, amphotericin, voriconazole	Survived
	37. Spinal for elective CS	11 days	A fumigatus	Antibiotics, late antifungal therapy	Died
	38. Spinal for elective CS, previous double valve replacement	2 days	Pseudomonas, ?A fumigatus	Antibiotics and voriconazole	Survived

Abbreviations: CS, cesarean section; CSE, combined spinal-epidural; CSF, cerebrospinal fluid; h/o TB, history of tuberculosis; IV, intravenous; LP, lumbar puncture; PCEA, patient-controlled epidural analgesia; PDPH, post-dural puncture headache; PI, povidone iodine.

should be given pending further information. The use of steroids is debatable, but usually recommended for community-acquired meningitis [44].

Causative organisms

Taking into account these and the numerous reported cases of post–spinal meningitis in surgical patients, in the great majority the causative organism is a viridans-type or α-hemolytic *Streptococcus*, often identified as *Streptococcus salivarius* [4,30,31,35,37,38,44]. These organisms are normally of low virulence and, as the name implies, live harmlessly in the upper air passages, as well as the vagina, but they like a watery environment and the cerebrospinal fluid provides a suitable culture medium. By the same token they are disinclined to grow on culture plates, but prefer broth, hence the frequency with which they are apparently missed, or dismissed as contaminants merely because they are commensals [35,44]. Nevertheless, once carried to the subarachnoid space by special conveyance, cause meningitis they certainly do.

In some cases, β-hemolytic *Streptococcus* or *Pseudomonas* have been isolated; the latter also loves a watery medium. A recent case was described of Herpes simplex meningitis following cesarean section [48], but the type of anesthesia was not reported and the authors failed to respond to a written request for clarification.

A cluster of cases of meningoencephalitis occurring in July 2005 in previously fit women who had undergone cesarean section in Sri Lanka, half of whom died, caused great concern and some initial perplexity. The quality of anesthesia and the aseptic technique were immaculate and it was not until a fungal infection was confirmed at the first autopsy that subsequent lives could be saved by antifungal treatment [45,46]. The *Aspergillus* does not normally cause meningitis except in the immunocompromised; like *Streptococcus viridans* it requires a means of entry to the CSF. The source of the infection turned out to be syringes used for spinal anesthesia that had been donated following the tsunami and stored in an unsuitable warehouse, at 41°C and 75% humidity.

There is a clear distinction between the range of organisms causing nosocomial meningitis and those causing community-acquired meningitis (*Neisseria meningitidis*, *Streptococcus pneumoniae*, or *Haemophilus influenzae*). Among the cases in Table 2, the odd exception [22,41] proves the rule.

Risk factors

Among the 36 cases of anesthesia-related meningitis described here, 21 followed spinals, 6 followed CSEs, and 3 followed accidental dural puncture. Thus 30 of 36 followed known dural puncture. Of the six cases following epidural blockade, two probably had primarily *epidural* infection (cases 11 and 28), two insertions were difficult and probably involved undetected dural damage (a well-recognized possibility, even with "normal" epidurals), and two were caused by a Group B *Streptococcus* (cases 16 and 22), a more virulent organism also to be found in the patient's bloodstream and vagina. Nevertheless, in an Iowa study of 73 parturients with β-hemolytic streptococcal infection, the *only one* to develop meningitis had been given spinal anesthesia [49]. Survey findings [4,17,49] as well as case reports [44] would support dural puncture as a prerequisite for nosocomial meningitis, substantiating the view that, in the cases following apparently normal epidural analgesia, there was undetected dural puncture.

Clearly a contaminated needle may carry organisms from the operator's unmasked upper air passages [40,44] or from the patient's skin, into the CSF, but as dural puncture may be associated with the entry of blood into the cerebrospinal fluid, the source of organisms may also be the patient's bloodstream [24,29,30]. Bacteremia is therefore a contributory factor.

It is noticeable that the great majority of parturients with nosocomial meningitis have labored. Despite the occurrence of meningitis among surgical patients, no obstetric cases were found in the Swedish survey, where spinal and CSE anesthesia are rarely used during labor [4]. Meningitis appears *surprisingly rare* when spinals are used for elective caesarean section. There are five possible reasons.

1. The spinal is sited in the OR, a cleaner environment than the delivery suite.
2. The patient is not thrashing about in an amniotic fluid-soaked bed.
3. In the OR the anesthesiologist is more likely to wear a mask.
4. Unlike vaginal delivery, elective cesarean section is not normally associated with streptococcal bacteremia.
5. An antibiotic is always given immediately after delivery by cesarean section.

As among surgical patients [4], immunocompromise is a theoretic risk factor, although the parturients in the cases cited in Table 2 were apparently fit beforehand.

There is no evidence that vaginal delivery per se, even with genital tract sepsis, but without neuraxial anesthesia, is a sufficient risk factor for meningitis [49,50]. The implication would seem to be that the dura should not be punctured *during labor* if an epidural would do instead.

Epidural abscess and related infection

Epidural abscess is a recognized complication of epidural catheterization, but it may also occur spontaneously [18]. It arises infrequently among obstetric patients, as it is seen with greatest frequency among the elderly and immunocompromised [3,4]. Cases have been reported sporadically following neuraxial blockade in obstetric patients [40,51–65]; they are summarized in Table 3. One was reported as meningitis, but was actually an

Table 3
Case reports of epidural abscess in obstetric patients

Author	Procedure	Catheter duration	Onset	Findings	Treatment	Comments and outcome
Crawford 1975 [51] UK	Epidural for labor	Labor only	16 days	Bacteremic infection of hematoma β hemolytic Streptococcus	Laminectomy	Developed subacute bacterial endocarditis
Ngan Kee et al [52] New Zealand	Epidural, early labor, twins, for CS. Difficult insertion	52 h	5 days	Neuro deficit 6 days. MRI Staphylococcus aureus from vagina and abscess	Cefuroxime; then cefotaxime + rifampicin; laminectomy 8 days	Recovered gradually
Borum et al [53] USA	Epidural for labor and tubal ligation	27 h	4 days	Local inflammation; mild deficit; MRI: abscess, S aureus	Surgery and drainage 6 days	Recovered
Kindler et al 1996 [54] Switzerland	Epidural for labor, difficult insertion, severe preeclampsia	88 h	10 days	Local inflammation; CT; Mass; S aureus	Immediate surgery flucloxacillin	Recovered
Jenkin et al [55] Australia	Epidural for CS; diabetic	?Operation only	6 days	Group B Streptococcus, present in vagina	Surgery; penicillin, gentamycin	Minimal residual leg weakness
Dysart and Balakrishnan [56] New Zealand	CSE for CS; good asepsis; no antibiotic	48 h	9 days	S aureus in blood. Mild neurological deficit.	Ceftriaxone, gentamycin and metronidazole; then flucloxacillin and rifampicin	Gradually recovered with conservative treatment

Reference	Procedure	Duration	Onset	Presentation	Treatment	Outcome
Dhillon and Russell [57] UK	Epidural for labor; good asepsis; blood in catheter	6.5 h	8 days	Local swelling, mild neuro deficit; pus extending from subcutaneous to epidural space; *Streptococcus pneumoniae*	Surgery 9 days; flucloxacillin, penicillin	Recovered
Collier and Gatt [58] Australia	Epidural for labor; CS, postop analgesia	84 h	10 days	Lumbar puncture failed; MRI: abscess; no neurological deficit. No organism identified	Cephalothin, ceftriaxone, metronidazole	Slowly recovered
Rathmell et al [59] USA	CSE for labor after car accident, vaginal delivery	72 h	7–10 days	Local inflammation, slight neurological deficit, MRI abscess; *S aureus*	Laminectomy 10 days; cephalexin	Recovered
Unseld and Eisinger [60] Germany	Epidural for labor, two insertions	Brief	3 days	Neurological deficit. MRI: abscess; *Pseudomonas aeruginosa*	Abscess drained after 14 days	Recovered despite delay
Rohrbach and Plotz [61] Germany	Epidural for labor Immunological impairment?	Labor		MRI: abscess	Immediate surgical drainage; prolonged antibiotics	Recovered
Trautman et al[a] [40] Germany	Epidural for twin labor and delivery; mask worn	?24 h	2 days	Neurological deficit; LP grew *S aureus* (from anesthesiologist's nose); MRI: abscess	Repeated surgical drainage 4 days; ceftriaxone, netilmycin, ofloxacin	Paraparesis unchanged

(continued on next page)

Table 3 (*continued*)

Author	Procedure	Catheter duration	Onset	Findings	Treatment	Comments and outcome
Evans and Misra [62] UK	Epidural for twin labor, vaginal delivery; mask not worn	12 + h	1 week	Eventual neuro deficit. MRI: abscess. *S aureus*	Laminectomy after 12 days. Flucloxacillin > 6 weeks	Recovery slow and incomplete
Veiga Sanchez [63] Uruguay	Epidural CS	24 h	5 + days	Radiculitis. MRI: osteomyeltis and epidural abscess	Ceftriaxone	Gradually improved without drainage
Schroeder et al [64] Germany	Epidural for labor. Good asepsis	6 h	5 days	CT inconclusive; MRI abscess; *S aureus*. Mild sensory deficit	Laminectomy 6 days, ceftriaxone, rifampicin, metronidazole. Later clindamycin	Quick recovery
Chiang et al [65] Taiwan	CSE for CS, PCEA	72 h	3 days	Local inflammation + abscess on MRI. Presumed MRSA	Oxacillin, vancomycin, fusidic acid	Recovered without surgery

Abbreviations: CS, cesarean section; CSE, combined spinal epidural; LP, lumbar puncture; MRSA, methicillin-resistant *Staphylococcus aureus*; PCEA, patient-controlled epidural analgesia.
[a] see Table 2.

epidural abscess [40]. All followed epidural catheterization, in three cases as part of a CSE. None followed spinal anesthesia alone.

Clinical features and management

In the assembled cases the catheters remained in situ for a median of 24 hours (see Table 3) and the median time to presentation was 6 days, with the range of 2 to 16 days. Reviewing the world literature including non-obstetric cases, onset times have ranged from 1 to 60 days with the majority less than 5 days [66]. The presenting symptom is backache, usually extremely severe, with marked local tenderness, and sometimes radiating root pain. There may be evidence of inflammation with fluid leak at the insertion site. A blood count reveals raised C-reactive protein and white count [66]. Neurologic deficit may follow, in the form of leg weakness, paresthesiae, bladder disturbance, and other evidence of cauda equina syndrome. Fever and signs of inflammation serve to differentiate epidural abscess from hematoma. MRI allows early diagnosis, while blood culture may identify the organism before or without surgical interference. Diagnostic lumbar puncture is contraindicated.

Full neurologic recovery is dependent on age and also on early detection and treatment [62,66]. Once neurologic changes are present, surgical intervention is usually considered essential to recovery, although four of the women featured in Table 3 [56,58,64,65], with admittedly mild neurologic deficit, recovered fully with conservative treatment only. In three cases, recovery was incomplete despite surgical intervention [40,55,62]. Successful percutaneous needle drainage of an epidural abscess has been reported [67], although only laminectomy can ensure that all loculations are drained under direct vision. Antibiotic treatment needs to be continued for 2 to 4 weeks [68].

Epidural-related infection

Inflammation at the site of catheter insertion, along the track and adjacent to, but not apparently involving, the epidural space, is also described. Eight such reports involving various sites [24,69–75], some including many patients [73], are summarized in Table 4. Catheterization had usually been prolonged to allow postoperative patient-controlled analgesia. A recently published report described both a subdural abscess after a CSE and infection in the subcutaneous tissues of an apparently misplaced blood patch [74].

All such conditions are associated with back pain and signs of inflammation, and presumably pose a threat of spread to the epidural space. Moreover, paraspinal abscess may itself be associated with neurologic deficit [69,70].

Causative organisms

The great majority of epidural abscesses is caused by *Staphylococcus aureus* [66], with the occasional *Streptococcus* and *Pseudomonas* (see Table 3).

Table 4
Case reports of epidural-related infection in obstetric patients

Author	Procedure	Catheter duration	Onset	Findings and organism	Treatment	Comments and outcome
Ready and Helfer[a] [24] USA	Epidural for CS	48 h	5 days	*Streptococcus faecalis*; diagnosed as meningitis but actually epidural "inflammation"	Gentamycin, ceftazidime, vancomycin, penicillin G	Recovered
Kinahan and Douglas. 1995 [69] Canada	Epidural analgesia for labor, re-sited due to blood in catheter; vaginal delivery	10 h	4 days	MRI: Piriformis pyomyositis; vagina grew group **B** *Streptococcus* and *Enterococcus*. Neurologic deficit	Ampicillin; "IV antibiotics"	Recovered
Raj and Foy 1998 [70] New Zealand	Epidural analgesia for labor, instrumental vaginal delivery	Labor	19 days	h/o pelvic arthropathy; neurologic deficit; paraspinal abscess grew *Mycobacterium tuberculosis*	Surgical drainage and decompression. Tuberculosis therapy	Probably coincidental. Recuperated
Hill et al 2001 [71] New Zealand	Epidural analgesia for labor	24 h	2–4 days	*Staphylococcus aureus* paraspinal abscess	Surgery 2 days	Recovered
Bajwa et al 2002 [72] USA	Spinal for CS	None	7 days	Discitis; biopsy grew *Streptococcus bovis*	Vancomycin	Possibly unrelated

Reference	Anesthesia			Presentation	Treatment	Outcome
Cohen et al 2003 [73] USA	PCEA ropivacaine, epinephrine, fentanyl	n/k	2–3 days	12 cases of epidural site infection		
Collis et al 2005 [74] UK	Epidural 3 attempts, for labor	4 h	2–6 days	Superficial discharge; MRI: subdural abscess, *S aureus*	Laminectomy and decompression. Vancomycin, fusidate, cefotaxime	Recovered
	Epidural 2 attempts, for labor	6.5 h	<1 day	Head and backache and inflamed buttock; MRI: subcutaneous infected blood patch. *Escherichia coli* in blood	Blood patch, apparently misplaced. Vancomycin; ciprofloxacin	Persistent back pain
Huang et al 2005 [75] Taiwan	Spinal for CS. Separate epidural for PCEA. Mask but no hand wash, PI	58 h	Gradual onset; presented 20 days	Local inflammation; MRI: paraspinal abscess	Gentamycin, teicoplanin; oxacillin. Surgical drainage	Recovered

Abbreviations: CS, cesarean section; h/o, history of; IV, intravenous; n/k, not known; PCEA, patient-controlled epidural analgesia; PI, povidone iodine.
[a] see Table 2.

Epidural-related infections have been caused by a variety of organisms (see Table 4).

Potential routes of infection

The catheter track

The catheter track appears to be the most important route of entry. Inflammation may be noted at the catheter entry point before the onset of more serious symptoms, implicating the catheter track rather than its contents [54,59]. Organisms may come from the patient's own skin. Bacteria, particularly *Staphylococcus epidermidis*, reside in large numbers in the deeper recesses of hair follicles, and are hard to eradicate by antiseptic skin preparation [76,77].

The bloodstream

Cases such as those involving a β-hemolytic *Streptococcus* [51,55] may have resulted from blood-borne infection alighting on a nidus in the form of a catheter or hematoma in the epidural space.

Equipment

Infection following a brief period of catheterization [57,60,64] suggests that epidural equipment may have contaminated the epidural space. The strain of *S aureus* may show the source to be the nose of the operator [40].

The injectate

The injectate is a potential route of infection if it does not contain a bacteriostatic local anesthetic such as racemic bupivacaine. Although rarely implicated as the source of infection, infusions of opioid alone or of ropivacaine or levobupivacaine, which have less antibacterial activity than bupivacaine [78–81], have been used for postoperative analgesia in many reported cases [24,52,54,58,59,64,73].

Possible risk factors

Prolonged catheterization

This is a self-evident risk for epidural site infection [3,18,52,66,82]. It is hardly surprising that catheters are progressively more likely to become contaminated over time.

Immunocompromise

Diabetes, steroid treatment and malignancy feature regularly in surveys of epidural infection and abscess [3,4,52,66,82,83], although less commonly among parturients. This topic is covered more fully by an excellent review [83].

Traumatic catheter insertion

Difficult insertion with multiple attempts, breaks in sterile technique, and subsequent need for manipulation, are frequently mentioned [3,52,54,57,60].

It is easy to see how multiple attempts can disturb both the aseptic technique and organisms deep in the skin.

Blood in the epidural space

A hematoma is a potential nidus for infection but seems to be implicated infrequently [51]. The risk of infecting the epidural space with a blood patch is considered by some so great as to necessitate prior blood culture. Concern about the danger of introducing infection with an autologous blood patch in the presence of maternal fever led Cesur and colleagues [84] to use allogeneic blood to treat a post–dural puncture headache in a pyrexial patient. Nevertheless, a Medline search for *epidural abscess* AND *epidural blood patch* yields zero at the time of writing, while the only recorded instance of an infected blood patch is one that appears to have been misplaced or to have leaked into the subcutaneous fat [74]. It has been mooted that the presence of HIV infection might contraindicate blood patch, but the virus is so prevalent throughout the body that this fear appears groundless [85,86].

Infection elsewhere

After dural puncture, the presence of bacteremia is a risk factor for meningitis [87] and, as would seem intuitive, adjacent infection is a risk for epidural abscess [51,52]. Among surgical patients, inflammation at the epidural entry point has been found to be increased in frequency when there is an infected wound elsewhere in the body [88,89], although Jakobsen and colleagues [88] conclude that a distant abscess or infected wound should not contraindicate epidural analgesia. Chorioamnionitis might be considered a risk for meningitis rather than abscess. Although a common threat, chorioamnionitis may be accompanied by bacteremia in only 2.5% of sufferers [88] and has not apparently been implicated in neuraxial infection [90–92].

Lying in a wet contaminated bed

Lying in a wet contaminated bed is generally considered a risk for parturients [44,54,93], and in a similar vein, hyperhidrosis has been cited in cases of epidural abscess [65,94].

Unsuitable dressing on an indwelling epidural catheter entry point

The prevalence of lying in a wet contaminated bed would suggest the advisability of an occlusive dressing. Doubt has been cast on the wisdom of such a policy, however [54,73], as it may be associated with an increase in sepsis [95]. A chlorhexidine-impregnated patch dressing may be more suitable [96]. The subject is further addressed in the recommendations that follow.

Absence of antibacterial local anesthetic agent

It has been postulated that the comparatively low infection rate associated with prolonged epidural compared with intravenous catheterization may in part be attributable to the use of antibacterial local anesthetics in the former [97]. However, opioids alone and single-enantiomer local anesthetics, which have little antibacterial action, are now used increasingly commonly (see *Potential routes of infection*). For prolonged epidural catheterization it would seem logical to add a local anesthetic with antibacterial activity to an opioid.

The etiology and risk factors for meningitis and epidural abscess are summarized and compared in Table 5.

Measures to prevent neuraxial infection

Measures to prevent neuraxial infection have now happily become the focus of increased attention, with several reviews in recent years that repay attention [77,83,96–98]. It is frequently mourned that measures we are asked to use are not evidence-based. Unlike infection related to surgical wounds or central venous catheterization, neuraxial infection is too rare for evidence about its prevention to be obtainable from randomized trials. Extrapolation from other fields (often misleading), indirect evidence, logic, and common sense may be the best available tools, while oft despised case reports are frequently quoted and indeed may be the only "evidence" about some risk factors.

Table 5
Summary of etiologic factors for meningitis and epidural abscess

	Meningitis	Epidural abscess
Entry	• Via dural puncture, from contaminated equipment or the patient's blood	• Along the catheter track or, less so, down its lumen • *Staphylococcus aureus*
Usual causative organism	• Viridans type *Streptococcus*	• Patient's skin and bed • Contaminated epidural equipment
Possible source of infection	• Operator's mouth • Talking without a mask • Blood-borne • Vagina	• Injectate • *Rarely* blood-borne • Prolonged catheterization
Risk factors	• Dural puncture + labor ± vaginal delivery • No face mask • Vaginal infection • Bacteremia • Poor aseptic technique • Immunocompromise?	• Immunocompromised: steroids, diabetes, AIDS • Multiple attempts at insertion • Poor aseptic technique • Lying in a wet contaminated bed • Absence of bactericidal local anesthetic

The following, in the order in which they must be practiced, are candidates for inclusion in the armamentarium against neuraxial infection:

Wear hat and mask

The value of masks (sometimes redundantly called face masks, whether for giving inhalational anesthesia or as worn by staff) is commonly misunderstood. Randomized trials have demonstrated that the omission of masks in the OR does not increase wound infection, but this has no relevance to the insertion of neuraxial blocks. Moreover, the authors of a reliable study [99] did not dare include prosthetic surgery, which should tell us something. Reviews of the need to wear masks may concentrate on protection for staff or surgical wound infection, but often overlook completely their place in anesthetic procedures [100]. That many anesthesiologists fail to wear masks and believe them to be useless [17,101,102] is not evidence of their ineffectiveness in preventing neuraxial infection. Among case reports of nosocomial meningitis, a mask is not mentioned, not worn ("as it is of doubtful value" [28] or because it "contributes little to prevent infection during spinal or epidural anesthesia" [31] or is not considered part of a "full aseptic technique" [29]) or mentioned in the wrong order ("Following surgical scrub, the anesthesiologist put on sterilized gloves, a surgical gown, and a mask." [103]—such an order of events defies the imagination).

Commensals in the upper air passages *do not cause wound infection*, but as well as endangering prostheses, they repeatedly cause nosocomial meningitis, particularly when a mask is not worn by the anesthesiologist [4,18,44,77,104]. Such a complication is normally too rare to designate as an outcome of a randomized trial. This is where both indirect evidence and common sense come in. A mask can readily and efficiently diminish the dispersion of bacteria from the mouth and nose [105,106]. Not talking during insertion is not an option for the compassionate obstetric anesthesiologist.

Hubble and colleagues [107] found that, during dummy operations, bacterial counts in laminar flow theaters increased fourfold when hats were omitted, 15-fold when masks were omitted, and 22-fold when neither were worn. There is therefore indirect evidence to support wearing a hat as well as a mask.

In the face of all the evidence, it is clearly mandatory to wear a mask for spinal insertion, and because of the possibility of accidental dural puncture, not to mention Staphylococci in the nose, for epidural insertion also. Masks must be correctly applied, of good quality, and changed regularly, at least between patients [108]. The cost of a mask is a fraction of the cost of dural puncture, let alone that of a case of meningitis [44].

Remove prostheses and baubles from the hands

It belies belief that anyone would wear jewelry and false fingernails when preparing to conduct a sterile procedure, yet they apparently do [102]. Not surprisingly, such addenda make cleaning the hands less efficient [109].

Wash hands in alcohol or carry out a surgical scrub

This procedure is considered more important than wearing sterile gloves [77,98]. Studies have shown that an alcohol-based gel is more effective at eliminating microflora than an antimicrobial soap [109], that various alcoholic preparations are most effective at eliminating *Escherichia coli* but that chlorhexidine has a longer lasting effect [110] and that 4% chlorhexidine is more effective and longer lasting than 10% povidone iodine [111].

Don sterile gloves without touching the outside with bare hands

A *sterile gown*, although part of the surgical ritual of "full aseptic precautions," is rarely worn for spinal insertion, but usually worn for epidural siting in the United Kingdom to avoid contaminating a catheter that is destined to remain some time in the patient. This is an expensive addition to the ritual, and impossible to evaluate, but can only be safer than not doing so. There is little dissent about sterile gloves [102], although they are no substitute for hand washing [77,96].

Clean the patient's back widely, twice, with chlorhexidine in alcohol

Many studies have addressed how best to clean the patient's skin and keep it clean; they are comprehensively reviewed elsewhere [96]. Guidelines developed for skin preparation for surgery and for central venous and arterial catheterization [112] have been adapted, in part, as recommendations for neuraxial anesthesia [96].

As with hand disinfection, chlorhexidine outperforms povidone iodine consistently. Sakuragi and colleagues [113] showed that 0.5% chlorhexidine in ethanol, unlike 10% povidone iodine, could completely inhibit growth of methicillin-resistant *Staphyloccous aureus* in vitro. A study from France comparing 0.25% chlorhexidine (with benzalkonium and 4% benzyl alcohol) and 10% povidone iodine [114] and another from the United States comparing 2% aqueous chlorhexidine and 10% povidone iodine [115] showed the superiority of chlorhexidine in preventing central venous and arterial catheter-related sepsis and bacteremia.

In the field of epidural insertion results are similar. Thus, Kinirons and colleagues [116] showed that 0.5% chlorhexidine in alcohol was more efficient and longer lasting than 10% povidone iodine in inhibiting catheter colonization in prolonged use, although Kasuda and colleagues [117] found no difference between the agents for short-term catheterization. Organisms residing deep in the hair follicles are a potential source of epidural infection [76]. Sato and colleagues [76] found that, with its greater penetrative power, 0.5% chlorhexidine in alcohol was significantly better than 10% povidone iodine at inhibiting growth of organisms in human skin sampled at lumbar laminectomy. Yentur and colleagues [118] confirmed that skin preparation with 10% povidone iodine cannot prevent contamination of epidural needles and catheters during insertion. Moreover, open bottles of 10% povidone iodine do not maintain their sterility [119]. Of direct clinical relevance is the observation by Cameron and colleagues [120] that switching between povidone iodine and chlorhexidine for skin preparation was associated with remarkable changes in epidural insertion–site infection (Fig. 1), while site infection was associated with epidural abscess. Fig. 1 suggests that even *alcoholic* iodine is less efficient than alcoholic chlorhexidine.

Alcohol is rapid and effective and improves the efficacy of both chlorhexidine and iodine, whether as Duraprep [93] or the old-fashioned iodine tincture [121], but chlorhexidine has consistently superior residual activity. Whether given as 0.5% alcoholic solution or by aqueous spray, reduced skin colonization is still observed hours later at epidural catheter removal [122].

Antiseptic solutions reduce bacterial counts exponentially, thus if the count is high before skin preparation, it will still be relatively high after a single application; two applications are therefore not only more effective, they may also be strongly indicated [123].

It is therefore important to spray or paint at least twice, allowing the solution to dry between applications, a routine that is widely practiced [76,108,110,122,124,125]. Alcoholic preparations dry rapidly, so if the first coat is applied by the anesthesiologist before preparing the sterile equipment, dual application need not delay proceedings for a mother in pain. Moreover, if a spray is used it may be applied by an assistant with further time saving.

Neither povidone iodine nor chlorhexidine is licensed for skin preparation before neuraxial anesthesia [96]. Yet because chlorhexidine injected directly into the anterior chamber of a rat's eye has been associated with degeneration of adrenergic nerves [126], it is supposed that minute amounts of skin prep passing into a patient's subarachnoid space could pose a material threat. Thus, despite its numerous glaring disadvantages (Table 6), iodine is still preferred to chlorhexidine in some quarters. The best expert

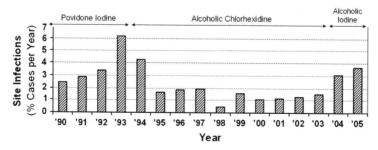

Fig. 1. Annual incidence of epidural insertion site infection, showing skin preparation solution used before epidural insertion. (*Reproduced from* Cameron CM, Scott DA, McDonald WM, et al. A review of neuraxial epidural morbidity. Anesthesiology 2007;106:997–1002; with permission.)

Table 6
Properties of chlorhexidine and povidone iodine compared

	Chlorhexidine	Povidone iodine
Speed of onset	Quick	Slow, several minutes
Accelerated by alcohol	Yes	Yes
Duration[a]	Effect extended "several hours"	"Limited...requires reapplication every 24 h"
Skin reaction	Rare	Yes, erythema, urticaria, vesicular lesions
Effective in presence of blood or pus	Yes	No
Bacterial resistance	Rare	Yes, particularly Staphylococcus aureus
Approved for skin prep before neuraxial block	No	No
CNS adverse events described	No	No
Stays sterile in container	Yes	No

   [a] Studies consistently demonstrate a more prolonged effect with chlorhexidine. The explanation of these apparently contradictory statements has been sought but is unknown.
   Data from Hebl JR. The importance and implications of aseptic techniques during regional anesthesia. Reg Anesth Pain Med 2006;31:311–23.

opinion recommends otherwise [96], while it would seem wise to keep any skin prep solution off the cart on which the sterile equipment is prepared.

Avoid contaminating equipment that will enter the patient

Common sense suggests it is wise to apply sterile drapes securely to the area and, if possible, to use a no-touch technique for any elements that will enter the subarachnoid space.

Apply a suitable dressing to the catheter entry point

Evidence-based guidelines relating to dressing central and peripheral venous catheters [112] are probably, in the main, applicable to prolonged epidural catheterization. A meta-analysis suggests that application of a transparent polyurethane film as an *intravenous* catheter dressing *is* associated with an increase in local sepsis and bacteremia [95], although the guidelines [112] appear to misquote these findings. Moreover, no amount of occlusion can exclude the bacteria already resident in the patient's skin [76]. More suitable would appear to be a chlorhexidine-impregnated patch dressing, which not only reduces skin colonization, it also absorbs blood and exudate, which would otherwise provide a favorable culture medium [96].

In a high-risk situation, avoid prolonged catheterization and prescribe antibiotics

The risk of epidural abscess is increased by prolonged catheterization, by immunocompromise, and by multiple attempts at insertion. It would seem

---

Box 2. Summary of recommendations to minimize infection when siting neuraxial blocks

1. Remove hand jewelry and avoid wearing artificial nails
2. Wear a hat and an effective mask, changed between patients
3. Wash hands thoroughly, preferably alcohol wash
4. Don powder-free sterile gloves; avoid touching the outside of the gloves with bare hands
5. Clean the patient's skin with alcoholic chlorhexidine spray or paint widely, twice
6. Ensure the area is securely draped and avoid contaminating equipment
7. For prolonged catheterization, consider including a local anesthetic with antibacterial activity
8. Avoid prolonged epidural catheterization in the presence of immunocompromise and after multiple attempts at insertion

---

logical, therefore, to avoid prolonged epidural catheterization when other risk factors are present. If it is felt that the benefits of epidural analgesia outweigh the risks, then there is circumstantial evidence that suitable antibiotics reduce the chances of infection, although early administration may be crucial [3,77,97]. Inclusion of racemic bupivacaine would be an added safeguard (see *Possible risk factors*).

A more cautious approach suggests: "No amount of preparation … can maintain sterility throughout the time that an epidural catheter may remain in situ. No skin dressing, occlusive or otherwise, can prevent entry via a catheter site of bacteria resident in the patient's skin. If there is the slightest contraindication to prolonged catheterization, the moral is simple: *take it out*"[50].

In relation to the risk of nosocomial meningitis, an approach of extreme caution would be, where possible, to avoid dural puncture during labor without good reason, particularly in the presence of genital tract infection or other risks. Antibiotics may also play a role in preventing meningitis after dural puncture.

Recommendations for the prevention of neuraxial infection are summarized in Box 2.

References

[1] Kreis O. On spinal narcosis during labour. Special centennial article First published in 1900 in Zentalblatt fur Gynakologie and translated into English for: Int J Obstet Anesth 2000;9: 174–8.
[2] Lee LA, Posner KL, Domino KB, et al. Injuries associated with regional anesthesia in the 1980s and 1990s. Anesthesiology 2004;101:143–52.
[3] Wang LP, Hauerberg J, Schmidt JF. Incidence of spinal epidural abscess after epidural analgesia: a national 1-year survey. Anesthesiology 1999;91:1928–36.

[4] Moen V, Dahlgren N, Irestedt L. Severe neurological complications after central neuraxial blockades in Sweden 1990–1999. Anesthesiology 2004;101:950–9.

[5] Auroy Y, Benhamou D, Bargues L, et al. Major complications of regional anesthesia in France: the SOS regional anesthesia hotline service. Anesthesiology 2002;97:1274–80.

[6] Crawford JS. Some maternal complications of epidural analgesia for labour. Anaesthesia 1985;40:1219–25.

[7] Ong BY, Cohen MM, Esmail A, et al. Paresthesias and motor dysfunction after labor and delivery. Anesth Analg 1987;66:18–22.

[8] Scott DB, Hibbard BM. Serious non fatal complications associated with extradural block in obstetric practice. Br J Anaesth 1990;64:537–41.

[9] Scott DB, Tunstall ME. Serious complications associated with epidural/spinal blockade. Int J Obstet Anesth 1995;4:133–9.

[10] Holdcroft A, Gibberd FB, Hargrove RL, et al. Neurological problems associated with pregnancy. Br J Anaesth 1995;75:522–6.

[11] Paech MJ, Godkin R, Webster S. Complications of obstetric epidural analgesia and anaesthesia: a prospective analysis of 10995 cases. Int J Obstet Anesth 1998;7:5–11.

[12] Albright GA, Forster RM. The safety and efficacy of combined spinal and epidural analgesia/anesthesia (6,002 blocks) in a community hospital. Reg Anesth Pain Med 1999; 24:117–25.

[13] Holloway J, Seed PT, O'Sullivan G, et al. Paraesthesiae and nerve damage following combined spinal epidural and spinal anaesthesia. Int J Obstet Anesth 2000;9:151–5.

[14] Ruppen W, derry S, McQuay H, et al. Incidence of epidural hematoma, infection and neurologic injury in obstetric patients with epidural analgesia/anesthesia. Anesthesiology 2006;105:394–9.

[15] Horlocker TT, McGregor DG, Matsushige DK, et al. A retrospective review of 4767 consecutive spinal anesthetics: central nervous system complications. Anesth Analg 1997; 84:578–84.

[16] Dahlgren N, Tornebradt K. Neurological complications after anaesthesia. A follow-up of 18 000 spinal and epidural anaesthetics performed over three years. Acta Anaesthesiol Scand 1995;39:872–80.

[17] Videira RLR, Ruiz-Neto PP, Neto MB. Post spinal meningitis and asepsis. Acta Anaesthesiol Scand 2002;46:639–46.

[18] Loo CC, Dahlgren G, Irestedt L. Neurological complications in obstetric regional anaesthesia. Int J Obstet Anesth 2000;9:99–124.

[19] Gibbons RB. Chemical meningitis following spinal anesthesia. JAMA 1969;210:900–2.

[20] Phillips OC. Aseptic meningitis following spinal anesthesia (Comment on anonymous case report). Anesth Analg 1970;49:866–71.

[21] Corbett JJ, Rosenstein BJ. Pseudomonas meningitis related to spinal anesthesia. Report of three cases with a common source of infection. Neurology 1971;21:946–50.

[22] Neumark J, Feichtinger W, Gassner A. Epidural block in obstetrics followed by aseptic meningitis. Anesthesiology 1980;52:518–9.

[23] Berga S, Trierweiler MW. Bacterial meningitis following epidural anesthesia for vaginal delivery: a case report. Obstet Gynecol 1989;74:437–9.

[24] Ready LB, Helfer D. Bacterial meningitis in parturients after epidural anesthesia. Anesthesiology 1989;71:988–90.

[25] Roberts SP, Petts HV. Meningitis after obstetric anaesthesia. Anaesthesia 1990;45:376–7.

[26] Sansome AJT, Barnes GR, Barrett RF. An unusual presentation of meningitis as a consequence of inadvertent dural puncture. Int J Obstet Anesth 1991;1:35–7.

[27] Bugedo G, Valenzuela J, Munoz H. [Aseptic meningitis following spinal anesthesia. Report of a case]. Rev Med Chil 1991;119:440–2 [in Spanish].

[28] Lee JJ, Parry H. Bacterial meningitis following spinal anaesthesia for Caesarean section. Br J Anaesth 1991;66:383–6.

[29] Davis L, Hargreaves C, Robinson PN. Postpartum meningitis. Anaesthesia 1993;48:788–9.

[30] Newton JA, Lesnik IK, Kennedy CA. *Streptococcus salivarius* meningitis following spinal anesthesia. Clin Infect Dis 1994;18:840–1.

[31] Lurie S, Feinstein M, Heifetz C, et al. Iatrogenic bacterial meningitis after spinal anesthesia for pain relief in labor. J Clin Anesth 1999;11:438–9.

[32] Harding SA, Collis RE, Morgan BM. Meningitis after combined spinal-extradural anaesthesia in obstetrics. Br J Anaesth 1994;73:545–7.

[33] Stallard N, Barry P. Another complication of the combined extradural-subarachnoid technique. Br J Anaesth 1995;75:370–1.

[34] Goldstein MJ, Parker RL, Dewan DM. Status epilepticus amauroticus secondary to meningitis as a cause of postpartum cortical blindness. Reg Anesth 1996;21:595–8.

[35] Cascio M, Heath G. Meningitis following a combined spinal-epidural technique in a labouring term parturient. Can J Anaesth 1996;43:399–402.

[36] Donnelly T, Koper M, Mallaiah S. Meningitis following spinal anaesthesia—a coincidental infection? Int J Obstet Anesth 1998;7:170–2.

[37] Bouhemad B, Dounas M, Mercier FJ, et al. Bacterial meningitis following combined spinal-epidural analgesia for labour. Anaesthesia 1998;53:292–5.

[38] Duflo F, Allaouchiche B, Mathon L, et al. Méningite bactérienne aprés anesthésie rachidienne et péridural combinée en obstétrique. Ann Fr Anesth Reanim 1998;17:1286.

[39] Choy JC. Mortality from peripartum meningitis. Anaesth Intensive Care 2000;28:328–30.

[40] Trautmann M, Lepper PM, Schmitz FJ. Three cases of bacterial meningitis after spinal and epidural anesthesia. Eur J Clin Microbiol Infect Dis 2002;21:43–5.

[41] Pinder AJ, Dresner M. Meningococcal meningitis after combined spinal-epidural analgesia. Int J Obstet Anesth 2003;12:183–7.

[42] Vernis L, Duale C, Storme B, et al. Perispinal analgesia for labour followed by patient-controlled infusion with bupivacaine and sufentanil: combined spinal-epidural vs. epidural analgesia alone. Eur J Anaesthesiol 2004;21:186–92.

[43] Thomas T, Cooper G. In: Why mothers die 1997–1999. Confidential enquiries into maternal deaths in the United Kingdom. London: RCOG Press; 2001. p. 147.

[44] Baer ET. Post-dural puncture bacterial meningitis. Anesthesiology 2006;105:381–93.

[45] Rodrigo N, Perera KNT, Ranwala R, et al. Aspergillus meningitis following spinal anaesthesia for caesarean section in Colombo, Sri Lanka. Int J Obstet Anesth 2007;16:256–60.

[46] Gunaratne PS, Wijeyaratne CN, Seneviratne HR. Aspergillus meningitis in Sri Lanka— a post-tsunami effect? N Engl J Med 2007;356:754–6.

[47] Yaniv LG, Potasman I. Inatrogenic meningitis: an increasing role for resistant viridans streptococci? Case report and review of the last 20 years. Scand J Infect Dis 2000;32:693–6.

[48] Godet C, Beby-Defaux A, Agius G, et al. Maternal Herpes simplex virus type 2 encephalitis following Cesarean section. J Infect 2003;47:174–5.

[49] White CA, Koontz FP. Hemolytic streptococcus infections in postpartum patients. Obstet Gynecol 1973;41:27–32.

[50] Reynolds F. Infection as a complication of neuraxial blockade. Int J Obstet Anesth 2005;14:183–8.

[51] Crawford JS. Pathology in the extradural space. Br J Anaesth 1975;47:412–5.

[52] Ngan Kee WD, Jones MR, Thomas P, et al. Extradural abscess complicating extradural anaesthesia for caesarean section. Br J Anaesth 1992;69:647–52.

[53] Borum SE, McLeskey CH, Williamson JB, et al. Epidural abscess after obstetric epidural analgesia. Anesthesiology 1995;82:1523–6.

[54] Kindler C, Seeberger M, Siegmund M, et al. Extradural abscess complicating lumbar extradural anaesthesia and analgesia in an obstetric patient. Acta Anaesthesiol Scand 1996;40:858–61.

[55] Jenkin G, Woolley IJ, Brown GV, et al. Post partum epidural abscess due to group B *Streptococcus*. Clin Infect Dis 1997;25:1249.

[56] Dysart RH, Balakrishnan V. Conservative management of extradural abscess complicating spinal-extradural anaesthesia for caesarean section. Br J Anaesth 1997;78:591–3.

[57] Dhillon AR, Russell IF. Epidural abscess in association with obstetric analgesia. Int J Obstet Anesth 1998;6:118–21.

[58] Collier CB, Gatt SP. Epidural abscess in an obstetric patient. Anaesth Intensive Care 1999; 27:662–6.

[59] Rathmell JP, Garahan MB, Alsofrom GF. Epidural abscess following epidural analgesia. Reg Anesth Pain Med 2000;25:79–82.

[60] Unseld H, Eisinger I. [Epidural abscess following repeated epidural catheter placement for delivery]. Anaesthesist 2000;49:960–3 [in German].

[61] Rohrbach M, Plotz J. [Epidural abscess following delivery with peridural analgesia. The question of prevention]. Anaesthesist 2001;50:411–5 [in German].

[62] Evans PR, Misra U. Poor outcome following epidural abscess complicating epidural analgesia for labour. Eur J Obstet Gynecol Reprod Biol 2003;109:102–5.

[63] Veiga Sanchez AR. [Vertebral osteomyelitis and epidural abscess after epidural anesthesia for a cesarean section]. Rev Esp Anestesiol Reanim 2004;51:44–6 [in Spanish].

[64] Schroeder TH, Krueger WA, Neeser E, et al. Spinal epidural abscess—a rare complication after epidural analgesia for labour and delivery. Br J Anaesth 2004;92:896–8.

[65] Chiang HL, Chia YY, Chen YS, et al. Epidural abscess in an obstetric patient with patient-controlled epidural analgesia—a case report. Int J Obstet Anesth 2005;14:242–5.

[66] Kindler CH, Seeberger MD, Staender SE. Epidural abscess complicating epidural anesthesia and analgesia. Acta Anaesthesiol Scand 1998;42:614–20.

[67] Tabo E, Ohkuma Y, Kimura S, et al. Successful percutaneous drainage of epidural abscess with epidural needle and catheter. Anesthesiology 1994;80:1393–5.

[68] Royakkers AANM, Willigers H, van der Ven AJ, et al. Catheter-related epidural abscesses—don't wait for neurological deficits. Acta Anaesthesiol Scand 2002;46:611–5.

[69] Kinahan AM, Douglas MJ. Piriformis pyomyositis mimicking epidural abscess in a parturient. Can J Anaesth 1995;42:240–5.

[70] Raj V, Foy J. Paraspinal abscess associated with epidural in labour. Anaesth Intensive Care 1998;26:424–6.

[71] Hill JS, Hughes EW, Robertson PA. A *Staphylococcus aureus* paraspinal abscess associated with epidural analgesia in labour. Anaesthesia 2001;56:871–8.

[72] Bajwa ZH, Ho C, Grush A, et al. Discitis associated with pregnancy and spinal anesthesia. Anesth Analg 2002;94:415–6.

[73] Cohen S, Uzum N, Aptekin B. Aseptic precautions for inserting an epidural catheter. Anaesthesia 2003;58:930.

[74] Collis RE, Harris SE. A subdural abscess and infected blood patch complicating labour analgesia. Int J Obstet Anesth 2005;14:246–51.

[75] Huang YY, Zuo Z, Yuan HB, et al. A paraspinal abscess following spinal anaesthesia for caesarean section and patient-controlled epidural analgesia for postoperative pain. Int J Obstet Anesth 2005;14:252–5.

[76] Sato S, Sakuragi T, Dan K. Human skin flora as a potential source of epidural abscess. Anesthesiology 1996;85:1276–82.

[77] Hebl JR, Horlocker TT. You're not as clean as you think. The role of asepsis in reducing infectious complications related to regional anesthesia. Reg Anesth Pain Med 2003;28: 376–9.

[78] Zaidi S, Healy TEJ. A comparison of the antibacterial properties of six local analgesic agents. Anaesthesia 1977;32:69–70.

[79] Pere P, Lindgren L, Vaara M. Poor antibacterial effect of ropivacaine: comparison with bupivacaine. Anesthesiology 1999;91:884–6.

[80] Hodson M, Gajraj R, Scott NB. A comparison of the antimicrobial activity of levobupivacaine vs bupivacaine: an *in vitro* study with bacteria implicated in epidural infection. Anaesthesia 1999;54:699–702.

[81] Goodman EJ, Jacobs MR, Bajaksouzian S, et al. Clinically significant concentrations of local anesthetics inhibit *Staphylococcus aureus* in vitro. Int J Obstet Anesth 2002;11:95–9.

[82] Du Pen SL, Petereon DG, Williams A, et al. Infection during chronic epidural catheterization: diagnosis and treatment. Anesthesiology 1990;73:905–9.

[83] Horlocker TT, Wedel DJ. Regional anesthesia in the immunocompromised patient. Reg Anesth Pain Med 2006;31:334–45.

[84] Cesur M, Alici HA, Erdem AF, et al. Epidural blood patch with allogeneic blood for post-dural puncture headache. Int J Obstet Anesth 2005;14:261–2.

[85] Gershon RY, Manning-Williams D. Anesthesia and the HIV-infected parturient: a retrospective study. Int J Obstet Anesth 1997;6:76–81.

[86] Shapiro HM. Opposer: epidural blood patch is contraindicated in HIV-positive patients. Int J Obstet Anesth 1994;3:168–9.

[87] Carp H, Bailey S. The association between meningitis and dural puncture in bacteremic rats. Anesthesiology 1992;76:667–9.

[88] Jakobsen KB, Christensen MK, Carlsson PS. Extradural anaesthesia for repeated surgical treatment in the presence of infection. Br J Anaesth 1995;75:536–40.

[89] Bengtsson M, Nettelblad H, Sjoberg F. Extradural catheter-related infections in patients with infected cutaneous wounds. Br J Anaesth 1997;79:668–70.

[90] Bader AM, Gilbertson L, Kirz L, et al. Regional anesthesia in women with chorioamnionitis. Reg Anesth 1992;17:84–6.

[91] Gibbs RS, Castillo MS, Rodgers PJ. Management of acute chorioamnionitis. Am J Obstet Gynecol 1980;136:709–13.

[92] Goodman EJ, DeHorta E, Taguiam JM. Safety of spinal and epidural anesthesia in parturients with chorioamnionitis. Reg Anesth 1996;21:436–41.

[93] Birnbach DJ, Meadows W, Stein DJ, et al. Comparison of povidone iodine and DuraPrep, an iodophor-in-isopropyl alcohol solution, for skin disinfection prior to epidural catheter insertion in parturients. Anesthesiology 2003;98:164–9.

[94] Masanobu I, Shigeru S, Masayuki S, et al. Epidural abscess in a patient with dorsal hyperhidrosis. Can J Anesth 2003;50:450–3.

[95] Hoffmann KK, Weber DJ, Samsa GP, et al. Transparent polyurethane film as an intravenous catheter dressing. A meta-analysis of the infection risks. JAMA 1992;267:2072–6.

[96] Hebl JR. The importance and implications of aseptic techniques during regional anesthesia. Reg Anesth Pain Med 2006;31:311–23.

[97] Wedl DJ, Horlocker TT. Regional anesthesia in the febrile or infected patient. Reg Anesth Pain Med 2006;31:324–33.

[98] Hepner DL. Gloved and masked—will gowns be next? The role of asepsis during neuraxial instrumentation. Anesthesiology 2006;105:241–3.

[99] Tunevall TG. Postoperative wound infections and surgical face masks: a controlled study. World J Surg 1992;16:147–8.

[100] Skinner MW, Sutton BA. Do anaesthetists need to wear surgical masks in the operating theatre? A literature review with evidence-based recommendations. Anaesth Intensive Care 2001;29(4):331–8.

[101] Panikkar KK, Yentis SM. Wearing of masks for obstetrical regional anaesthesia. A postal survey. Anaesthesia 1996;51:398–400.

[102] Sellors JE, Cyna AM, Simmons SW. Aseptic precautions for inserting an epidural catheter: a survey of obstetric anaesthetists. Anaesthesia 2002;57:593–6.

[103] Kasai T, Yaegashi K, Hirose M, et al. Aseptic meningitis during combined continuous spinal and epidural analgesia. Acta Anaesthesiol Scand 2003;47:775–6.

[104] Baer ET. Introgenic meninigitis: the case for face masks. Clin Infect Dis 2000;31:519–21.

[105] McLure HA, Talboys CA, Yentis SM, et al. Surgical face masks and downward dispersal of bacteria. Anesthesia 1998;53:624–6.

[106] Phillips BJ, Fergusson S, Armstrong P, et al. Surgical facemasks are effective in reducing bacterial contamination caused by dispersal from the upper airway. Br J Anaesth 1992;69:407–8.

[107] Hubble MJ, Weale AE, Perez JV, et al. Clothing in laminar flow operating theatres. J Hosp Infect 1996;32:1–7.

[108] Couzigou C, Vuong TK, Botherel AH, et al. Iatrogenic *Streptococcus salivarius* meningitis after spinal anaesthesia: need for strict application of standard precautions. J Hosp Infect 2003;53(4):313–4.

[109] McNeil SA, Foster CL, Hedderwick SA, et al. Effect of hand cleansing with antimicrobial soap or alcohol-based gel on microbial colonization of artificial fingernails worn by health care workers. Clin Infect Dis 2001;32(3):367–72.

[110] Ayliffe GA, Babb JR, Davies JG, et al. Hand disinfection: a comparison of various agents in laboratory and ward studies. J Hosp Infect 1988;11:226–43.

[111] Cremieux A, Reverdy ME, Pons JL, et al. Standardized method for evaluation of hand disinfection by surgical scrub formulations. Appl environ microbiol 1989;55:2944–8.

[112] O'Grady NP, Alexander M, Dellinger EP, et al. Guidelines for the prevention of intravascular catheter-related infections. Available at: http://www.cdc.gov/mmwr/preview/mmwrhtml/rr5110a1.htm. Accessed July 13, 2007.

[113] Sakuragi T, Yanagisawa K, Dan K. Bactericidal activity of skin disinfectants on methicillin-resistant *Staphylococcus aureus*. Anesth Analg 1995;81:555–8.

[114] Mimoz O, Pieroni L, Lawrence C, et al. Prospective, randomized trial of two antiseptic solutions for prevention of central venous or arterial catheter colonization and infection in intensive care unit patients. Crit Care Med 1996;24(11):1818–23.

[115] Maki DG, Ringer M, Alvarado CJ. Prospective randomised trial of povidone-iodine, alcohol, and chlorhexidine for prevention of infection associated with central venous and arterial catheters. Lancet 1991;338:339–43.

[116] Kinirons B, Mimoz O, Lafendi L, et al. Chlorhexidine versus povidone iodine in preventing colonization of continuous epidural catheters in children: a randomized, controlled trial. Anesthesiology 2001;94(2):239–44.

[117] Kasuda H, Fukuda H, Togashi H, et al. Skin disinfection before epidural catheterization: comparative study of povidone-iodine versus chlorhexidine ethanol. Dermatology 2002; 204(Suppl 1):42–6.

[118] Yentur EA, Luleci N, Topcu I, et al. Is skin disinfection with 10% povidone iodine sufficient to prevent epidural needle and catheter contamination? Reg Anesth Pain Med 2003;28(5): 389–93.

[119] Birnbach DJ, Stein DJ, Murray O, et al. Povidone iodine and skin disinfection before initiation of epidural anesthesia. Anesthesiology 1998;88:668–72.

[120] Cameron CM, Scott DA, McDonald WM, et al. A review of neuraxial epidural morbidity. Anesthesiology 2007;106:997–1002.

[121] Little JR, Murray PR, Traynore PS, et al. A randomized trial of povidone-iodine compared with iodine tincture for venipuncture (*sic*) site disinfection: effects on rates of blood culture contamination. Am J Med 1999;107:119–25.

[122] Robins K, Wilson R, Watkins EJ, et al. Chlorhexidine spray versus single use sachets for skin preparation before regional nerve blockade for elective caesarean section: an effectiveness, time and cost study. Int J Obstet Anesth 2005;14:189–92.

[123] Reynolds F. Infection as a complication of neuraxial blockade. In reply. Int J Obstet Anesth 2006;15:85–6.

[124] Benhamou D, Mercier FJ, Dounas M. Hospital policy for prevention of infection after neuraxial blocks in obstetrics. Int J Obstet Anesth 2002;11:265–9.

[125] Ritter MA, French ML, Eitzen HE, et al. The antimicrobial effectiveness of operative-site preparative agents: a microbiological and clinical study. J Bone Joint Surg Am 1980;62: 826–8.

[126] Henschen A, Olson L. Chlorhexidine-induced degeneration of adrenergic nerves. Acta Neuropathol 1984;63(1):18–23.

ANESTHESIOLOGY
CLINICS

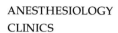

Anesthesiology Clin
26 (2008) 53–66

Major Obstetric Hemorrhage

Frederic J. Mercier, MD, PhD[a],*,
Marc Van de Velde, MD, PhD[b]

[a]*Department of Anesthesia and Intensive Care, Hopital Antoine Beclere—APHP
and Universite Paris-Sud, 157 rue de la Porte de Trivaux,
92141 Clamart Cedex BP 405, France*
[b]*Department of Anaesthesiology, University Hospitals Gasthuisberg,
Katholieke Universiteit Leuven, Herestraat 49, B-3000 Leuven, Belgium*

Major obstetric hemorrhage remains the leading cause of maternal mortality and morbidity worldwide [1]. In addition, even in many developed countries, it is also the maternal complication for which the highest rate of substandard care and potential avoidance are observed [2]. It is thus important to have a thorough knowledge of the pathophysiology, etiology, and therapeutic options of major obstetric hemorrhage. However, the key point is a well-defined and multidisciplinary approach that aims to act quickly and avoid omissions or conflicting strategies that are likely to occur in this stressful situation. This strategy, based on national or international guidelines, has to be discussed and agreed on in every maternity unit and finally written down as a local consensual procedure.

Antepartum hemorrhage

Antepartum hemorrhage is a relatively frequent problem, occurring in 5% to 6% of pregnant women [1]. Many cases originate from benign pathology and will not result in significant maternal or fetal morbidity [1]. Approximately half of the cases result from unknown origin [3]. Despite earlier claims, recent evidence suggests that antepartum hemorrhage of unknown origin does produce more premature labor and delivery and, subsequently, more fetal and neonatal problems [3]. Cases with abnormal placentation, usually placenta previa or placental abruption, can result in serious complications for both mother and child.

* Corresponding author.
E-mail address: frederic.mercier@abc.aphp.fr (F.J. Mercier).

1932-2275/08/$ - see front matter © 2008 Elsevier Inc. All rights reserved.
doi:10.1016/j.anclin.2007.11.008   *anesthesiology.theclinics.com*

Antepartum hemorrhage can result in postpartum hemorrhage (PPH). PPH results from one or a combination of four basic processes: uterine atony, retained placental products, genital-tract trauma, or coagulation abnormalities, though this last process is rarely the primary cause of early (<24 hour) PPH (see this section below).

Abruptio placentae

Placental abruption is defined as the separation of the placental bed from the decidua basalis before delivery of the fetus. The classic presentation is that of vaginal blood loss, uterine tenderness, and increased uterine activity [1]. Sometimes concealed blood loss (up to 1–2 L, then usually associated with fetal death) occurs in a retroplacental hematoma, resulting in danger-ous underestimation of the true blood loss. Placental abruption can cause coagulopathy, which occurs in 10% of cases. However, if fetal demise occurs, the incidence is much higher (up to 50%). Route and timing of delivery are determined by maternal and fetal compromise. Sometimes, expectant management may be considered because of early gestational age, if there is no worrying coagulation disorders and no other maternal or fetal problem. However, as a general rule, prompt delivery must be considered when placental abruption occurs.

Placenta previa

When the placenta implants in advance of the fetal presenting part, placenta previa is diagnosed. Three types of placenta previa are defined, depending on the relationship between the cervical os (rather than the fetal-presenting part itself) and the placenta: total, partial, or marginal. It occurs in 0.5% of pregnancies, usually in association with prior uterine scarring such as a previous cesarean (C-section), uterine surgery, or a previous placenta previa. Painless vaginal blood loss is the classic sign. The first episode of bleeding usually stops spontaneously and does not result in fetal compromise.

Placenta accreta/increta/percreta

Placenta accreta vera is defined as an abnormally adherent placenta, without invasion in the myometrium. Placenta increta invades the myome-trium and placenta percreta perforates the uterine muscle and invades the serosa or the surrounding pelvic structures, usually the bladder (Fig. 1). As a result of the increasing rate of C-sections, the incidence of placenta accreta is increasing. The combination of a placenta previa and a previous uterine scar increases the risk significantly. Chattopadhyay and colleagues and Clark and colleagues [4,5] noted that when the uterus is unscarred, the incidence of placenta accreta is 5% in case of placenta previa. With a previous C-section, the incidence increased to 10%, and when more

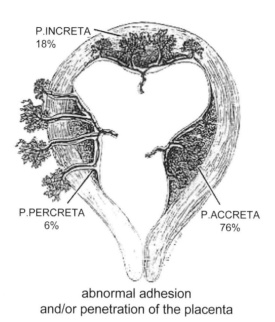

abnormal adhesion
and/or penetration of the placenta

Fig. 1. Placenta accreta. (*From* Kamani AA, Gambling DR, Christilaw J, et al. Anesthetic management of patients with placenta accreta. Can J Anaesth 1987;34:613–7; with permission.)

than one previous C-section was performed, more than 50% of patients had placenta accreta. Ultrasonography and MRI may be useful when abnormal placentation is suspected. However, they both have a poor sensitivity and the diagnosis is often made on opening the abdomen and uterus [6].

Uterine rupture

Previous C-section is the major risk factor for uterine rupture [7]. In the study by Ofir and colleagues [8], the incidence was 0.2%, whereas it was 10 times less in parturients with an unscarred uterus. In the latter situation, the bleeding is classically more frequent and severe than during rupture of a scarred uterus [9]. Conversely, in the more frequent setting of a scarred uterus, uterine rupture may be incomplete and pain infrequent, and an abnormal fetal heart rate pattern can be the only presenting symptom along with anarchic uterine contractions or hypertonus. The diagnosis is confirmed by manual uterus exploration or laparotomy. However, the most recent study by Ofir and colleagues [8] has challenged this concept and found no significant differences in maternal or perinatal morbidity between rupture of a scarred versus an unscarred uterus. Although this etiology is rare, it plays an important role in maternal mortality and severe morbidity related to ante- or peripartum bleeding [9].

Vasa previa

When the cord is inserted velamentous, fetal vessels transverse the fetal membranes ahead of the fetal presenting part. Rupture of the membranes can result in a tear of these fetal vessels, leading to an exsanguinated fetus. It is a rare condition occurring in 1 in 2500 deliveries. If minimal blood loss accompanies fetal distress, one should suspect the diagnosis. As fetal blood content is very small (roughly 250 mL), even this small amount of bleeding will result in fetal death within only a few minutes if immediate C-section is not performed. Thus, it is one of the rare situations where true, immediate C-section (under general anesthesia) is needed to try to save the fetus.

Amniotic fluid embolism

Another cause of peripartum hemorrhage is amniotic fluid embolism [10]. Peripartum hemorrhage results from often rapid and dire coagulopathy. Amniotic fluid embolism occurs in 1 in 10,000 pregnancies, but might be more common than previously believed because of undiagnosed "moderate" forms. Indeed, although amniotic fluid embolism usually presents itself with cardiorespiratory collapse and usually followed by cardiac arrest, coagulopathy that usually occurs soon after the initial presenting symptoms can sometimes be the only symptom. Thus, in all cases, immediate delivery is needed (even if the fetus is already dead), and copious postpartum bleeding resulting from major coagulation disorders and uterine atony must be anticipated.

Postpartum hemorrhage

Primary PPH is defined as blood loss of greater than 500 mL within 24 hours of delivery and affects about 5% of deliveries. However, this definition cannot be used in clinical practice because assessment of blood loss is inaccurate; thus, any abnormal bleeding (in rate or duration) after delivery should trigger at once the diagnosis of PPH. There are many known risk factors for PPH, before or during labor, but their odds ratio or sensitivity/specificity are too low on which to base a strategy to prevent PPH, except for placenta previa/accreta [11–13]. In other words, every parturient has to be considered at risk and thus every maternity unit needs to be prepared to deal with PPH. The three most common causes of PPH are uterine atony, retained placenta, and cervical/vaginal lacerations. Taken together, they represent roughly 95% of all causes of PPH.

Retained placenta

This is the second most important etiology of PPH (roughly 20%–30% of cases), but it must be systematically investigated first, because uterine atony is frequently associated and can be misleading. It is suggested by the finding of an absent or incomplete placenta. If delivery of the placenta has not taken place, it must lead without delay to manual removal of the placenta, under anesthesia whenever possible, to ensure uterus emptying. Otherwise, manual uterine exploration has to be performed, even if inspection of the placenta suggests no retained products of conception (Fig. 2).

Uterine atony

Uterine atony is the leading cause of PPH, observed alone in 50% to 60% of cases; it presents as painless continuous bleeding, often developing slowly at the beginning. Blood can be concealed in the uterus and not exteriorized until external compression of the uterine fundus is performed. The other key diagnostic criterion is abdominal palpation of a soft and oversized uterus. Prevention relies on active management of the third stage of labor—that is, application of controlled traction on the umbilical cord and countertraction on the uterus just above the pubic symphysis, plus slow prophylactic injection of oxytocin (5–10 IU) when the anterior shoulder is delivered (active management of the placental stage) [14] or right after placenta delivery [15]. Treatment is based on bladder emptying and oxytocin (10–20 IU; ± uterine massage). When these measures are not quickly effective (see Fig. 2 and organizational aspects below), cervical/vaginal lacerations must be

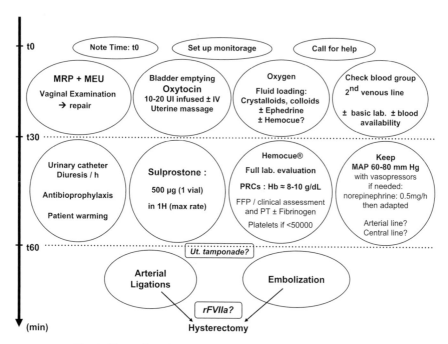

Fig. 2. Hemorrhage in the labor ward. Step management for PPH.

searched for and then be followed by rapid implementation of prostaglandin treatment if bleeding still persists.

Cervical/vaginal lacerations

This is the third cause of PPH (roughly 10% of cases), and it is more likely to occur after instrumental extraction, fetal macrosomia, or quick labor and delivery before full cervical dilation. Diagnosis is also suggested when retained placenta and uterine atony have been discarded. It is made by performing a thorough examination of the vagina and cervix with appropriate valves and thus requires perfect analgesia/anesthesia. In fact, this diagnosis is often made much too late (the bleeding can be concealed in the vaginal wall or pelvis), when the parturient displays hemodynamic instability, coagulation disorders, and increasing pelvic pain.

Episiotomy can also lead to significant bleeding if not quickly repaired.

Uterine inversion

This is a rare iatrogenic event ($<1/1000$) where the internal surface of the uterus is partially or completely exteriorized into the vagina. It is favored by uterine atony and may occur when excessive umbilical traction or abdominal pressure has been applied. The diagnosis is usually obvious. Clinical features include abdominal pain and often severe hemodynamic instability that appears far in excess of what could be solely anticipated from bleeding. Immediate uterine reversion must be performed by the obstetrician and can be facilitated by short-time tocolysis (trinitrine as first line), using usually a potent IV vasopressor at the same time to counteract hypotension (phenylephrine or adrenaline).

Coagulation disorders

Coagulation disorders can be the cause or the consequence of PPH. Many causes can be listed (congenital, such as von Willebrand disease, or acquired, such as HELLP syndrome, disseminated intravascular coagulopathy, anticoagulation therapy, etc). In fact, coagulation disorders are rarely a true triggering cause of PPH, contrary to the causes mentioned in the text above.

Planning for obstetric hemorrhage—organizational aspects

The effective management of obstetric hemorrhage relies on very simple but often overlooked principles that all concur to timely treatment:

- Simultaneous, coordinated, multidisciplinary management (ie, obstetricians, anesthesiologists, hematologists, laboratory and blood bank technicians, radiologists).
- Consensual and practical definition of hemorrhage: any abnormal bleeding (in rate or duration) should trigger at once the diagnosis of

hemorrhage. This is particularly important after delivery where the border between physiologic bleeding and PPH must be clear-cut to avoid any treatment delay.

- Consensual, preplanned, step management available as a written operational protocol.

A summarized example of step management for PPH derived from American and French guidelines is given in Fig. 2 [1,12]:

- As a first step, the obstetric team needs to focus on the search and basic treatment of the three most common causes of PPH: retained placenta (manual removal of the placenta and manual uterine exploration), uterine atony (bladder emptying and IV oxytocin ± uterine massage), and cervical/vaginal lacerations (examination of the vagina and cervix with appropriate valves, and repair as needed). Simultaneously, the anesthetic team provides basic resuscitation and adequate analgesia for these obstetric interventions.
- The second step is implemented as soon as the first step has proven ineffective at stopping the bleeding and no later than 30 minutes after initial PPH diagnosis, to improve effectiveness [16]. It mainly relies on prostaglandin administration, either IV prostaglandin E_2 (PGE_2) sulprostone [16,17] or intramuscular 15-Methyl prostaglandin $F_{2\alpha}$ ($PGF_{2\alpha}$) carboprost [1,18]; uterine tamponade can also be useful. More advanced resuscitation and monitoring are also usually needed and provided by the anesthetic team at this stage (see Fig. 2 and transfusion therapy section, below).
- The third step is considered within an additional 30 minutes (and no longer than after 1 hour) if the second step has also failed to stop bleeding. It relies on invasive therapy, either surgical artery ligation ± B-lynch suture or radiologic embolization (see details in the following paragraphs).
- The last step is hysterectomy; meanwhile, the use of recombinant activated factor VII (rFVIIa) can be considered (see details below).

Of course, this systematic step-by-step approach of PPH treatment has to be adapted to the individual situation, rate of bleeding, or specific etiologies, but it is useful in most circumstances to gain time, avoid omissions, and prevent conflicting strategies within the multidisciplinary team.

Invasive therapy

Several invasive options are available to control PPH when medical treatment is unsuccessful at controlling bleeding: uterine balloon tamponade, arterial embolization, uterine compression sutures, and internal iliac artery ligation. A systematic literature review performed by Doumouchstis and colleagues [19] showed that uterine embolization and B-Lynch sutures were effective in 91% of cases, whereas uterine tamponade and iliac artery ligation were successful in 84% of cases. The place of rFVIIa is still a matter of debate (see specific section below); however, the implementation of these invasive treatments should never be significantly delayed. If these options fail, peripartum hysterectomy remains the only way to stop bleeding and save lives.

Uterine balloon tamponade

Uterine packing has long been the treatment of choice to manage PPH; it is safe, quick, and effective in a majority of cases [20]. More recently, uterine balloon tamponade has been favored. An overall success rate of 84% has been reported [19,21]. It is easily performed by relatively inexperienced personnel and requires no (or only minimal) anesthesia. Various balloon devices have been used, with the Sengstaken-Blakemore esophageal catheter being the most frequently employed [19].

Uterine arterial embolization

Another less radical approach to control bleeding is the use of uterine artery embolization. It has become a well-recognized alternative method of treatment in the conservative management of PPH in association with local or medical treatment, or in the event of their failure. This therapeutic approach avoids morbidity associated with peripartum hysterectomy and preserves fertility. It is also a possible additional approach when arterial ligation or hysterectomy fails to control bleeding [22].

In 1979, Brown and colleagues [23] described for the first time the use of transcatheter uterine artery embolization to control PPH. Since then, several reports have demonstrated its safety and efficacy both in the treatment of major hemorrhage as well as in its prevention. The reported success rate of uterine artery embolization in the literature is more than 90% [24–27]. In most patients, fertility is preserved and normal menstruation returns almost 100% [27]. Minor complications such as pain and transient inflammation with fever are rare (0%–10%) [27]. More severe complications such as pelvic infection, pulmonary embolism, or uterus and bladder necrosis have been reported but are extremely rare [28,29].

Although transfer to the radiology suite may be sometimes possible even when major hemorrhage occurs and the patient is hemodynamically unstable, transfer is usually only done when vital signs are stable because facilities equipped to handle major bleeding are often much better in the operating room. In addition, transfer duration to radiology plus speed and expertise of the intervening radiologist are of paramount importance when this radiologic option is considered. Placement of arterial catheters and occlusion balloons before delivery is currently the treatment option of choice whenever major hemorrhage is highly suspected. These balloons can be used to reduce blood loss significantly while the patient is prepared to undergo embolization.

B-Lynch suture

When confronted with major uncontrollable obstetric hemorrhage, several surgical options are available to the surgeon. Since its first description in 1997, the so-called B-Lynch uterine compression suture has been used successfully to control bleeding following failed conservative management [30]. Indeed, up until May 2005, 46 cases were published and in only two patients did the technique fail to control bleeding, resulting in a subsequent hysterectomy [31]. This technique also allows uterus conservation for subsequent menstrual function and pregnancies and seems to be devoid of long-term sequelae [31]. Ideally, a formal randomized trial should be performed to demonstrate its superiority over hysterectomy. Most likely this will not occur, as such a trial will be difficult to set up and implement; moreover, it might be considered unethical.

Surgical iliac (or uterine) artery ligation

When uterine tamponade and arterial embolization fail, a laparotomy to perform iliac artery ligation is an option to preserve the uterus. It can also be performed as a first invasive option, during C-section delivery, or when the patient is hemodynamically unstable or if embolization is not readily available. A success rate of 84% has been described [19]. Joshi and colleagues [32] more recently reported that iliac artery ligation failed to arrest bleeding in up to 39% of women in a series of 88 patients. However, in the present authors' analysis of the overall literature, these arterial ligation techniques (either iliac or uterine, depending mainly on local experience) have a very good success rate ($\geq 90\%$), provided that they are implemented quickly (ie, as soon as more standard measures have proven ineffective; see Fig. 2) [33,34].

The procedure is technically challenging, particularly for surgical iliac artery ligation, and carries well-documented risks such as post-ischemic lower motor neuron damage, acute intestinal obstruction, claudicatio pain, and peripheral nerve ischemia [35–38]. Nonetheless, it has the advantage of quick implementation and availability in all maternity units, provided it has been accurately taught during obstetric or surgical training courses. When arterial ligation fails, hysterectomy is usually necessary. This may carry a higher risk of morbidity when compared with emergency hysterectomy performed without prior iliac artery ligation [39].

Hysterectomy

As a last resort, but decided on quickly when all other interventions have failed, peripartum emergency hysterectomy may be required to control bleeding and save lives. Habek and Becarevic reported a 0.08% incidence of peripartum hysterectomy in a recently published study [40]. In a recent population-based descriptive study using the United Kingdom obstetric surveillance system, all cases of peripartum hysterectomy were identified over a 1-year period [41]. Of the 315 cases recorded, most occurred following uterine atony and morbidly adherent placentation. In a significant number of these women who had had a hysterectomy, prior surgical or medical treatment had failed, including B-Lynch sutures, arterial embolization, and the administration of activated factor VII.

Transfusion therapy and resuscitation

Massive blood loss often requires blood transfusion. Concerns for potential transmission of infectious disease have led to a reevaluation of red blood cell transfusion indications. Although it was customary to transfuse below a hemoglobin of less than 10 g/dL, new consensus guidelines concluded that, perioperatively, a healthy patient only requires transfusion of less than 7 g/dL [42]. Intuitively, the increased metabolism associated with pregnancy suggests that pregnant patients tolerate anemia less then nonpregnant patients. Indeed, Karpati and colleagues [43] demonstrated a high incidence of myocardial ischemia, determined by tropinin measurements, in PPH patients. Hypotension, tachycardia, and the need for cathecholamines were independent risk factors to develop ischemia. Transfusion should be initiated with red blood cells in all obstetric patients with signs of inadequate oxygen-carrying capacity and in most obstetric patients with a hemoglobin of less than 7 g/dL, or when blood loss is ongoing and the hemoglobin is around 7 g/dL. If hemorrhage is accompanied by coagulation disorders, 15 to 20 mL/kg of fresh frozen plasma should be given as first-line treatment and target hemoglobin should be set higher, above 8 g/dL, to improve overall coagulation activity [44]. Transfusion of platelet concentrates is recommended to treat active bleeding associated with thrombocytopenia below 50 G$\bullet$L^{-1} [12].

Recent outcome studies in (non-obstetric) massive hemorrhage actually suggest that morbidity and mortality are reduced when transfusion is initiated earlier and when a fresh frozen plasma:red blood cell ratio of 1:1 is used instead of the lower 0.5:1 classic ratio [45,46]. In massive bleeding, it is of paramount importance to have adequate IV access if needed by placing a central venous (jugular or femoral) large-bore multiple line (echographic venous location is often useful in hypovolemic patients when a portable device is readily available). The use of a rapid transfusion device plus a skin-warming device also helps preventing hypothermic-induced coagulopathy and hypovolemic-induced acidemia. An arterial (radial or femoral) line allows precise and beat-to-beat blood pressure measurement and facilitates blood sampling for laboratory evaluation. It can be used also to adjust vasopressor therapy (norepinephrine) at minimal rate in addition to fluid and transfusion therapy when needed for maintenance of mean arterial pressure between 60 and 80 mmHg (see Fig. 2) [12]. Large-spectrum antibioprophylaxis is added to these advanced resuscitation measures to reduce the high infectious risk linked to massive bleeding management.

Intraoperative cell salvage

The use of intraoperative cell salvage in peripartum hemorrhage is still controversial, although major obstetric anesthesia societies now regard it as an acceptable alternative to allogeneic transfusion [47]. At present, the main reason of opposition is concern that the implementation of this technique may result in delay compared with homologous/allogeneic transfusion during emergency obstetric hemorrhage [48]. Conversely, proponents say that every spared allogeneic unit of red blood cells is important to reduce administration errors, transmitted infections, immunologic reactions, and blood supply shortage [47,49]. It has been recently calculated that intraoperative cell salvage might, theoretically, reduce exposure to appropriately transfused allogeneic erythrocytes in about 20% of C-section delivery patients [50]. Although there are no large, randomized controlled studies to rule out any risk of coagulopathy or even iatrogenic amniotic fluid embolus, experimental and clinical data now strongly suggest that it is very unlikely to exist. Indeed, modern autologous techniques, in combination with leukocyte depletion filter, remove virtually all fetal squames and phospholipid lamellar bodies; in addition, extensive clinical experience is similarly reassuring [47].

Intraoperative cell salvage (or preoperative autologous donation in scheduled cases) has an undisputed role in obstetrics in patients with high risk such as placenta previa/accreta, massive fibroids, or rare blood type or unusual antibodies. Intraoperative cell salvage can be also useful in the treatment of Jehovah's Witnesses or in geographic areas where allogeneic blood supply is particularly problematic. In institutions where cell-saver devices are available routinely for non–obstetric-scheduled surgery, use of intraoperative cell salvage for unexpected peripartum bleeding can also be useful, provided that "attempting to set the cell saver up in a crisis will not divert staff away from vital resuscitation" [48].

Recombinant factor VIIA (NovoSeven)

The first report of the use of rFVIIa for PPH was released in 2001, but more widespread case reports and small series were only published in 2003 and 2004 [51–55]. They suggested that rFVIIa was often effective at stopping or reducing the bleeding, particularly when other conventional treatments (see above) had failed. The dosage used varied roughly from 20 to 120 mcg/kg, without clear evidence of a dose-response relationship [54,55]. To date, there is still no randomized controlled study published to ascertain the efficacy of this treatment in PPH, but a multicenter one is ongoing in France to look at early versus delayed use of rFVIIa (ie, before or after implementation of surgical artery ligation or embolization) [56]. In addition, a European registry currently in press has collected 108 cases and reported an overall 80% success rate (most common recorded dose ≤ 90 mcg/kg), with very few adverse events noted as possibly related to rFVIIa administration [57]. Nonetheless, because of lack of level 1 evidence, the use, dosage, and timing of rFVIIa are still a matter of debate. Recently, European guidelines have pointed out that "rFVIIa may be considered as treatment for life-threatening post-partum hemorrhage, but should not be considered as a substitute for, nor should it delay, the performance of a life-saving procedure such as embolization or surgery, nor the transfer to a referring center" [58].

References

[1] Mayer D, Spielman FJ, Bell EA. Antepartum and postpartum hemorrhage. In: Chestnut DH, editor. Obstetric anesthesia. Principles and practice. 3rd edition. Philadelphia: Elsevier Mosby; 2004. p. 662–82.

[2] Bouvier-Colle MH, Ould El Joud D, Varnoux N, et al. Evaluation of the quality of care for severe obstetrical haemorrhage in three French regions. BJOG 2001;108:898–903.

[3] Chan CC, To WW. Antepartum hemorrhage of unknown origin—what is its clinical significance? Acta Obstet Gynecol Scand 1999;78:186–90.

[4] Chattopadhyay SK, Kharif H, Sherbeeni MM. Placenta previa and accreta after previous caesarean section. Eur J Obstet Gynecol Reprod Biol 1993;52:151–6.

[5] Clark SL, Koonings PP, Phelan JP. Placenta previa/accreta and prior cesarean section. Obstet Gynecol 1985;66:89–92.

[6] Lam G, Kuller J, McMahon M. Use of magnetic resonance imaging and ultrasound in the antenatal diagnosis of placenta accreta. J Soc Gynecol Investig 2002;9:37–40.

[7] Miller DA, Goodwin TM, Gherman RB, et al. Intrapartum rupture of the unscarred uterus. Obstet Gynecol 1997;89:671–3.

[8] Ofir K, Sheiner E, Levy A, et al. Uterine rupture: differences between a scarred and an unscarred uterus. Am J Obstet Gynecol 2004;191:425–9.

[9] Camann WR, Biehl DH. Antepartum and postpartum hemorrhage. In: Hughes SC, Levinson G, Rosen MA, editors. Shnider and Levinson's anesthesia for obstetrics. 4th edition. Philadelphia: Lippincott Williams & Wilkins; 2002. p. 361–71.

[10] Arkoosh VA. Amniotic fluid embolism. In: Hughes SC, Levinson G, Rosen MA, editors. Shnider and Levinson's anesthesia for obstetrics. 4th edition. Philadelphia: Lippincott Williams & Wilkins; 2002. p. 361–71.

[11] Combs CA, Murphy EL, Laros RK Jr. Factors associated with postpartum hemorrhage with vaginal birth. Obstet Gynecol 1991;77:69–76.

[12] Goffinet F, Mercier FJ, Teyssier V, et al. Post partum haemorrhage: recommendations for clinical practice by the CNGOF (December 2004). Gynecol Obstet Fertil 2005;33:268–74.

[13] Reyal F, Sibony O, Oury JF, et al. Criteria for transfusion in severe postpartum hemorrhage: analysis of practice and risk factors. Eur J Obstet Gynecol Reprod Biol 2004;112:61–4.

[14] Prendiville WJ, Elbourne D, McDonald S. Active versus expectant management in the third stage of labour [review]. Cochrane Database Syst Rev 2000;3:CD000007.

[15] Jackson KW Jr, Allbert JR, Schemmer GK, et al. A randomized controlled trial comparing oxytocin administration before and after placental delivery in the prevention of postpartum hemorrhage. Am J Obstet Gynecol 2001;185:873–7.

[16] Goffinet F, Haddad B, Carbonne B, et al. Practical use of sulprostone in the treatment of hemorrhages during delivery. J Gynecol Obstet Biol Reprod 1995;24:209–16.

[17] Baumgarten K, Schmidt J, Horvat A. Uterine motility after post-partum application of sulprostone and other oxytocics. Eur J Obstet Gynecol Reprod Biol 1983;16:181–92.

[18] Hayashi RH, Castillo MS, Noah ML. Management of severe postpartum hemorrhage with a prostaglandin F2 alpha analogue. Obstet Gynecol 1984;63:806–8.

[19] Doumouchstis SK, Papageorghiou AT, Arulkumaran S. Systematic review of conservative management of postpartum hemorrhage: what to do when medical treatment fails? Obstet Gynecol Surv 2007;62(8):540–7.

[20] Maier RC. Control of postpartum hemorrhage with uterine packing. Am J Obstet Gynecol 1993;169:317–21.

[21] Dabelea VG, Schultze PM, McDuffie RS. Intrauterine balloon tamponade in the management of postpartum haemorrhage. J Obstet Gynaecol 2006;107:38S.

[22] Sproule MW, Bendomir AM, Grant KA, et al. Embolisation of massive bleeding following hysterectomy, despite internal iliac artery ligation. Br J Obstet Gynaecol 1994;101:908–9.

[23] Brown BJ, Heaston DK, Poulson AM, et al. Uncontrollable postpartum bleeding: a new approach to hemostasis through angiographic arterial embolization. Obstet Gynecol 1979; 54:361–5.

[24] Deux JF, Bazot M, LeBlanche AF, et al. Is selective embolization of uterine arteries a safe alternative to hysterectomy in patients with postpartum hemorrhage? AJR 2001;177:145–9.

[25] Mitty HA, Sterling KM, Alvarez M, et al. Obstetric hemorrhage: prophylactic and emergency arterial catheterization and embolotherapy. Radiology 1993;188:183–7.

[26] Hong TM, Tseng HS, Lee RC, et al. Uterine artery embolization: an effective treatment for intractable obstetric haemorrhage. Clin Radiol 2004;59:96–101.

[27] Soncini E, Pelicelli A, Larini P, et al. Uterine artery embolization in the treatment and prevention of postpartum hemorrhage. Int J Gynaecol Obstet 2007;96:181–5.

[28] Cottier JP, Fignon A, Tranquart F, et al. Uterine necrosis after arterial embolization for postpartum hemorrhage. Obstet Gynecol 2002;100:1074–7.

[29] Porcu G, Roger V, Jacquier A, et al. Uterus and bladder necrosis after uterine artery embolisation for postpartum haemorrhage. Br J Obstet Gynaecol 2005;112:122–3.

[30] B-Lynch C, Coker A, Lawal AH, et al. The B-Lynch surgical technique for the control of massive postpartum hemorrhage: an alternative to hysterectomy? Five cases reported. Br J Obstet Gynaecol 1997;104:372–85.

[31] Price N, B-Lynch C. Technical description of the B-Lynch brace suture for treatment of massive postpartum hemorrhage and review of published cases. Int J Fertil Womens Med 2005;50:148–63.

[32] Joshi VM, Otiv SR, Majumber R, et al. Internal iliac artery ligation for arresting postpartum haemorrhage. BJOG 2007;114:356–61.

[33] Lédée N, Ville Y, Musset D, et al. Management in intractable obstetric haemorrhage: an audit study on 61 cases. Eur J Obstet Gynecol Reprod Biol 2001;94:189–96.

[34] O'Leary JA. Uterine artery ligation in the control of postcesarean hemorrhage. J Reprod Med 1995;40:189–93.

[35] Evans S, McShane P. The efficacy of internal iliac artery ligation in obstetric hemorrhage. Surg Gynecol Obstet 1985;160:250–3.

[36] Fernandez H, Pons JC, Chambon G, et al. Internal iliac artery ligation in post-partum hemorrhage. Eur J Obstet Gynecol Reprod Biol 1988;28:213–20.

[37] Allahbadia G. Hypogastric artery ligation: a new perspective. J Gynecol Surg 1993;9:35–42.

[38] Shin RK, Stecker MM, Imbesi SG. Peripheral nerve ischaemia after internal iliac artery ligation. J Neurol Neurosurg Psychiatr 2001;70:411–2.

[39] Dildy GA 3rd. Postpartum hemorrhage: new management options. Clin Obstet Gynecol 2002;45:330–44.

[40] Habek D, Becarevic R. Emergency peripartum hysterectomy in a tertiary obstetric center: 8-year evaluation. Fetal Diagn Ther 2007;22:139–42.

[41] Knight M, UKOSS. Peripartum hysterectomy in the UK: management and outcomes of the associated hemorrhage. BJOG 2007;doi: 10.1111/j.1471–0528.2007.01507.x.

[42] Consensus conference. Perioperative red blood cell transfusion. J Am Med Assoc 1988;260: 2700–3.

[43] Karpati PC, Rossignol M, Pirot M, et al. High incidence of myocardial ischemia during postpartum hemorrhage. Anesthesiology 2004;100:30–6.

[44] Jansen AJ, van Rhenen DJ, Steegers EA, et al. Postpartum hemorrhage and transfusion of blood and blood components. Obstet Gynecol Surv 2005;60:663–71.

[45] Johansson PI, Stensballe J, Rosenberg I, et al. Proactive administration of platelets and plasma for patients with a ruptured abdominal aortic aneurysm: evaluating a change in transfusion practice. Transfusion 2007;47:593–8.

[46] Gonzalez EA, Moore FA, Holcomb JB, et al. Fresh frozen plasma should be given earlier to patients requiring massive transfusion. J Trauma 2007;62:112–9.

[47] Catling S. Blood conservation techniques in obstetrics: a UK perspective. Int J Obstet Anesth 2007;16:241–9.

[48] Clark V (opposer). Controversies in obstetric anaesthesia. Facilities for blood salvage (cell saver technique) must be available in every obstetric theatre. Int J Obstet Anesth 2005;14:50–52.

[49] Thomas D (proposer). Controversies in obstetric anaesthesia. Facilities for blood salvage (cell saver technique) must be available in every obstetric theatre. Int J Obstet Anesth 2005;14:48–50.

[50] Fong J, Gurewitsch ED, Kang HJ, et al. An analysis of transfusion practice and the role of intraoperative red blood cell salvage during cesarean delivery. Anesth Analg 2007;104(3): 666–72.

[51] Franchini M, Lippi G, Franchi M. The use of rFVIIa in obstetric and GYN haemorrhage. BJOG 2007;114:8–15.

[52] Bouwmeester FW, Jonkhoff AR, Verheijen R, et al. Successful treatment of life threatening postpartum hemorrhage with recombinant activated factor VII. Obstet Gynecol 2003;101: 1174–6.

[53] Brice A, Hilbert U, Roger-Christoph S, et al. Recombinant activated factor VII as a life-saving therapy for severe postpartum haemorrhage unresponsive to conservative traditional management [Intérêt du facteur VII activé recombinant dans l'hémorragie de la délivrance sévère réfractaire à la prise en charge conservatrice conventionnelle]. Ann Fr Anesth Reanim 2004;23:1084–8 [in French].

[54] Boehlen F, Morales MA, Fontana P, et al. Prolonged treatment of massive postpartum haemorrhage with recombinant factor VIIa: case report and review of the literature. BJOG 2004;111:284–7.

[55] Ahonen J, Joleka R. Recombinant factor VIIa for life-threatening post partum haemorrhage. Br J Anaesth 2005;94:592–5.

[56] U.S. National Institutes of Health. ClinicalTrials.gov. Available at: http://clinicaltrials. gov/ct/show/NCT00370877;jsessionid=422EC32CA6B5E533AB8841B645036340?order=38. Accessed February 12, 2008.

[57] Alfirevic Z, Elbourne D, Pavord S, et al. The use of recombinant activated factor VII in primary postpartum hemorrhage: the Northern European Registry 2000–2004. Obstet Gynecol 2007;110:1270–8.

[58] Vincent JL, Rossaint R, Riou B, et al. Recommendations on the use of recombinant activated factor VII as an adjunctive treatment for massive bleeding—a European perspective. Crit Care 2006;10:R120.

ANESTHESIOLOGY
CLINICS

Anesthesiology Clin
26 (2008) 67–74

The Historical Narrative: Tales of Professionalism?

Douglas R. Bacon, MD, MA

Department of Anesthesiology, College of Medicine, Mayo Clinic,
200 First Street SW, Rochester, MN 55905, USA

Stories from time constitute history. While there is a both a formal form to the telling of these narratives, and the informal family tales told when gathered around the holiday table, or the professional legacy handed down from attending to resident, all are history, for the word story is the critical component to history. The content of these stories delineates much of what the teller values. In a family, the stories of one unsuccessful member may be used to illustrate proper behavior or to teach a lesson—although the listeners may not conceptualize the lesson, they often internalize it. More often, the family stories illustrate success or notable accomplishments: positive behavioral lessons for future generations. Indeed, it is these family tales that give a sense of identity and history to the listener and can make the often-dry recitation of facts done in formal history classes come alive.

So it is with the history of obstetric anesthesia. While the cast of characters is not genetically related to the readers, except in very rare cases, the stories told serve a purpose. These narratives are repeated because they speak to issues with which anesthesiologists still struggle. The argument may be framed differently, as in the case of the nineteenth century argument against labor analgesia on religious grounds, which was transformed in the latter half of the twentieth century as a social objection. No matter how the argument is framed, physicians have countered it and, in so doing, have demonstrated tenets of professionalism. It is these examples that help frame the current concept of professional behavior and more importantly have to some extent framed societal expectations of the obstetric anesthesiologist. The challenge is to interpret the history of obstetric anesthesia in light of the modern definition of professionalism as delineated in the the Physician Charter [1].

E-mail address: bacon.douglas@mayo.edu

doi:10.1016/j.anclin.2007.12.001 *anesthesiology.theclinics.com*

Discovery

William Thomas Green Morton on October 16, 1846, demonstrated that ether could induce insensibility to the surgeon's knife. A jaw tumor was removed from Gilbert Abbot by John Collins Warren at the Massachusetts General Hospital in front of an audience of medical professionals. The news of this public demonstration traveled quickly, given the nature of communication in the 1840s. On December 16, 1846, the information in the form of a letter arrived in London. On December 19, the first ether anesthetic was given in the United Kingdom for the removal of a tooth. On December 21, the famous surgeon Robert Liston amputated the leg of a butler, and uttered the famous words, "This Yankee dodge beats mesmerism hollow" [2].

James Young Simpson, the professor of midwifery in Edinburgh, Scotland, was among the first to use ether for the relief of labor pain. On January 19, 1847, he used ether to ameliorate the pain of labor. This first case, that of a young woman with rickets and a severely deformed pelvis, was at grave risk of dying and there was no hope for a live birth. By using ether, the mother survived the complicated delivery pain-free. That same January day, Simpson was appointed the Queen's Physician in Scotland [3].

Simpson continued to provide anesthesia in childbirth for both complicated and normal deliveries; however, he rapidly became dissatisfied with ether and sought a more pleasant, rapid-acting anesthetic. At the suggestion of David Waldie, he experimented with chloroform, which had first been prepared in 1831. On the evening of November 4, 1847, Simpson and his friends inhaled it after dinner at a party in Simpson's home. They promptly fell unconscious and, when they awoke under the table and clearly off their dining room chairs, were delighted with their success. Within 2 weeks, Simpson submitted his first account of chloroform's use to *The Lancet* [4].

In the nineteenth century, the relief of obstetric pain had significant social and religious consequences, which made anesthesia during childbirth a contentious subject. The battle centered on whether relieving labor pain was contrary to God's will. The pain associated with childbirth was believed to be a Devine punishment for Original Sin. Shortly after giving his first obstetric anesthetics, Simpson published a pamphlet entitled *Answers to the Religious Objections Advanced Against the Employment of Anesthetic Agents in Midwifery and Surgery and Obstetrics*, which argued against these religious prohibitions. In this work, Simpson acknowledged the Book of Genesis as source of this reaction, and noted that God had promised to relieve the daughters of Eve of this pain. Additionally, Simpson believed that labor pain had anatomic causes and therefore could be studied scientifically. Simpson argued that the upright position of humans necessitated strong pelvic muscles to support the abdominal contents. Therefore, the uterus necessarily developed strong musculature to overcome the resistance of the pelvic floor to deliver the infant. Great contractile power necessarily caused great pain. In the end, Simpson's pamphlet most likely did not change the prevailing viewpoints about controlling labor pain. Simpson's writings did, however, articulate many concepts that his contemporaries were debating [5].

Obstetrical anesthesia in general, and chloroform specifically, gained considerable respect after Queen Victoria had chloroform for labor analgesia. The Queen's consort, Prince Albert, interviewed John Snow, a London physician, before Snow was called to Buckingham Palace to administer chloroform at the request of the Queen's obstetrician. During the monarch's labor, Snow gave analgesic doses of chloroform on a folded handkerchief, creating a technique soon named *chloroform à la reine*. Victoria loathed the pain of childbirth and commented in her journal, "Dr. Snow gave that blessed chloroform and the effect was soothing, quieting, and delightful beyond measure" [6]. The Queen abruptly terminated the religious debate over the appropriateness of anesthesia for labor, for as head of the Church of England her endorsement of the practice eliminated religious debate, at least within "her" church. Four years later, Snow was to give a second anesthetic to the Queen, who was determined to have chloroform analgesia during her last confinement. Snow's daybook states that by the time he arrived, Prince Albert had begun the anesthetic [7].

A small digression: professionalism

This oft-repeated story of two of the "giants" of anesthesia history, James Young Simpson and John Snow, and the reigning British monarch, Queen Victoria, is familiar to almost anyone with a passing interest in obstetric anesthesia. Why is knowledge of these events ubiquitous? This narrative speaks to anesthesiologists particularly, because it stresses several elements of professionalism, and our need to be viewed within the context of appropriate physician behavior. In an effort to create a workable framework that can be used for medical education, The Physician Charter was created by a consortium of US and European physicians. This definition consists of three fundamental principles and 10 professional responsibilities. The three fundamental principles are primacy of patient welfare, patient autonomy, and social justice. The 10 professional responsibilities phrased as commitments are professional competence, honesty with patients, patient confidentiality, maintaining appropriate relations with patients, improving quality of care, improving access to care, distribution of finite resources, scientific knowledge, maintaining trust by managing conflicts of interest, and professional responsibilities [1].

Simpson's role can be used to illustrate the Charter's Principle of Patient Welfare. Simpson knew that his first patient would most likely die if she delivered the child she was carrying. At the time, Simpson knew that ether would relieve her pain, which would be in her best interest. As the Charter defines patient welfare, dedication to serving the patient's best interest is paramount. Snow, in giving Queen Victoria chloroform labor analgesia, pushed back against societal forces because it was in the best interest of his patient.

In defining professionalism, the Physician Charter also discusses commitments. Simpson's role in the narrative history speaks clearly to the commitment to scientific knowledge. He sought out a new anesthetic agent when ether proved to be less than ideal for his purposes. Furthermore, Simpson was also dedicated to improving patient care. He saw a need, especially in complicated confinements, to use a new agent and technique to optimize outcome. It is unclear whether his first patient would have survived delivery without ether, but the implication is that she would have. John Snow, as the first physician to limit his practice to anesthesia, studied both ether and chloroform and determined the best way to administer these agents for labor analgesia and anesthesia if necessary. *Chloroform à la reine* became the accepted technique for labor analgesia for many decades after Queen Victoria's delivery. Finally, both physicians, in publishing and lecturing on their techniques before medical societies, demonstrated their commitment to professional responsibilities. By sharing their knowledge and teaching others they worked to maximize patient care and to have their work in the new field scrutinized by others.

Rectal ether

James Taylor Gwathmey, MD, an anesthesiologist who worked in the New York Lying-in Hospital, became interested in the technique of rectal ether and applying it to obstetrics. Gwathmey wanted to find a way of relieving labor pain that did not endanger the mother or child, and that was simple and inexpensive to administer. Furthermore, he wanted only commercially available, standardized drugs to be used, and this method should be possible to use at home as well as in hospital. Ideally, the mother would be in a state of relaxation and analgesia, yet conscious. Gwathmey's method was based on a mixture of ether in oil method instilled into the rectum, which had been extensively used in surgery. After considerable study, numerous formulae had been developed to predict dosage. Gwathmey proved the technique's utility in several hundred cases of childbirth before publishing his results. Gwathmey's technique was simple. He avoided mixing ether in water due to failure of the method, as the ether parted from the saline rapidly resulting in explosive losses. Gwathmey found that an oil/ether mixture in a 1:3 ratio worked best. After the instillation of rectal ether, analgesia occurred in 45 minutes and lasted from 2 to 6 hours. Most multipara patients required one or two instillations [8].

Outside of publishing his results, Gwathmey frequently communicated with the leading obstetric anesthetist of the time. In "selling" rectal ether, Gwathmey described this technique as having few undesirable side effects: no nausea, no vomiting, and no stage of excitement. The ether was easy to administer and to teach to nursing staff. Fetal outcome was excellent with a healthy, crying baby [9]. Charles Hunt of Eugene, Oregon, developed a questionnaire that was sent to 180 leading obstetricians, as he felt that the replies would be representative of the most careful and better trained obstetricians of the country. One hundred and twenty replies were received. Eighty-seven percent of those who answered had been using this method over a number of years, representing high popularity and wide acceptance of this technique. Eighty-two percent were favorably impressed [8].

In 1930, Gwathmey [10] was able to report the results of 20,000 cases from the Lying-In Hospital and three other New York institutions. Rectal ether had resulted in no increase in morbidity and mortality for either mother or the baby. Furthermore, labor was not prolonged and hemorrhages after delivery were less than with ether inhalation. Fetal outcome remained excellent with a crying child at birth. After analyzing over 50,000 records covering the two 4-year periods before and after introduction of the rectal ether, there was no increase in stillbirths, forceps delivery, or cesarean section. By 1942, more than 100,000 cases of oil-ether anesthesia in obstetric cases had been reported in the United States with the consensus of opinion that the method was safe for the mother and child. The only strict contraindication was the presence of lesions of the bowel. Rectal ether in oil was routinely used in patients with nephritis, eclampsia, and cardiac disease without untoward results [10].

Like his predecessor, Gwathmey [10] demonstrates several integral elements of professionalism. In searching for a technique that would be easily applicable to the vast majority of patients, Gwathmey, in addition to serving the principle of patient welfare, clearly demonstrates a commitment to improving access to care. The fact that his technique could be used in the home as well as the hospital with minimal side effects, allowed a greater number of women access to labor analgesia. An argument can be made that Gwathmey also had a commitment to a just distribution of finite resources. Again, the simplicity of the technique allowed many practitioners to administer this form of analgesia. Anesthesiologists were rare; access to their services was limited. Thus, rectal oil-ether analgesia allowed this resource to be stretched a bit further so that more patients were able to have analgesia during labor.

Epidural analgesia and anesthesia

The development of continuous epidural anesthesia and analgesia is derived from the history of continuous spinal anesthesia, and the search for a technique whereby the epidural space could be quickly and easily identified. Epidural, or peridural anesthesia, as it was originally described, can be traced to Jean-Anthanase Sicard and Fernand Cathelin, who in

1901 independently published their accounts of this form of anesthesia. Their approach was through the sacral hiatus, giving what would currently be described as a caudal anesthetic [11]. Fidel Pages, in the early 1920s, described the intraspinous approach to the epidural space. He reported satisfactory anesthesia for intra-abdominal procedures. In the early 1930s, Dogliotti [12], building on the discovery of negative pressure in the epidural space, described a practical technique for lumbar segmental anesthesia. Building on Doglotiti's work, Alberto Gutierrez, in 1932, described the hanging drop technique to identify the epidural space [13,14].

In 1931, Aburel [15] placed a silk ureteral catheter in the epidural space and used this catheter for labor analgesia. During the Second World War, in the United States, Hingson [16] was assigned to care for the pregnant wives of Coast Guard seamen. Hingson wanted a method that would provide analgesia for these women. Unaware of Aburel's work, Hingson took a Lemmon Malleable Needle, used for continuous spinal anesthesia and placed it sacrally, deep to the peridural ligament. Safe and effective, this method of painless childbirth became popular as continual caudal anesthesia [16]. In 1949, Curbello [17] modified Edward Touhey's continuous spinal silk catheter and placed it into the epidural space, creating the first continuous epidural block. By 1962, the first polyvinyl catheters with a closed tip were manufactured and introduced, making the continuous epidural a much easier block to correctly perform [18].

Controversy concerning epidural analgesia in labor continued. Opponents to the practice claimed it increased the number of instrumental deliveries. Proponents claimed it did not, and by the early 1990s, the combination of dilute local anesthetic and narcotic was demonstrated to be no different than any other form of obstetric pain relief [19]. Currently, epidural analgesia has been combined with subarachnoid narcotics to ease the pain of labor. Combined spinal-epidural anesthesia has become one of the leading techniques on obstetric floors in the early twenty-first century [20].

The story of the search for and discovery of epidural anesthesia demonstrates the professionalism of a number of physicians. The commitment to scientific knowledge is an integral part of this story. Each physician contributed a small modicum of knowledge, yet then sum of the parts has become standard care for those requesting and needing epidural analgesia. The commitment to improving quality of care is seen in the number of different techniques developed; a continual search for that which is best. Finally, the commitment to professional responsibility is seen in that each physician not only built upon the work of the others, but worked with colleagues to develop these techniques. The demonstration of Touhey's silk ureteral technique for continuous spinal triggered Curbello to use the same catheter in the epidural space. Yet, without Touhey's demonstration, Curbello might not have ever tried continuous epidural anesthesia!

Virginia Apgar

In 1949, when E.M. Papper [21] became chairman of anesthesiology at Columbia University in New York City, Virginia Apgar was displaced as chair. By mutual agreement, Apgar was assigned to the obstetric suite to improve anesthesia and outcomes for both the mother and child. Charged by Papper to put together an obstetric and neonatal group, she took up the challenge with vigor [21]. In 1952, over breakfast a medical student had asked Apgar if there was a method for evaluating the newborn, and she had replied there was none. As the conversation progressed, Apgar quickly outlined a system to evaluate newborns on the back of a napkin. Published in 1953, the score has been in use for more than 50 years, helping to resuscitate newborns. Interestingly, one of the fist uses of the score was to prove that there were few effects of regional as opposed to general anesthesia on newborns [22].

Apgar's work clearly demonstrates several elements of professionalism. The principle of the primacy of patient welfare, in this case the newborn, is demonstrated through Apgar's dedication to improving the care of all children. Clearly there is an element of the commitment to improving patient care, as the evaluation system identified those children in need of resuscitation.

Summary

The historical narrative is a story told to illustrate a point, however subconsciously. The "giants" of obstetric anesthesia—Simpson, Snow, Apgar—and countless other less well-known physicians all contributed to the history of obstetric anesthesia. We remember them by retelling this history to illustrate elements of professionalism and how we as a profession wish to act. The Physician Charter is an excellent first approximation of a workable definition of this quality, which can and does change over time. By using the three principles and 10 professional responsibilities as a template, the past comes alive as a teaching method to each and every obstetric anesthesiologist.

References

[1] ABIM Foundation, ACP_ASIM Foundation, European Federation of Internal Medicine. Medical professionalism in the new millennium: a physician charter. Ann Intern Med 2002;136:243–6.

[2] Fenster JM. Ether day. New York: HarperCollins; 2001. p. 118–9.

[3] Stratmann L. Chloroform: the quest for oblivion. Phoenix Mill (UK): Sutton Publishing Limited; 2003. p. 35.

[4] Sykes K, Bunker J. Anaesthesia and the practice of medicine: historical perspectives. London: The Royal Society of Medicine Press Ltd; 2007. p. 16–9.

[5] Caton D. What a blessing she had chloroform. New Haven (CT): Yale University Press; 1999. p. 103–6.

[6] Queen Victoria. Journal of Queen Victoria. In: Strauss MB, editor. Familiar medical quotations. Boston: Little Brown; 1968. p. 17.

[7] Johansen PV, Paneth N, Rachman S, et al. Cholera, chloroform, and the science of medicine: a life of John Snow. New York: Oxford University Press; 2003. p. 368–9.

[8] Hunt CE. Analgesia in obstetrics by the Gwathmey synergistic method. North West Medicine 1929;28:82–7.

[9] Multiple Letters between John S. Lundy, M.D. and James T. Gwathmey 1924–1927. The Collected papers of john S. Lundy. Rochester (MN): Mayo Foundation Archive.

[10] Gwathmey JT. The story of oil-ether colonic anesthesia. Anesthesiology 1942;3:171–5.

[11] Bromage PR. Epidural analgesia. Philadelphia: W.B. Saunders; 1978. p. 1–7.

[12] Dogliotti AM. Anesthesia. Chicago: S.B. Debour; 1939. p. 529–44.

[13] Lund PC. Peridural analgesia and anesthesia. Springfield: Charles C Thomas; 1966. p. 3–10.

[14] Aldrete JA, Auad OA, Gutierrez VP, et al. Alberto Gutierrez and the hanging drop. Reg Anesth Pain Med 2005;30(4):397–404.

[15] Aburel E. L'anesthesielocale continue (prolongee) en obstetrique. Bulletin de la Societe d'Obstetrique et Gynecologie de Paris 1931;20:35–9 [in French].

[16] Hingson RA, Edwards WB. Continuous caudal analgesia: an analysis of the first ten thousand confinements thus managed with the report of the author's first thousand cases. JAMA 1943;123:538–46.

[17] Curbello MM. Continuous peridural segmental anesthesia by means of a utreteral catheter. Anesth Analg 1949;28:13–23.

[18] Lee JA. A new catheter for continuous extradural analgesia. Anaesthesia 1962;17:248–50.

[19] Vertommen JD, Vandermeulen E, Van Aken H, et al. The efffects of the addition of sufentanil to 0.125% bupivacaine on the quality of analgesia during labor and on the incidence of instumental deliveries. Anesthesiology 1991;74:809–14.

[20] Gogarten W, Van Aken H. A century of regional analgesia in obestrics. Anesth Analg 2000; 91:773–5.

[21] Papper EM. The palate of my mind. In: Fink BR, Stephen CR, editors. Careers in anesthesiology. Park Ridge (IL): The Wood Library-Museum of Anesthesiology; 1997. p. 136.

[22] Calmes SH. Dr. Virginia Apgar: the effect of Dr. Ralph Waters on her career. In: Morris LE, Schroeder ME, Warener ME, editors. Ralph Milton Waters, M.D. mentor to a profession. Park Ridge (IL): The Wood Library-Museum of Anesthesiology; 2004. p. 96.

ELSEVIER
SAUNDERS

Anesthesiology Clin
26 (2008) 75–88

ANESTHESIOLOGY
CLINICS

Vasopressors in Obstetrics

Jason Reidy, MBBS, FRCA[a,b],
Joanne Douglas, MD, FRCPC[a,b],*

[a]Department of Anesthesiology, Pharmacology and Therapeutics,
University of British Columbia, Vancouver, BC, Canada
[b]Department of Anesthesia, BC Women's Hospital and Health Centre,
4500 Oak Street, Vancouver, BC, Canada V6H 3N1

Hypotension is a common side effect when neuraxial analgesia/anesthesia is administered to the obstetric population. The incidence of hypotension is generally less with neuraxial analgesia for labor and greater when neuraxial block is administered for surgical intervention because surgical intervention requires a higher, more intense block. Generally speaking, spinal anesthesia, because of its more rapid onset, is associated with a higher incidence of more severe hypotension (up to 90%) than epidural anesthesia [1]. The hypotensive effects of neuraxial anesthesia are compounded by the physiologic changes of pregnancy and may result in a variety of unpleasant symptoms for the mother, such as nausea, vomiting, dizziness, and, if sustained, can negatively impact the fetus. Multiple-gestation pregnancy is no longer considered a risk factor for a higher incidence of hypotension than singleton pregnancy [2].

Maternal hypotension

Hypotension following neuraxial anesthesia for cesarean section (CS) is the result of several factors. Sympathectomy leads to a decrease in systemic vascular resistance, venous return, and cardiac output. The reduced cardiac output can be due to the decrease in venous return or bradycardia associated with higher blocks. These factors combined with aorto-caval compression in late pregnancy can lead to profound hypotension. Normal pregnancy may be associated with autonomic imbalance making pregnant women with

* Corresponding author. Department of Anesthesia, BC Women's Hospital and Health Centre, 4500 Oak Street, Vancouver, BC, Canada V6H 3N1.
    E-mail address: jdouglas@cw.bc.ca (J. Douglas).

1932-2275/08/$ - see front matter © 2008 Elsevier Inc. All rights reserved.
doi:10.1016/j.anclin.2007.11.005 *anesthesiology.theclinics.com*

a relatively overactive sympathetic nervous system more prone to hypotension during neuraxial anesthesia [3].

Uterine blood flow is directly dependent on maternal blood pressure and maternal hypotension may have deleterious effects on the fetus. If sustained, it may lead to fetal compromise and possibly death. Milder, less prolonged hypotension may result in fetal/neonatal acidosis [4,5]. Oxygenation of the fetus in some animals is maintained mainly by a large blood supply to the uteroplacental circulation, offering a margin of safety to the fetus during maternal hypotension [6]. In sheep, fetal acidosis does not occur until the uterine blood flow is reduced by more than 60% [7].

Neonatal acidosis is partly determined by the duration and extent of hypotension associated with neuraxial anesthesia [8]. In a recent meta-analysis comparing spinal to epidural anesthesia for CS, Reynolds and Seed [9] suggested that spinal anesthesia is not the ideal anesthetic for CS because of the risk of neonatal acidosis. However, a large prospective analysis of CS outcome did not find any association between spinal anesthesia and neonatal acidosis [10].

Methods that increase central blood volume (intravenous fluids, mechanical increase in preload) are generally ineffective in preventing hypotension [11]. On the other hand, vasopressors are effective in preventing and treating maternal hypotension secondary to neuraxial anesthesia but the choice of vasopressor has been debated.

History

In the 1950s and 1960s there were several clinical reports that investigated different methods of treating spinal-induced hypotension [12,13]. In a 1962 study, intramuscular prophylactic methoxamine was more effective than intramuscular ephedrine in preventing and treating hypotension but it was associated with a higher incidence of hypertension [13]. These studies led to animal research into vasopressor effects on the fetal placental unit that suggested that ephedrine was the most effective agent in preventing and treating hypotension with minimal effects on the fetus/neonate [14–16]. In particular, uterine blood flow was maintained more favorably with beta-agonists than with alpha-agonists. This research led to the adoption of ephedrine as the vasopressor of choice to treat maternal hypotension from neuraxial anesthesia [17]. In these animal studies, the ewes received no anesthesia, general anesthesia, a combination of general and neuraxial anesthesia, or the doses of vasopressor used were greater than those used clinically. In these early animal studies, only one used spinal anesthesia alone [17]. Therefore, although ephedrine became the vasopressor of choice, the results do not necessarily reflect what would occur during neuraxial anesthesia in humans.

In 1988, Ramanathan and Grant [18] challenged the concept that ephedrine was better than phenylephrine to treat hypotension following epidural anesthesia for CS. They concluded that neither transient maternal hypotension nor the use of phenylephrine to treat hypotension caused fetal acidosis. Further clinical studies have confirmed the effectiveness of phenylephrine in preventing and treating hypotension in normal pregnancies and thus in many centers phenylephrine has become the vasopressor of choice.

The situation in the compromised fetus may be more problematic. Erkinaro and colleagues [19] looked at the effects of phenylephrine and ephedrine on neonatal lactate concentrations following maternal hypoxia and hypotension in the sheep model. Ephedrine restored maternal hemodynamics to baseline without deterioration in fetal lactate concentration but the phenylephrine group had a continued deterioration in fetal lactate concentration despite restoration of maternal hemodynamics to supranormal levels. There is a need for further investigation to determine the best vasopressor when uteroplacental circulation is compromised.

Treatment of hypotension

Today phenylephrine and ephedrine are the vasopressors of choice to prevent and treat hypotension following neuraxial anesthesia for CS. The relative potency ratio for phenylephrine:ephedrine is 80:1 in the prevention of post–spinal hypotension at CS [20].

Ephedrine

Ephedrine has been the gold standard for the treatment of hypotension in obstetric anesthesia because of its good safety record, ready availability, and familiarity to most obstetric anesthesiologists. Ephedrine is a sympathomimetic that has both a direct (alpha- and beta-receptor agonist) and an indirect mechanism of action (release of norepinephrine from presynaptic nerve terminals). Ephedrine's effects on the maternal cardiovascular system are twofold and are mainly secondary to its indirect action. Not only does ephedrine cause an increase in myocardial contractility and heart rate and hence cardiac output, via the $beta_1$-receptors, it also causes peripheral vasoconstriction and raises the blood pressure, via alpha-receptors. Ephedrine has a slow onset of action making it difficult to titrate an appropriate bolus dose.

In animal studies, ephedrine preserves uteroplacental blood flow during pregnancy when compared with $alpha_1$-receptor agonists [21]. It is hypothesized that this effect of ephedrine is secondary to its beta effect and the relative lack of sympathetic innervation of the uteroplacental circulation, as compared with the nonpregnant state [22]. However, in normal, healthy parturients undergoing spinal anesthesia for CS treatment of hypotension with ephedrine, compared with phenylephrine, it is associated with an increased incidence of neonatal acidosis [8,23].

Ephedrine crosses the human placenta [24] and may have an effect on fetal heart rate and heart rate variability [25], possibly secondary to increased circulating fetal catecholamines [26]. Ephedrine may stimulate alpha-adrenergic receptors in brown fat increasing carbon dioxide production through an alteration of fetal metabolism. This may cause neonatal acidosis. This possible reason for acidosis was confirmed in a study by Cooper and colleagues [27] who compared infusions of ephedrine alone and ephedrine/phenylephrine. In the ephedrine group, acidotic neonates had a 77% greater arteriovenous pCO_2 difference than nonacidotic neonates.

Although the studies demonstrating adverse fetal acid-base outcomes are compelling, there is no evidence that ephedrine use results in adverse neonatal outcome in normal, healthy pregnancies. The use of ephedrine in the compromised fetus may be more clinically significant.

Phenylephrine

Phenylephrine is a short-acting, potent vasoconstrictor that causes an increase in both systolic and diastolic blood pressure. Hypotension, secondary to neuraxial anesthesia, is due to vasodilatation. Phenylephrine counteracts this vasodilatation directly, restoring baseline blood pressure. Traditionally, phenylephrine was used as a second line vasoconstrictor in obstetrics because of concerns that it caused vasoconstriction in the uteroplacental circulation.

Phenylephrine is an alpha-adrenoceptor agonist that exerts its action via $alpha_1$-adrenoceptors in the peripheral circulation. It has minimal action at beta-adrenoceptors and thus does not have a positive chronotropic effect like ephedrine. In fact, it tends to have a negative chronotropic effect secondary to an increase in venous return and a decrease in maternal cardiac output, the significance of which is unknown [1]. Bradycardia, secondary to phenylephrine, may require treatment with M_2-muscarinic antagonists (eg, atropine).

While many believe that phenylephrine is the vasopressor of choice, it has been investigated only in the elective cesarean population. There is little evidence to categorically support its use during nonelective CS for delivery of a premature fetus, a compromised fetus, or in a mother with preexisting hypertension [1].

Other vasoconstrictors

Metaraminol is a mixed alpha- and beta-agonist, but its alpha effects predominate at clinical doses. Ngan Kee and colleagues [28] demonstrated that metaraminol was superior to ephedrine at maintaining both maternal blood pressure and fetal pH during spinal anesthesia for CS. The doses of vasoconstrictors in this study were large and the benefits may have been exaggerated. Metaraminol is not widely used.

Methoxamine is a pure alpha-agonist vasoconstrictor. Wright and colleagues [29] compared ephedrine and methoxamine in CS under epidural anesthesia. They found that the ephedrine group had a higher systolic blood pressure at delivery than the methoxamine group and that methoxamine caused significant, but transient changes in resistance to uterine blood flow. Fetal outcomes were similar between the groups.

Angiotensin II is a potent vasoconstrictor with a short half-life, which affects the uterine vasculature less than other vasconstrictors [30]. Ramin and colleagues [31] demonstrated a benefit to using angiotensin II over ephedrine when comparing fetal pH after prophylactic infusions of the two drugs at CS. It is not widely used in obstetric anesthesia.

Vasopressor administration

Prophylaxis

Intramuscular vasopressor prophylaxis has obvious limitations in terms of timing of administration (Table 1). Older studies found that intramuscular ephedrine (25 or 50 mg) was not consistently effective in preventing hypotension during CS under epidural or spinal anesthesia and could result in maternal hypertension and fetal acidosis [13,34,35]. Intramuscular phenylephrine (1.5 mg) has been used to reduce the incidence of spinal-induced hypotension in nonpregnant patients undergoing hip fracture repair [36]. However, the dose and the exact timing necessary to achieve this consistently are debatable and the study may not translate to the obstetric population.

Studies have looked at the effectiveness of a prophylactic ephedrine bolus on the incidence of maternal hypotension [37,38]. Ngan Kee and colleagues [38] found that a 30-mg bolus of ephedrine administered over 30 seconds following intrathecal injection did not completely eliminate maternal hypotension, nausea, vomiting, and fetal acidosis. Shearer and colleagues [37] found that a 10-mg dose of intravenous ephedrine did not alter the incidence of maternal hypotension. Thus, a single, prophylactic, intravenous bolus of ephedrine is ineffective and other techniques to prevent hypotension should be used.

Several studies have looked at prophylactic infusions of ephedrine to prevent maternal hypotension following neuraxial anesthesia for CS with varying degrees of effectiveness depending on the dose and rate of administration [33,39–41]. These studies have shown that the higher the dose of ephedrine, the lower the incidence of maternal hypotension, but this may be accompanied by an increased incidence of side effects.

The rapid onset and short duration of action of phenylephrine has led to investigation of its use as an infusion. A comparison of prophylactic phenylephrine, infused at 100 µg/min with intermittent boluses of 100 µg of phenylephrine to treat hypotension (20% decrease from baseline), found a significantly lower systolic arterial blood pressure in the treatment group than the prophylactic group [42]. Fetal outcomes were similar. Aggressive, prophylactic control of maternal blood pressure at CS results in better outcomes in terms of maternal nausea and vomiting and fetal umbilical

Table 1
Doses of vasopressors used for hypotension prophylaxis

Study	Anesthesia	Aim	Ephedrine regimen	Phenylephrine regimen	Phenylephrine/ephedrine combination	Outcome
Ngan Kee et al [32]	Spinal, elective cesarean	To keep SBP at 100%, 90% or 80% of baseline value		100 µg/min infusion continued if SBP equal to or less than target for group		Umbilical artery pH highest in the 100% of baseline SBP group. Lowest incidence of nausea and vomiting in this group also.
Cooper et al [27]	Spinal, elective cesarean	Titrated to maintain SBP at baseline	3 mg/mL @ 20–40 mL/h	100 µg/mL @ 20–40 mL/h	50 µg/mL phenylephrine and 1.5 mg/mL ephedrine @ 20–40 mL/h	Less fetal acidosis in the phenylephrine and combination groups when compared with ephedrine alone.
LaPorta et al [26]	Spinal, elective cesarean	To maintain maternal SBP>100 mm Hg	5 mg IV bolus	40 µg IV bolus		Ephedrine group had higher neonatal catecholamine concentrations and lower umbilical artery pH.
Alahuhta et al [33]	Spinal, elective cesarean	Prophylaxis	5-mg bolus then infusion @ 50 mg/h	100 µg bolus then infusion @ 1 mg/h		Neonatal pH and Apgar scores similar between the groups.

Abbreviations: IV, intravenous; SBP, systolic blood pressure.

artery pH [32]. As well, hypotension did not occur after spinal anesthesia when a prophylactic phenylephrine infusion (100 μg/min) was combined with a rapid crystalloid co-load of up to 2 L [43].

Combination therapy

Combining phenylephrine and ephedrine may, in theory, provide good blood pressure control without the risk of reduced cardiac output or brady-cardia as well as minimizing ephedrine's adverse neonatal acid-base effects. Mercier and colleagues [44] compared an ephedrine/phenylephrine infusion with an ephedrine infusion alone and found that the incidence of hypotension in the combination group was half that in the ephedrine-alone group with a beneficial effect on umbilical artery pH. However, when Cooper and col-leagues [27] performed a randomized, double blind trial comparing ephedrine, phenylephrine, and ephedrine/phenylephrine infusions there was no decrease in the incidence of maternal nausea and vomiting or neonatal acidosis when the combination was used compared with phenylephrine alone. In fact, the addition of ephedrine to the phenylephrine infusion increased maternal nausea and vomiting.

Side effects of vasopressors

Ephedrine

In most parturients the side effects from ephedrine are generally mild (Table 2). For example, ephedrine use, compared with phenylephrine, is associated with a higher incidence of maternal nausea and vomiting [27]. However, ephedrine may have significant cardiovascular side effects and should be used with caution in women with cardiovascular disease. Ephed-rine increases myocardial oxygen consumption and irritability, secondary to catecholamine release. As catecholamines reduce the myocardial effective refractory period, ephedrine may increase the likelihood of dysrhythmias [45]. There is one case of self-limiting ventricular tachycardia at CS following ephedrine boluses [46]. As well, ephedrine has been implicated in the genesis of coronary artery spasm [47] and myocardial infarction [48] under spinal anesthesia in nonpregnant patients with normal coronary angiography. Tachyphylaxis occurs with ephedrine so repeated doses may become ineffective [49].

Phenylephrine

Phenylephrine causes reflex bradycardia, secondary to an increase in pre-load, which may require treatment with atropine. Phenylephrine increases the myocardial effective refractory period and raises the ventricular fibrillation threshold in dogs. Thus, phenylephrine may be protective against dysrhythmias [45]. However, Lai and Jenkins [50] reported a case of

Table 2
Advantages and disadvantages of ephedrine/phenylephrine for prophylaxis and treatment of hypotension

	Advantages	Disadvantages
Ephedrine	Long duration of action	Tachycardia
	Long history of use in obstetrics	Dysrhythmias
		Tachyphylaxis
		Limited effect on vasodilation
		Slow onset
		Long duration
		Difficult to titrate
		Increases maternal oxygen demand
		Decreases fetal pH
Phenylephrine	Potent	Bradycardia
	Rapid onset	May require anticholinergic
	Short duration of action	Decreased cardiac output secondary to bradycardia
	Easy to titrate	Packaged in concentrated form—open to dilution errors
	Direct vasoconstrictor	
	Decreases nausea/vomiting	
Combination	Benefits of phenylephrine and ephedrine	Disadvantages of both

ventricular bigeminy during a phenylephrine infusion at CS under spinal anesthesia that they attributed to the phenylephrine. Bigeminy persisted throughout the duration of the phenylephrine infusion without any cardiovascular compromise. Spinal anesthesia can be associated with dysrhythmias [51] and cardiac arrest [52]. The reduction in atrial filling, secondary to decreased venous return, may be arrhythmogenic [53].

There are case reports of hypersensitivity reactions to topical phenylephrine in ophthalmic patients [54] but there are no similar reports in the obstetric literature. Block height may be affected by the choice of vasopressor [55]. The clinical significance of this is debatable.

Other situations

Preeclampsia

Physiological changes in normal pregnancy lead to an overall state of vasodilatation and a decrease in response to vasoconstrictors [56]. In preeclampsia there is an increase in peripheral vascular resistance secondary to endothelial changes [57] and, in part, an increase in sympathetic outflow [3]. This may make the parturient with severe preeclampsia more prone to hypotension when neuraxial anesthesia is used.

In the past, spinal anesthesia was not recommended for CS in women with severe preeclampsia. However, several prospective trials have demonstrated that spinal anesthesia is safe in this patient population [56–62]. In studies comparing healthy pregnant women to women with preeclampsia, the incidence of hypotension following spinal anesthesia was lower and less severe in women with preeclampsia compared with healthy pregnant women [58]. There is no evidence that this lower incidence is secondary to a lower uterine mass (due to prematurity or intrauterine growth restriction) [56].

Little has been written about the use of vasopressors to treat hypotension following spinal anesthesia in women with preeclampsia. Some authors recommend using a smaller dose than would be used in the normal parturient to avoid the risks of "overshoot" of blood pressure. In published, prospective trials of spinal anesthesia in women with severe preeclampsia, ephedrine, in bolus doses of 3 to 6 mg, was the vasopressor used (Table 3). The choice of vasopressor in this patient group needs further investigation to determine the optimum drug and dose [63]. The need to avoid hypotension at CS must be balanced by the need to avoid hypertension as a result of increased sensitivity to vasoconstrictors.

Maternal hemorrhage

Occasionally, vasopressors are used in situations other than the treatment of neuraxial-induced hypotension. Vasopressin, an endogenous hormone secreted by the posterior pituitary gland, acts on the peripheral vasculature to cause vasoconstriction. Vasopressin may be applied locally to prevent or decrease bleeding during termination of pregnancy or placenta accreta [64].

Table 3
Spinal for severe preeclampsia and vasopressor use

Study	No. severe preeclampsia	Incidence of hypotension	Vasopressor dose	IV Fluids preload
Wallace et al [61]	27	22%	Ephedrine 5 mg	1000 mL RL
Karinen et al [59]	6	? Overall 51%, included mild preeclampsia	Ephedrine 5 mg	1000 mL RL
Sharwood-Smith et al [62]	11	55%	Ephedrine 6 mg q2 min	250 mL RL
Aya et al [58]	30	53%	Ephedrine 6 mg q2 min	1500–2000 mL RL
Aya et al [56]	65	24.6%	Ephedrine 6 mg q2 min	1500–2000 mL RL preload
Visalyaputra et al [57]	53	51%	Ephedrine 3 mg if SBP 100–120 mm Hg, 6 mg if SBP <100 mm Hg	500 mL HES, RL 100 mL/h preload
Dyer et al [60]	35	?	Ephedrine 5 mg q1 min	<750 mL RL

Abbreviations: RL, Ringer's lactate; SBP, systolic blood pressure; HES, hetastarch.

However, vasopressin has been associated with myocardial ischemia and caution is warranted in women with known cardiovascular disease. Vasopressors are also used as a temporizing measure to restore blood pressure during maternal resuscitation from hemorrhage. This allows more definitive therapy to be administered to correct the underlying cause of the hemorrhage such as intravenous fluids, blood, blood products, oxytocics (including prostaglandins), and surgery.

Future

More studies are necessary to help refine vasopressor administration during spinal anesthesia for CS to gain the most benefit for the mother and her fetus. In particular, research is necessary when the CS is performed for a compromised fetus.

Recent evidence points to genetic variability in the $beta_2$-adrenoceptor, with 10 different polymorphs [65]. Some of these polymorphs are associated with a change in the function of the receptor and differing hemodynamic responses to either the neuraxial anesthesia or the treatment of the hypotension. This may provide an area for future investigation to optimize the management of post–spinal hypotension.

Heart rate variability (HRV) analysis, a measure of sympathetic activity, may help predict which women are more likely to develop hypotension and to tailor vasopressor use appropriately [66,67]. In one study, Hanss and colleagues [66] found that women with a high sympathetic baseline before spinal anesthesia were more likely to sustain severe hypotension. Whether this will lead to the routine use of HRV is uncertain at present.

Summary

Hypotension is a common, treatable side effect of neuraxial anesthesia, which has significant side effects for the mother and demonstrable biochemical effects in the fetus. Reviews of current literature reveal that treatment of post–spinal hypotension during CS with ephedrine is no longer the standard because of the higher incidence of neonatal acidosis [16,23]. It is hypothesized that this acidosis is secondary to an increase in fetal metabolism caused by placental transfer of ephedrine and not because of a reduction in uterine blood flow. The clinical significance of neonatal acidosis in the elective cesarean population is questionable, as there have not been any measurable negative clinical outcomes.

There is limited evidence to support a significant reduction in maternal nausea and vomiting when phenylephrine is used alone, as compared with either phenylephrine or a combination of ephedrine and phenylephrine. There does not appear to be any benefit from the combination of the two drugs. The meta-analysis by Lee and colleagues [23] did not find a significant difference in efficacy of phenylephrine and ephedrine in managing maternal hypotension or in clinical neonatal outcome. It is clear that a shift in management of hypotension in the obstetric population is in order, but we can only speculate on the benefits for the compromised fetus because of the lack of available information in that patient population.

References

[1] Khaw KS, Ngan Kee WD, Lee SWY. Hypotension during spinal anaesthesia for caesarean section: implications, detection, prevention and treatment. Fetal and Maternal Medicine Review 2006;17(2):157–83.

[2] Ngan Kee WD, Khaw KS, Ng FF, et al. A prospective comparison of vasopressor requirement and hemodynamic changes during spinal anesthesia for cesarean delivery in patients with multiple gestation versus singleton pregnancy. Anesth Analg 2007;104(2):407–11.

[3] Lewinsky RM, Riskin-Mashiah S. Autonomic imbalance in preeclampsia: evidence for increased sympathetic tone in response to the supine-pressor test. Obstet Gynecol 1998;91: 935–9.

[4] Roberts SW, Leveno KJ, Sidawi JE, et al. Fetal acidemia associated with regional anesthesia for elective cesarean delivery. Obstet Gynecol 1995;85:79–83.

[5] Mueller MD, Brühwiler H, Schüpfer GK, et al. Higher rate of fetal acidemia after regional anesthesia for elective cesarean delivery. Obstet Gynecol 1997;90:131–4.

[6] Wilkening RB, Meschia G. Comparative physiology of placental oxygen transport. Placenta 1992;4:230–7.

[7] Skillman CA, Plessinger MA, Woods JR, et al. Effect of graded reductions in uteroplacental blood flow on the fetal lamb. Am J Physiol 1985;32:559–65.

[8] Ngan Kee WD, Lee A. Multivariate analysis of factors associated with umbilical arterial pH and standard base excess after caesarean section under spinal anaesthesia. Anaesthesia 2003; 58:125–30.

[9] Reynolds F, Seed PT. Anaesthesia for caesarean section and neonatal acid-base status: a meta-analysis. Anaesthesia 2005;60:636–53.

[10] Bloom SL, Spong CY, Weiner SJ, et al. Complications of anesthesia for cesarean delivery. Obstet Gynecol 2005;106:281–7.

[11] Cyna AM, Andrew M, Emmett RS, et al. Techniques for preventing hypotension during spinal anaesthesia for caesarean section. The Cochrane Database of Systematic Reviews 2007;Volume 2.

[12] Kennedy RL, Friedman DL, Katchka DM, et al. Hypotension during obstetrical anesthesia. Anesthesiology 1959;20:153–5.

[13] Moya F, Smith B. Spinal anesthesia for CS. Clinical and biochemical studies of effects on maternal physiology. JAMA 1962;179:609–14.

[14] Ralston DH, Shnider SM, de Lorimer AA. Effects of equipotent ephedrine, metaraminol, mephentermine and methoxamine on uterine blood flow in the pregnant ewe. Anesthesiology 1974;40:354–70.

[15] James FM III, Greiss FC Jr, Kemp RA. An evaluation of vasopressor therapy for maternal hypotension during spinal anesthesia. Anesthesiology 1970;33:25–33.

[16] Halpern SH, Chochinov M. The use of vasopressors for the prevention and treatment of hypotension secondary to regional anesthesia for CS. In: Halpern SH, Douglas MJ, editors. Evidence-based obstetric anesthesia. Malden: Blackwell Publishing; 2005. p. 101–7.

[17] Shnider AM, de Lorimer AA, Holl JW, et al. Vaspressors in obstetrics. Am J Obstet Gynecol 1968;7:911–9.

[18] Ramanathan S, Grant GJ. Vasopressor therapy for hypotension due to epidural anesthesia for CS. Acta Anaesthesiol Scand 1988;32:559–65.

[19] Erkinaro T, Mäkikallio K, Kavasmaa T, et al. Ephedrine and phenylephrine for the treatment of maternal hypotension in a chronic sheep model of increased vascular resistance. Br J Anaesth 2006;96(2):231–7.

[20] Saravanan S, Kocarev M, Wilson RC, et al. Equivalent dose of ephedrine and phenylephrine in the prevention of post-spinal hypotension in caesarean section. Br J Anaesth 2006;96(1):95–9.

[21] Tong C, Eisenach JC. The vascular mechanism of ephedrine's beneficial effect on uterine perfusion during pregnancy. Anesthesiology 1992;76:792–8.

[22] Kobayashi S, Endou M, Sakuraya F, et al. The sympathomimetic actions of l-ephedrine and d-pseudoephedrine: direct receptor activation or norepinephrine release? Anesth Analg 2003;97(5):1239–45.

[23] Lee A, Ngan Kee WD, Gin T. A quantitative, systematic review of randomized controlled trials of ephedrine versus phenylephrine for the management of hypotension during spinal anesthesia for cesarean delivery. Anesth Analg 2002;94:920–6.

[24] Hughes SC, Ward MG, Levinson G, et al. Placental transfer of ephedrine does not affect neonatal outcome. Anesthesiology 1985;63:217–9.

[25] Wright RG, Shnider SM, Levinson G, et al. The effect of maternal administration of ephedrine on fetal heart rate and variability. Obstet Gynecol 1981;57(6):734–8.

[26] LaPorta RF, Arthur GR, Datta S. Phenylephrine in treating maternal hypotension due to spinal anaesthesia for caesarean delivery: effects on neonatal catecholamine concentrations, acid base status and apgar scores. Acta Anaesthesiol Scand 1995;39:901–5.

[27] Cooper DW, Carpenter M, Mowbray P, et al. Fetal and maternal effects of phenylephrine and ephedrine during spinal anesthesia for cesarean delivery. Anesthesiology 2002;97(6):1582–90.

[28] Ngan Kee WD, Lau TK, Khaw KS, et al. Comparison of metaraminol and ephedrine infusions for maintaining arterial pressure during spinal anesthesia for elective CS. Anesthesiology 2001;95(2):307–13.

[29] Wright PMC, Iftikhar M, Fitzpatrick KT, et al. Vasopressor therapy for hypotension during epidural anesthesia for CS: effects on maternal and fetal flow velocity ratios. Anesth Analg 1992;75:56–63.

[30] Vincent RD Jr, Werhan CF, Norman PF, et al. Prophylactic angiotensin II infusion during spinal anesthesia for elective cesarean delivery. Anesthesiology 1998;88:1475–9.

[31] Ramin SM, Ramin KD, Cox K, et al. Comparison of prophylactic angiotensin II versus ephedrine infusion for prevention of maternal hypotension during spinal anesthesia. Am J Obstet Gynecol 1994;171:734–9.

[32] Ngan Kee WD, Khaw KS, Ng FF. Comparison of phenylephrine infusion regimens for maintaining maternal blood pressure during spinal anaesthesia for caesarean section. Br J Anaesth 2004;92:469–74.

[33] Alahuhta S, Räsänen J, Jouppila P, et al. Ephedrine and phenylephrine for avoiding maternal hypotension due to spinal anaesthesia for caesarean section. Int J Obstet Anesth 1992;1:129–34.

[34] Gutsche BB. Prophylactic ephedrine preceding spinal analgesia for CS. Anesthesiology 1976; 45:462–5.

[35] Rolbin SH, Cole AFD, Hew EM, et al. Prophylactic intramuscular ephedrine before epidural anaesthesia for caesarean section: efficacy and actions on the foetus and newborn. Can Anaesth Soc J 1982;29:148–53.

[36] Nishikawa K, Yamakage M, Omote K, et al. Prophylactic IM small-dose phenylephrine blunts spinal anesthesia-induced hypotensive response during surgical repair of hip fracture in the elderly. Anesth Analg 2002;95(3):751–6.

[37] Shearer VE, Ramin SM, Wallace DH, et al. Fetal effects of prophylactic ephedrine and maternal hypotension during regional anesthesia for CS. J Matern Fetal Med 1996;5:79–84.

[38] Ngan Kee WD, Khaw KS, Lee BB, et al. A dose-response study of prophylactic intravenous ephedrine for the prevention of hypotension during spinal anesthesia for cesarean delivery. Anesth Analg 2000;90:1390–5.

[39] King SW, Rosen MA. Prophylactic ephedrine and hypotension associated with spinal anesthesia for cesarean delivery. Int J Obstet Anesth 1998;7:18–22.

[40] Kang YG, Abouleish E, Caritis S. Prophylactic intravenous ephedrine infusion during spinal anesthesia for CS. Anesth Analg 1982;61:839–42.

[41] Olsen KS, Feilberg VL, Hansen CL, et al. Prevention of hypotension during spinal anaesthesia for caesarean section. Int J Obstet Anesth 1994;3:20–4.

[42] Ngan Kee WD, Khaw KS, Ng FF. Prophylactic phenylephrine infusion for preventing hypotension during spinal anesthesia for cesarean delivery. Anesth Analg 2004;98:815–21.

[43] Ngan Kee WD, Khaw KS, Ng FF. Prevention of hypotension during spinal anesthesia for cesarean delivery: an effective technique using combination phenylephrine infusion and crystalloid cohydration. Anesthesiology 2005;102(4):744–50.

[44] Mercier FJ, Riley ET, Fredericksen WL, et al. Phenylephrine added to prophylactic ephedrine infusion during spinal anesthesia for elective CS. Anesthesiology 2001;95:668–74.

[45] Tisdale JE, Patel RV, Webb CR, et al. Proarrhythmic effects of intravenous vasopressors. Ann Pharmacol 1995;29:269–81.

[46] Kluger MT. Ephedrine may predispose to arrhythmias in obstetric anaesthesia [letter]. Anaesth Intensive Care 2000;28(3):336.

[47] Hirabayashi Y, Saitoh K, Fukuda H, et al. Coronary artery spasm after ephedrine in a patient with high spinal anesthesia. Anesthesiology 1996;84:221–4.

[48] Wahl A, Eberli FR, Thomson DA, et al. Coronary artery spasm and non-Q-wave myocardial infarction following intravenous ephedrine in two healthy women under spinal anaesthesia. Br J Anaesth 2002;89:519–23.

[49] Liles JT, Dabisch PA, Hude KE, et al. Pressor responses to ephedrine are mediated by a direct mechanism in the rat. J Pharmacol Exp Ther 2006;316:95–105 [check abbreviation].

[50] Lai FM, Jenkins JG. Ventricular bigeminy during phenylephrine infusion used to maintain normotension during caesarean section under spinal anaesthesia. Int J Obstet Anesth 2007; 16:288–90.

[51] Shen C-L, Ho Y-Y, Hung Y-C, et al. Arrhythmias during spinal anesthesia for CS. Can J Anesth 2000;47:393–7.

[52] Lovstad RZ, Granhus G, Hetland S. Bradycardia and asystolic cardiac arrest during spinal anaesthesia: a report of five cases. Acta Anaesthesiol Scand 2000;44:48–52.

[53] Van Zijl DHS, Dyer RA, Scott Millar RN, et al. Supraventricular tachycardia during spinal anaesthesia for caesarean section. Int J Obstet Anesth 2001;10:202–5.

[54] Dewachter P, Mouton-Faivre C. Anaesthetists should be aware of delayed hypersensitivity to phenylephrine. Acta Anaesthesiol Scand 2007;51:637–9.

[55] Cooper DW, Jeyaraj L, Hynd R, et al. Evidence that intravenous vasopressors can affect rostral spread of spinal anesthesia in pregnancy. Anesthesiology 2004;101:28–33.

[56] Aya AGM, Vialles N, Tanoubi I, et al. Spinal anesthesia-induced hypotension: a risk comparison between patients with severe preeclampsia and healthy women undergoing preterm cesarean delivery. Anesth Analg 2005;101:869–75.

[57] Visalyaputra S, Rodanant O, Somboonviboon W, et al. Spinal versus epidural anesthesia for cesarean delivery in severe preeclampsia: a prospective randomized, multicenter study. Anesth Analg 2005;101:862–8.

[58] Aya AGM, Mangin R, Vialles N, et al. Patients with severe preeclampsia experience less hypotension during spinal anesthesia for elective cesarean delivery than healthy parturients: a prospective cohort comparison. Anesth Analg 2003;97:867–72.

[59] Karinen J, Rasanen J, Alahuhta S, et al. Maternal and uteroplacental haemodynamic state in pre-eclamptic patients during spinal anaesthesia for caesarean section. Br J Anaesth 1996;76: 616–20.

[60] Dyer RA, Els I, Farbas J, et al. Prospective, randomized trial comparing general with spinal anesthesia for cesarean delivery in preeclamptic patients with nonreassuring fetal heart trace. Anesthesiology 2003;99:561–9.

[61] Wallace DH, Leveno KJ, Cunningham FG, et al. Randomized comparison of general and regional anesthesia for cesarean delivery in pregnancies complicated by severe preeclampsia. Obstet Gynecol 1995;86:193–9.

[62] Sharwood-Smith G, Clark V, Watson E. Regional anaesthesia for caesarean section in severe preeclampsia: spinal anaesthesia is the preferred choice. Int J Obstet Anesth 1999;8:85–9.

[63] Macarthur A, Riley ET. Obstetric anesthesia controversies: vasopressor choice for post-spinal hypotension during cesarean delivery. Int Anesthesiol Clin 2007;45:115–32.

[64] Yang M-J, Tseng J-Y, Hsu W-L. Conservative surgical management of cesarean scar pregnancy with vasopressin. Int J Gynaecol Obstet 2007;97(2):154–5.

[65] Smiley RM, Blouin J-L, Negron M, et al. Beta$_2$-adrenoceptor genotype affects vasopressor requirements during spinal anesthesia for cesarean delivery. Anesthesiology 2006;104: 644–60.

[66] Hanss R, Bein B, Weseloh H, et al. Heart rate variability predicts severe hypotension after spinal anesthesia. Anesthesiology 2006;104:537–45.

[67] Chamchad D, Arkoosh VA, Horrow JC, et al. Using heart rate variability to stratify risk of obstetric patients undergoing spinal anesthesia. Anesth Analg 2004;99:1818–21.

ANESTHESIOLOGY
CLINICS

Anesthesiology Clin
26 (2008) 89–108

Obstetric Anesthesia: Outside the Labor and Delivery Unit

Paula A. Craigo, MD*,
Laurence C. Torsher, MD, FRCPC

*Department of Anesthesiology, Mayo Clinic, 200 First Street,
SW, Charlton 1-145, Rochester, MN 55905, USA*

The maternal mortality rate in the United States has stagnated for the past 2 decades. To further lower morbidity and mortality, we must take a broader perspective. When a pregnant woman is treated in a nonobstetric part of the hospital, care must adapt quickly to her special needs. Excessive concern as to medication, radiation, and litigation may render her care neither safe, timely, efficient, effective, nor patient-centered. Anesthesiologists can significantly improve the care of the pregnant patient by applying their uniquely broad-based skills, experience, and knowledge outside the labor unit.

A 25-five-year old woman collapses in a prenatal clinic and is successfully resuscitated from ventricular tachycardia. As she is prepared for cardiac catheterization, the pharmacy calls stating that at 12 weeks gestational age, she should not be receiving midazolam and fentanyl for sedation. The cath lab calls asking for help with sedation.

A young woman enters a large urban emergency department complaining of edema. Her blood pressure is 160/110 and she has 3+ proteinuria. She denies being sexually active and states her last menses was just 2 weeks prior. She is admitted to the internal medicine service for new-onset nephrotic syndrome. Pelvic examination reveals an enlarged uterus consistent with an early third trimester pregnancy.

A teenager early in her third trimester of pregnancy makes her fourth visit to the emergency room complaining of headache. After a small dose of meperidine for pain, she is found apneic. A CT scan shows a brain tumor compressing ventricles and midline shift.

In obstetric areas, protocols and personnel are exquisitely attuned to the issues affecting optimal care of the mother and fetus. Equipment and

* Corresponding author.
E-mail address: craigo.paula@mayo.edu (P.A. Craigo).

1932-2275/08/$ - see front matter © 2008 Elsevier Inc. All rights reserved.
doi:10.1016/j.anclin.2007.11.003   *anesthesiology.theclinics.com*

medications needed are immediately available. Similarly, nonobstetric areas have optimized care for the usual patient in their care, who is NOT pregnant. However, the pregnant woman is subject to the same illnesses and injuries as is her nonpregnant sister, and often requires treatment in a nonobstetric area. In this article we will examine how this "fish-out-of-water" phenomenon affects the care of pregnant women, and look at some strategies for addressing the issues that arise.

Most protocols and procedures written for nonobstetric areas assume patients are not pregnant. Patients who are pregnant or breast-feeding may be specifically excluded from coverage by these documents. Diagnostic errors are made when pregnancy-related entities are not considered, or when more familiar diagnoses are clung to when contradicting information is present. Caregivers may assume that a protocol is being instituted for a patient, not realizing that the protocol excludes pregnant or nursing women.

On the other hand, if pregnancy is known or suspected, care may crash to a halt. Asking, "Are there known dangers to the fetus in effective treatment of the mother?" is not the same as asking, "Is effective treatment of the mother known to be safe for the fetus?"

Providers may question every step that would normally be taken: is this *really* safe for the fetus? Since very few diagnostic and therapeutic modalities are known to be completely risk-free for the fetus, steps may be skipped, truncated, or replaced with less-effective options. While professional guidelines, Web sites, and drug-labeling information are being reviewed, care for the pregnant woman is delayed. When the provider consults medical information resources, scientific information is often insufficient to support a risk-benefit analysis of therapy in the pregnant woman [1]. With the best of intentions, substandard care may be delivered to the mother: appropriate medications withheld or given in ineffective doses, or needed diagnostic procedures postponed or replaced by less-informative tests. Professional guidelines and safety ratings have limits that may be misinterpreted by the nonobstetric specialist and are not a substitute for in-depth knowledge.

The specter of litigation hovers over this decision-making process: several highly publicized cases have demonstrated that, for success, the case against a physician does not have to have scientific merit; the plaintiff must simply be deserving of sympathy [2].

In this article, we will describe the primary management issues arising when a pregnant patient is treated in a nonobstetric area. We will look at the nonobstetric areas in which pregnant patients are likely to be cared for, discuss the issues with pharmacology and radiation, and then look at potential solutions that are on the horizon.

An approach to the pregnant patient

Individuals caring for the pregnant patient want to provide the best care for the woman and her fetus. They remind themselves of the multitude of physiological changes associated with pregnancy and the interventions that can potentially alter uterine blood flow and fetal well-being [3]. A caregiver can get so caught up in trying to optimize the myriad of physiological changes and fetal issues that larger maternal issues may be missed. The same principles of care that apply to the nonpregnant patient apply to the pregnant patient. The same illnesses and injuries befall pregnant and nonpregnant patients, and causes of mortality are very similar for the two groups of reproductive-aged women.

Examining primary causes of maternal morbidity and mortality may help identify areas in which practice can be improved, particularly when we look at all causes, not just those directly related to pregnancy. Pregnant women die from the same causes that kill nonpregnant women, plus those directly related to pregnancy. The United Kingdom has one of the longest-standing and most complete databases in the Confidential Enquiries into Maternal Deaths (CEMD). In the most recent report (2000–2002), indirect causes accounted for the majority of maternal deaths: psychiatric illness was the number one cause of maternal death, followed by cardiac disease [4].

The top three causes are usually quoted as hemorrhage, hypertension, and thromboembolic disease—but those are the top three causes *directly* related to pregnancy, not the most common causes of maternal death [5]. Looking at all entities, the top five causes of maternal death were, in order, suicide, cardiac disease, thromboembolism, central nervous system hemorrhage, and obstetric hemorrhage [4]. It is likely that our current databases underreport maternal morbidity and mortality resulting from entities indirectly related to pregnancy [6]. The top five causes of death in all females of reproductive age are accident, suicide, homicide, cancer, and cardiovascular events [7].

In most cases, faults in communication and teamwork contribute to negative outcomes [8]. The CEMD also noted that failure to appreciate the severity of maternal illness, failure to recognize and act on medical conditions outside the immediate experience of obstetric staff, failure of emergency department staff to recognize the severity of illness and obtain obstetric assessment, and suboptimal treatment as well as errors in diagnoses and treatment contributed to these maternal deaths [4].

Mortality is the tip of the iceberg—morbidity is vastly more common, but even less is known about it. Maternal deaths in the United States are neither reliably identified nor adequately evaluated. Recent steps such as linkage with fetal death and birth certificates improve identification. Standardized enhanced identification of cases has been urged [6].

Anesthesiologists tend to think of maternal mortality in terms of failure to intubate and pulmonary aspiration, complications of general anesthesia that account for most maternal deaths directly related to anesthesia [9]. However, direct anesthetic deaths are about as common as deaths from amniotic fluid embolism (six versus five cases, respectively) [4]. In addition, there is evidence that anesthetic-related deaths may be shifting from the time of induction of anesthesia to emergence and the postoperative period, which has implications for systems of care, rather than individual practitioners [10]. Although phenomenal strides were made over the middle of the twentieth century in decreasing pregnancy-related deaths, maternal mortality has not decreased any further over the past 20 years (Fig. 1) [11]. While efforts to make anesthesia as safe as possible should definitely continue, we will fail to make an impact on these deaths unless we broaden our outlook to include all preventable maternal injuries that may occur in areas in which we participate in care.

Maternal management challenges

Pregnant patients in nonobstetric areas

In a review of hospitalizations during pregnancy, Gazmararian and colleagues [12] noted that 8.7% of women were hospitalized during their pregnancy. As expected, pregnancy-related problems predominated and would most likely be managed on an obstetric or labor and delivery floor. However, 34% of the admissions were for problems that could result in the patient being admitted to a nonobstetric floor (Box 1). In addition, investigations and procedures resulting from any hospitalization are likely to occur in areas not commonly caring for pregnant patients.

The emergency department is the primary portal of entry for sick or injured patients. There are many reasons why the obstetric patient may face special problems in the emergency room even for illnesses that are

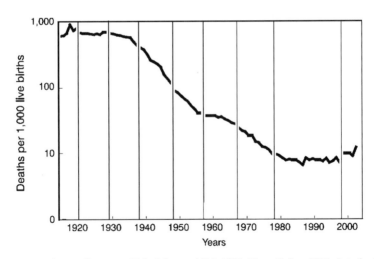

Fig. 1. Maternal mortality rates, United States, 1915–2003. Note: Before 1933, data for birth-registration states only. Line breaks are shown between successive *International Classification of Diseases* revisions. (*From* Hoyert DL. Maternal mortality and related concepts. National Center for Health Statistics. Vital Health Stat 2007;3(33):2.)

usually straightforward: there may be limited history available about the patient and her pregnancy; multiple services may be managing the patient simultaneously; the patient's pregnancy may not have been recognized, or the fact that the patient is pregnant not transmitted effectively among all personnel or from treatment area to area as she moves through the health care process; the patient may be in denial of her pregnancy [13].

Weiss [14] found that of all women hospitalized for injuries, 4.6% were pregnant. Transportation-related accidents, falls, poisoning, and assault, were the most common reasons for hospitalization, as well as the most common causes of injury-related hospitalizations for nonpregnant women of childbearing age. The anesthetic assessment and management of the pregnant trauma patient has been well reviewed elsewhere [15].

Pregnancy may disguise the nature of an illness or injury as well as its severity. Leukocytosis during pregnancy is common [16]. Third trimester cardiovascular exams may show signs usually indicative of early congestive heart failure, yet be normal for pregnancy [3]. In the event of hypovolemia, blood may be shifted from the placental to the maternal systemic circulation, preserving maternal cardiac output at the expense of fetal perfusion [3].

Medical and surgical services that do not routinely care for pregnant patients may change their usual approach to problem management because of concern about the fetus. This may result in suboptimal management. Patients with nonpregnancy-related indications for hospitalizations will frequently be admitted to a nonobstetric hospital floor, a setting that may be unprepared and out-of-step in caring for the pregnant patient. Few labor and delivery services have the volume or expertise to run an obstetric-based ICU. Consequently, pregnant patients will usually be in an ICU determined by their admitting problem, eg, cardiac care, neuro-ICU, and trauma.

Gastrointestinal endoscopy and bronchoscopy have evolved into integral diagnostic tools with a very low perceived risk. Much of the risk stratification, as well as perceived benefit, has arisen from the nonpregnant patient population. The data's applicability to the pregnant population is unclear [17]. Indications include significant gastrointestinal bleeding, severe nausea and vomiting or abdominal pain, difficult or painful swallowing, suspected colonic mass, severe diarrhea, and biliary disease or injury [17].

Primary issues with these procedures in the pregnant population are the need for sedation and airway management. In many institutions, light sedation is managed by the proceduralist, but deep sedation should trigger a request for anesthetic management. The American Society of Anesthesiologists has issued guidelines for nonanesthesiologists providing sedation, stating that certain types of patients including pregnant patients are at increased risk and consultation with appropriate specialists pre-procedurally decreases that risk [18]. However, they do NOT state that sedation should be withheld from the pregnant patient. Midazolam, as a benzodiazepine, is a Class D drug, although there is no evidence that nonchronic use of midazolam in the acute setting is associated with fetal anomaly [19].

Box 1. Obstetric and nonobstetric indications for hospitalization

Obstetric
Preterm labor
Hyperemesis
Pregnancy-associated hypertension
Premature rupture of the membranes
Cerclage, cervical incompetence
Placenta previa
Gestational diabetes
Fetal indication
Vaginal bleeding
Failed induction
Abruption
Uterine abnormalities

Nonobstetric
Kidney disorders
Other
Urinary tract infections
Noninfectious gastroenteritis
Abdominal pain
Gallbladder disorders
Asthma
Pneumonia
Trauma
Cardiovascular
Viral infections
Appendicitis
Adnexal and ovarian mass
Infectious gastroenteritis
Thrombophlebitis
Psychiatric problems
Tumor/leimyoma of uterus
Migraine
Bone/joint
Ovarian hyperfunction
Thyroid problems
Anemia
Drug dependency
Pancreatitis
Fever
Cellulitis
Varicella

Headache
Ulcerative colitis
HIV/AIDS
Poisoning
Uterine abnormalities
Sinusitis
Alcohol dependency

Listed in order of prevalence within each division.
Data from Gazmararian JA, Petersen R, Jamieson DJ, et al. Hospitalizations during pregnancy among managed care enrollees. Obstet Gynecol 2002;100:94.

Nonobstetric indications for hospitalization frequently will require surgical intervention. This would commonly be done in an operating room suite separate from a labor and delivery floor. As minimally invasive procedures are further developed, they may offer definite care with less maternal-fetal perturbation; however, it remains controversial whether or not laparoscopic techniques improve pregnancy outcomes. The trimester of pregnancy affects risk, as well as anesthetic and surgical management. In general, the second trimester is regarded as most opportune for those procedures that cannot be delayed until after delivery, because organogenesis is complete and the risk of preterm labor is lower than in the third trimester. In addition, the size of the uterus is less likely to interfere with surgical procedures [20].

Use of fetal monitoring during surgery is controversial. The most recent opinion of the American College of Obstetricians and Gynecologists (ACOG) recognized the highly emotional nature of this question, but made no recommendations beyond that of preoperative consultation by an obstetrician and a multidisciplinary team approach [21]. Obstetric consultation permits assessment of fetal status, gestational age, and the presence or absence of uterine contractions, as well as providing expert advice on therapeutic options and alternatives. Assessment and documentation of the fetal heart rate before and after the procedure seems wise, at least to detect pregnancies that are acutely at risk even before anesthesia and surgery begin. The pregnancy may not have been destined to a successful outcome to begin with, and the illness or injury may have had negative impact on the fetal status. While the American Society of Anesthesiologists has made no recommendations on care of the pregnant patient during nonobstetric surgery, anesthesia textbooks urge intraoperative fetal heart rate (FHR) monitoring as early as 16 weeks gestational age [22–24]. However, the literature is of little help to us in formulating an evidence-based opinion, as reflected in the ACOG statement [21,25].

There are two opposing viewpoints on intraoperative FHR monitoring. One approach sees the fetal heart rate as an additional monitor of the adequacy of uteroplacental perfusion that may provide data not obtainable from routine maternal monitors [26]. Uteroplacental flow is not autoregulated. If the mother is hypovolemic, blood will be shunted away from the uterus to support perfusion of the mother's vital organs. Particularly with the young, healthy mother, high sympathetic tone could maintain her perfusion pressures while robbing from the baby and not be reflected in maternal heart rate and blood pressure, only in the fetal heart rate [15]. General anesthesia with potent volatile agents blunts the sympathetic response [27]. It is not established whether maternal hemodynamic monitoring under anesthesia during significant hemorrhage is adequate to detect changes in maternal volume status that may affect fetal perfusion. Finally, use of the monitoring, even though its impact on outcome is not known, enables the care team to believe that everything possible was done in the event of a negative outcome.

The opposing approach looks at the difficulty of interpreting FHR monitoring during labor, the high frequency of false-positive patterns, the lack of study of FHR during surgery and anesthesia, the dearth of evidence that it improves fetal outcome in what is already a stressful time for the patient and her providers, and sees it as a complicating and distracting factor at best, or, at worst, a trigger for litigation alleging a failure to act in the face of heart rate patterns that retrospectively are held to account for an unsatisfactory outcome [25,28]. According to this viewpoint, the focus should be on optimal care of the mother, and intraoperative monitoring of FHR detracts from that focus, negating any theoretic benefit. This is consistent with the long-standing observation that neonatal outcome is determined by the nature and course of maternal illness, not by specifics of management, except as this affects maternal outcome [29].

Fetal heart variability and accelerations are reassuring signs of fetal well-being. Fetal heart variability is probably the most useful monitor to rule out asphyxia during labor; normal variability essentially ensures a pH above 7.0 and has largely supplanted scalp pH sampling [30]. Yet, variability is not present before 25 to 27 weeks, and commonly disappears with fetal sleep, maternal sedation, general anesthesia, or hypothermia [31]. A "flat-line" during general anesthesia has led to two reported unnecessary cesarean deliveries [26,32]. In one case report, FHR lost variability then dropped to 50 beats per minute during cardiopulmonary bypass and stayed there until maternal rewarming; the baby survived [33]. Even when this monitoring is used during labor, experts in the field so often disagree with each other that they have humorously been compared to the marine iguanas of the Galapagos Islands—"all on the same beach but facing different directions and spitting at one another constantly" (J. Parer, as quoted in *Williams Obstetrics*) [31].

FHR monitoring could be limited to evaluation of fetal oxygen supply, and not as a trigger for cesarean delivery. In the event of a nonreassuring pattern, conservative measures would be implemented to optimize maternal cardiac output as well as its transmission to the placental bed. Increased uterine displacement, fluid or blood resuscitation of the mother, reassessment of respiratory acid-base status, increased cardiac output as revealed by blood pressure, and enhanced oxygen delivery with increased oxygen saturation are possibilities [34]. In addition, repositioning of surgical instruments, uterine relaxation, and adjustment of surgical maneuvers that affect uterine perfusion (peritoneal insufflation, compression of the great vessels, and so forth) might lead to improvement.

However, many obstetricians feel that FHR monitoring places an onus on the team to deliver the child if these conservative maneuvers are not successful. This logically implies that not only does someone expert in reading the trace need to be continuously present, but that the personnel and instruments must be immediately available to affect urgent cesarean delivery and resuscitate the infant. Some anesthesiologists recommend stopping neurosurgery on the mother to allow cesarean section if nonreassuring FHR patterns are seen during surgery [35]. Stopping a procedure critical for the mother's life and health in order to deliver an anesthetized and probably premature infant based on the fetal heart rate may not benefit either party.

Delaying surgical procedures in order to assemble specialists and equipment or to transfer the mother to another center must be very carefully considered and it is paramount that necessary care not be trivially delayed.

Inaction and undertreatment of the pregnant woman

Caregivers may find themselves "frozen by the fetus," ie, so radically changing their management plans because of the presence of a fetus that they are functionally either denying care to the mother's illness, or undertreating it. In particular, drug therapy or radiologic diagnostic procedures in a pregnant woman can cause anxiety. This is driven by real concern for the mother and fetus as well as fear of litigation.

Fear of litigation

During the first trimester, fetal loss and teratogenesis are primary concerns. Every pregnancy begins with a 3% risk of anomaly and at least a 15% risk of miscarriage [2]. Thus a "risk-free" therapy or procedure would be expected to have similar risks, not less. This information is important for informed consent and counseling parents. Unfortunately, it also spurs providers to anxious inaction for fear that either fetal loss or malformation will occur and the medication, radiation, or procedure be blamed, although the association is temporal, not causal, and illness or injury certainly can play a role in negative outcomes. Unfortunately, cases of little scientific merit that have succeeded are well known to the medical community. In a particularly egregious example from the 1960s, a woman delivered a child with Trisomy 21 after a car accident; the other driver was held liable for the baby's disability [2].

As R.L. Brent points out in an excellent review [2], legal cases have more recently blamed malformations on specific agents (Bendectin, diagnostic ultrasound, electromagnetic fields, and progestational drugs) without scientific support. Irresponsible expert testimony, he argues, is a key aspect of these cases, and the ingredient potentially responsive to action from the medical community [2].

Bendectin was the only drug approved by the Food and Drug Administration (FDA) for nausea and vomiting of pregnancy, but thousands of law suits alleged it was teratogenic. In the 1970s, Bendectin was prescribed to approximately 30% of the 4 million pregnant women who delivered per year, with a baseline expected fetal anomaly rate of 120,000, 36,000 of whom would have been exposed to Bendectin—good news to some plaintiff attorneys [2].

Bendectin was removed from the market in 1982—not because it was proven unsafe, but because the costs of litigation and liability insurance exceeded the gross sales of the drug, and the manufacturer could no longer afford to produce it. With the removal of the drug, hospital admissions of pregnant women for refractory nausea and vomiting doubled [2]. In addition, many physicians became more hesitant to prescribe any drug during pregnancy.

Fear of litigation worsens reluctance to use drug therapy or radiologic tests in pregnant or nursing women. Other factors that increase concerns over the use of these two modalities will be discussed further.

Fear of medication

Over-the-counter, prescription, and herbal medications are often taken by pregnant patients [36]. Drug treatment of chronic conditions often cannot be safely discontinued; complications of pregnancy or intercurrent illnesses or injury may require drug therapy. However, 90% of the drugs approved for use in the United States between 1980 and 2000 have inadequate information available to perform a risk-benefit analysis [1]. Because of the significant role that drug administration plays in anesthetic management, we will look particularly closely at the forces influencing the safe use of medications in the pregnant or breast-feeding woman.

Until recent years, drugs under development were studied only in men, and not used by women, pregnant or not, until released to the public for use [37]. Research in the pregnant population certainly presents some daunting challenges. Pregnant and nursing women were, and are, excluded from studies because of concern over possible harm to the mother and/or the fetus, as well as the effect of metabolic and hormonal changes on study outcome. Institutional review boards may hesitate to approve these studies, be unfamiliar with the actual risks involved, and require extra documentation and review by specialists. Even when studies are approved, pregnant women might be less likely to agree to participate. After a drug is released to the market, data accumulate as the drug is used by nursing and pregnant women on an off-label basis.

Adding a new indication for a drug requires data from well-designed controlled trials in humans and reporting of adverse events and protocol changes is carefully regulated. Medical literature is not acceptable as the sole bases for a new application because of multiple concerns [38]. Thus, off-label use of drugs tends to flourish, particularly in the obstetric population, because of the absence of approved alternatives. This can negatively affect the woman's care.

Unless the package insert specifically approves the use of the drug in pregnant or breast-feeding women, some hospital committees may amend order sets to exclude these women. As an example, a protocol to treat nausea and vomiting may exclude pregnant and breast-feeding women because the package insert for the drug states it is "not approved" for use in this patient population. Although there are issues with the use of the medical literature to determine use of medications and devices [38], off-label uses of approved drugs are frequently the only available uses for the pregnant or breast-feeding woman. A drug routinely used off-label by obstetrics providers may be excluded from use when a pregnant or breast-feeding woman is cared for in a nonobstetric site, where nonobstetrics providers are less likely to be familiar with widely accepted off-label uses of drugs in pregnant and lactating women that have an established track record of safety and efficacy.

Lowering the dose of a drug is not without risk to mother and fetus. An increase in seizure activity as a result of a reduction in anticonvulsant medication, a thrombotic event due to inadequate anticoagulation, severe depression or even suicide after reduced dosing of antidepressant medication [39], clearly place the fetus as well as the mother at risk. As pregnancy progresses, some drugs even require an increased dose to achieve a therapeutic level [36].

Medical-legal challenges make even drugs with extensive track records of safe use at risk of sympathy awards to the family of a disfigured child, as was seen with Bendectin [2]. Drug manufacturers may modify labels with warnings that contradict the available scientific evidence, perhaps as a self-protective step. Enoxaparin was a possible replacement for warfarin for pregnant women with mechanical heart valves, as well as an alternative to unfractionated heparin, which is difficult to dose in pregnant women and associated with significant bone loss as well as thrombocytopenia. Unfortunately, early studies showed enoxaparin did not reliably prevent thrombotic complications in patients with mechanical heart valves, resulting in maternal and fetal death. However, the new label warned not only that the anticoagulant's efficacy in the valve group was questionable, but suggested teratogenesis after first-trimester use, making it difficult to use in women who would benefit from its therapeutic or prophylactic use for other indications [40]. In response, the American College of Obstetrician and Gynecologists published an opinion that enoxaparin did not present a teratogenic risk because such was not plausible (it does not cross the placenta). A study of more than 600 women showed only a 2.5% rate of congenital anomalies and the rarity and wide variety of anomalies reported did not create a pattern supportive of a particular pharmacologic trigger [41]. The label was subsequently changed.

Although the FDA has classified medications into risk classes (Box 2), the data are frequently based on animal studies with no or limited studies in humans, and its direct applicability to humans in the context of illness or surgery is unclear. The Australians have created a similar classification scheme (Table 1). It would be reasonable to expect that risk classification, drug labels, and international databases would agree. However, correlation is poor [1].

Fear of medication and fetal effects, although real, are frequently overstated, especially after the first trimester. With respect to anesthetic agents, analgesics, and cardiac medications, with the exception of angiotensin-converting enzyme (ACE) inhibitors, all others appear to be safe (risk class B and C), particularly in the second and third trimester. The ACE inhibitors, used chronically, will interfere with the fetal renin-angiotensin system resulting in oligohydramnios and fetal malformations, even fetal death (Table 2).

The administration of anesthetic drugs may in fact occur in one of the safest medical environments for the pregnant woman and her fetus. Acute administration of rapid-acting drugs during a limited time frame, with rapid total body clearance, titrated to effect, with usable and reliable end points in a highly monitored setting surrounded by skilled providers—represents a much more manageable scenario than what confronts many internists or obstetricians in their clinic.

Fear of radiation

Imaging is an integral part of the initial workup of patients, particularly after trauma, although renal, vascular, neurological, and cardiac problems frequently require studies as well. Studies may include routine x-rays,

---

Box 2. FDA's risk classes of medications

A – Human studies show no risk
B – Animal studies show risk but human studies do not
C – Animal studies show risk but no human studies conducted, or no studies at all
D – Evidence of human fetal risk
X – Studies have demonstrated animal or human fetal abnormalities and risk outweighs any possible benefit 21CFR §201.57

Data from Overview and Regulatory Issues Regarding Anesthetic Agents for Pediatric Patients presentation by Arthur Simone, MD, Ph.D. to the Anesthetic and Life Support Drugs Advisory Committee of the FDA March 23, 2007. Available at: http://www.fda.gov/ohrms/dockets/ac/07/slides/2007-4285s-01-simone.ppt. Accessed January 3, 2008.

Table 1
Australian pregnancy risk classification

A	Drugs that have been taken by a large number of pregnant women and women of childbearing age without any proven increase in the frequency of malformations or other direct or indirect harmful effects on the fetus having been observed.
B	Drugs that have been taken by only a limited number of pregnant women and women of childbearing age, without an increase in the frequency of malformation or other direct or indirect harmful effects on the human fetus having been observed.
	*B1: Studies in animals have not shown evidence of an increased occurrence of fetal damage.
	*B2: Studies in animals are inadequate or may be lacking, but available data show no evidence of an increased occurrence of fetal damage.
	*B3: Studies in animals have shown evidence of an increased occurrence of fetal damage, the significance of which is considered uncertain in humans.
C	Drugs that, owing to their pharmacological effects, have caused or may be suspected of causing harmful effects on the human fetus or neonate without causing malformations. These effects may be reversible. Accompanying texts should be consulted for further details.
D	Drugs that have caused, are suspected to have caused, or may be expected to cause an increased incidence of human fetal malformations or irreversible damage. These drugs may also have adverse pharmacological effects. Accompanying texts should be consulted for further details.

ultrasound, MRI, CT, and interventional studies. The risk of radiation is real, although often overestimated, particularly for diagnostic tests. In some situations, avoiding or delaying necessary imaging studies risks the life and health of both mother and fetus (Table 3).

Fetal risks of ionizing radiation include teratogenicity, growth restriction, and fetal loss (abortion). Delayed effects may include childhood leukemia. ACOG guidelines state that this risk begins at 1 to 2 rads (10 to 20 mGy) [42], although others state that exposure of less than 5 rads (50 mGy) has not been associated with increased fetal anomalies or loss [43]. The amount of radiation delivered to the fetus can vary significantly depending on the number of films, specific techniques, and shielding. Routine diagnostic studies with modern technique will not exceed the maximum accepted radiation exposure during pregnancy [43].

CT involves radiation, but is an excellent diagnostic modality acceptable in certain circumstances, such as appendicitis. Ultrasound and MRI do not use ionizing radiation. ACOG guidelines currently accept MRI in all three trimesters [42]. Ultrasound is an excellent initial imaging modality for the pregnant woman. Ultrasound identifies 60% of kidney stones, and is useful in diagnosing appendicitis. However CT or MRI may be required for a definitive diagnosis. ACOG has suggested that thoughtful imaging should not be denied the mother if it will contribute to treatment of her primary problem [42].

In one survey study, obstetricians and family practice physicians overestimated the teratogenic risk of radiography and CT during early pregnancy, and even recommended abortion in instances where the total ionizing radiation exposure was not sufficient to support such recommendations [44].

Table 2
Risk classification of drugs frequently used in anesthesia

Drug class		FDA class	ADEC
Analgesia	Acetaminophen	?	A
	Nitrous oxide	[a]Approved	—
	Ketorolac	C	C
	Ibuprofen	D	C
Antiarrhythmic	Amiodarone	D	C
Antibiotic	Ampicillin	B	A
	Keflex	B	A
Anticoagulation	Enoxaparin	B	C
	Heparin	C	C
	Warfarin	X	D
Anticonvulsant	Magnesium	A	—
Antiemetic	Ondansetron	B	B1
	Promethazine	C	C
	Droperidol	C	C
	Scopolamine	C	B2
Antihypertensive	Nifedipine	C	C
	Labetalol	C	C
	Esmolol	C	C
	Hydralazine	C	C
	Nitroprusside	C	C
	Captopril	C 1st trimester	D
		D 2nd trimester	
Volatile agents	Enflurane	B	A
	Desflurane	B	B3
	Sevoflurane	B	B2
	Halothane	C	A
	Isoflurane	C	B3
Induction	Ketamine	?	A
	Methohexital	B	B2
	Propofol	B	C
	Thiopental	C	A
	Etomidate	C	—
Muscle relaxants	Cisatracurium	B	—
	Atracurium	C	C
	Succinylcholine	C	—
	Mivacurium	C	B2
	Pancuronium	C	B2
	Rocuronium	C	B2
	Vecuronium	C	C
Opioid analgesics	Fentanyl	C	C
	Sufentanil	C	—
	Alfentanil	C	C
	Remifentanil	C	C
	Morphine	C	C
	Meperidine	C	C
	Codeine	C	A
Pressors	Vasopressin	C	B2
	Epinephrine	C	—
	Ephedrine	C	A
	Phenylephrine	C	—

Table 2 (*continued*)

Drug class		FDA class	ADEC
Local anesthetic	Lidocaine	B	—
	Ropivacaine	B	B1
	Bupivacaine	C	A
	Mepivacaine	C	A
	Chloroprocaine	C	—
	Tetracaine	C	—
Sedation	Midazolam	D	C
	Lorazepam	D	C
Stimulant	Caffeine	C	A

For ADEC pregnancy category classification, see Table 1. For FDA pregnanct category classification, see Box 2.

Abbreviations: ADEC, Australian Drug Evaluation Committee; FDA, Food and Drug Administration.

[a] Nitrous oxide is labeled for use as an analgesic during labor and delivery.

Data from Klasco RK, editor. DRUGDEX System (electronic version). Thomson Micromedex, Greenwood Village, Colorado, USA. Available at: http://www.thomsonhc.com. Accessed January 7, 2008.

Solutions

Pharmacology research

Concerns for the fetus have hampered research into these issues in the past; however, recently the horizon has opened and there is hope that

Table 3

Examples of common radiological exams and the fetal exposure associated with each of them

Exam	Dosage, mGy	Number of maternal exams that could hypothetically be performed and still be <50 mGy
Cervical spine (AP and lat)	<0.001	50,000
Chest (PA and lat)	<0.001	50,000
Abdomen	1–3	16–50
IVP	6	8
CT head	0	Very large
CT chest	0.2	250
CT angiogram coronaries	0.1	500
CT abdomen	4	12
CT abdomen and pelvis	25	2
CT angiogram of aorta (chest through pelvis)	34	1

Exposure of <50 mGy is considered to be safe by both American College of Obstetrics and Gynecology as well as the American College of Radiology. The risk of fetal damage is increased above 150 mGy. 1 rad = 10 mGy.

Abbreviations: AP, anteroposterior; lat, lateral; PA, posteroanterior; IVP, intravenous pyelogram.

Data from McCollough CH, Schueler BA, Atwell TD, et al. Radiation exposure and pregnancy: when should we be concerned? Radiographics 2007;27(4):909–17.

more information will be forthcoming to guide physicians. The National Institute of Child Health and Human Development (NICHD) initiated the OB Pharmacology Research Units Network in 2003 [45]. In addition to advancing the knowledge of drugs in pregnancy, the Network will be "...a proof-of-concept platform for future labeling studies...to demonstrate that clinical investigations can be performed ethically in pregnant women" [45]. To further collect applicable data, the FDA has begun requiring some drug manufacturers to initiate registries tracking the pharmaceutical exposure of pregnant women to drugs [46]. Changing the structure of information is being considered in order to make it more useful to practitioners [38].

Need for consideration of pregnant patients in policies hospital-wide

As multidisciplinary efforts proceed in improving communication, systems, and team work, personnel with expertise in the management of obstetric patients may find more opportunity to make all parts of the hospital work for the pregnant patient. This needs to be more than simply saying, "This policy does not apply to pregnant or breast-feeding patients." Anesthesiologists can make a difference in the safety of obstetric patients. This requires moving beyond preventing injury directly related to obstetric anesthesia, and applying experience, knowledge, and skill in resuscitation, surgical care, and emergency management to the wider arena of obstetric care outside the labor unit.

Multidisciplinary education

Many critical care and internal medicine specialists have limited experience with the obstetric patient. In addition, when emergencies occur on the labor and delivery suite, the responding teams may compound lack of experience with unfamiliarity with the location, as well as particular characteristics of available personnel and equipment. The CEMD noted that at one maternal cardiac arrest, the code team could not locate the labor and delivery unit [4].

Hospital rapid response and code teams mandated by the Joint Commission are unlikely to have obstetric expertise. The anesthesiologist, if present, may be the only one with skill and experience in this area. If the focus is on communication, resource management, and pooling of skill and experience, these teams have much to offer. However, it is important that care is not guided by protocols that fail to take into account specific issues of pregnancy.

Multidisciplinary education supports growth in teamwork and communication. First, practitioners with differing education and experience backgrounds come together to learn a unified body of knowledge that enables them to care for a particular group of patients. Second, these practitioners recognize that each has a valuable contribution to make that cannot be ignored, enhancing teamwork and communication.

Some specialties, eg, family practice, emergency medicine, and anesthesiology, are trained in the management of all age groups, including the pregnant woman. Emergency medicine and anesthesiology have enhanced skill in resuscitation.

In the event of maternal cardiovascular collapse without response to resuscitative efforts within 4 minutes, immediate operative delivery should be considered. Decompressing the uterus may offer the best chances for maternal survival by removing obstruction to venous return and the low-pressure circuit of the placenta from the maternal vascular tree.

General resuscitation courses such as Advanced Cardiac Life Support (ACLS) and Advanced Trauma Life Support (ATLS) have added a component concerned with the pregnant patient. Two courses, ALSO (*Advanced Life Support in Obstetrics*) and MOET (*Managing Obstetric Emergencies and Trauma*), focus entirely on the obstetric patient and fetus, and are probably the most well known of the six programs recently reviewed [47].

MOET was founded by two obstetricians and two obstetric anesthesiologists in the United Kingdom and is not yet offered in the United States. It is intended for obstetricians, emergency physicians, and anesthesiologists. A structured approach is offered for management of nonobstetric emergencies in the pregnant woman (such as major trauma) as well as pregnancy-related emergencies [47]. The course might be described as a combination of strategies to manage obstetric emergencies as well as an adaptation for the injured pregnant patient of the topics found in ATLS [48]. The ALSO course, originated by the American Academy of Family Physicians, focuses on emergencies in the perinatal period, primarily in labor and delivery units. It is offered to residents in obstetrics and family medicine in the United States. ALSO is taught in the United Kingdom and in more than 25 developing countries. In the United Kingdom, the course is offered to junior obstetricians, midwives, and general practitioners [47].

Summary

In addition to the pregnancy-related emergencies, pregnant women may be stricken by any illness or injury affecting women who are not pregnant. When the acute onset of an illness that is not related to pregnancy strikes, the woman may require medical care in an area in which no obstetrics provider is available. It is important that all physicians grasp the principles of managing these women.

The textbook *Williams Obstetrics* offers a rational approach: "A woman should never be penalized because she is pregnant …What therapy would be given if she was not pregnant?… If a proposed medical or surgical regimen is altered because the woman is pregnant, can the alteration be justified?" [20]. Although it is vitally important to be aware of changes due to pregnancy and the effects of the intervention on the mother and fetus, one cannot allow these concerns to result in substandard management of the other maternal problems. A healthy mother is a healthy fetal environment.

What is the role of the anesthesiologist in these situations? Anesthesiologists provide anesthesia for cesarean birth, analgesia for labor and vaginal delivery, help with resuscitation and management of the critically ill woman, as well as providing anesthesia for procedures mandated by hemorrhage, traumatic birth injury, and so forth.

The anesthesiologist has training and experience in the care of both the mother and her newborn. In addition to providing anesthesia and analgesia for procedures, the anesthesiologist provides a key service in resuscitation. At any maternal emergency, having an individual present with resuscitation skills suitable for both mother and infant, who can provide anesthesia support for emergency delivery, and is experienced with massive transfusion and ventilator management, would be the ideal situation. Likewise, when hospital systems are being developed, the anesthesiologist is likely to have experience with all the systems that are required to manage the acutely ill or injured parturient. Anesthesiologists must recognize the valuable contribution that can be made working with hospital systems to better meet these needs. Participation on hospital committees and thoughtful support of other departments' activities may have more impact on avoidable maternal mortality and morbidity than any action we can take in our obstetric anesthesia practices.

Key points

After a century of exponential improvement, the maternal mortality rate in the United States has not changed in the past 2 decades.

In the developed nations, the most common causes of death in pregnant women are not directly related to pregnancy. To further lower morbidity and mortality, the arena for improvement must be seen from a broader perspective.

When a pregnant woman is treated in a nonobstetric part of the hospital, systems, protocols, order sets, equipment, and personnel may not adapt appropriately to her pregnancy, or may fail to treat her problem in a safe, timely, effective, efficacious, and patient-centered manner because of concerns about the fetus.

Choosing drugs and tests using ionizing radiation requires ability to analyze risk-benefit for the individual patient; however, particularly in regards to medications, information may be insufficient or confusing. Litigation further clouds the picture.

Anesthesiologists have an opportunity to significantly improve the care of the pregnant patient through participation in hospital-wide systems by applying their uniquely broad-based skills, experience, and knowledge to the nonobstetric care of this special group.

References

[1] Lo WY, Friedman JM. Teratogenicity of recently introduced medications in human pregnancy. Obstet Gynecol 2002;100(3):465–73.

[2] Brent RL. How does a physician avoid prescribing drugs and medical procedures that have reproductive and developmental risks? Clin Perinatol 2007;34(2):233–62.

[3] Maternal physiology. In: Cunningham FG, Leveno KL, Bloom SL, et al, editors. Williams Obstetrics. 22nd edition. New York: McGraw-Hill Companies, Inc.; 2005. p. 121–50.

[4] Lewis G, editor. Why Mothers Die 2000–2002. London: RCOG Press; 2004.

[5] Chang J. Elam-Evans L.D. Berg C.J. et al. Pregnancy-related mortality surveillance—United States, 1991–1999. Surveillance Summaries, February 21, 2003. MMWR 2003;52:1–8.

[6] Deneux-Tharaux C, Berg C, Bouvier-Colle MH, et al. Underreporting of pregnancy-related mortality in the United States and Europe. Obstet Gynecol 2005;106(4):684–92.

[7] Centers for Disease Control and Prevention. Leading causes of death by age group, all females—United States, 2004. Available at: http://www.cdc.gov/women/lcod/04all.pdf. Accessed January 7, 2008.

[8] Joint Commission. Sentinel event root quality cause and trend data. Improving America's Hospitals: The Joint Commission's Annual Report on and Safety. 2007.

[9] Hawkins JL, Koonin LM, Palmer SK, et al. Anesthesia-related deaths during obstetric delivery in the United States, 1979–1990. Anesthesiology 1997;86(2):277–84.

[10] Mhyre JM, Riesner MN, Polley LS, et al. A series of anesthesia-related maternal deaths in Michigan, 1985–2003. Anesthesiology 2007;106(6):1096–104.

[11] Hoyert DL. Maternal mortality and related concepts. National Center for Health Statistics. Vital Health Stat 2007;3(33):1–10.

[12] Gazmararian JA, Petersen R, Jamieson DJ, et al. Hospitalizations during pregnancy among managed care enrollees. Obstet Gynecol 2002;100(1):94–100.

[13] Wessel J, Gauruder-Burmester A, Gerlinger C. Denial of pregnancy—characteristics of women at risk. Acta Obstet Gynecol Scand 2007;86(5):542–6.

[14] Weiss HB. Pregnancy-associated injury hospitalizations in Pennsylvania, 1995. Ann Emerg Med 1999;34(5):626–36.

[15] Hull SB, Bennett S. The pregnant trauma patient: assessment and anesthetic management. Int Anesthesiol Clin 2007;45(3):1–18.

[16] Mourad J, Elliott J, Erickson L, et al. Appendicitis in pregnancy: new information that contradicts long-held clinical beliefs. Am J Obstet Gynecol 2000;182(5):1027–9.

[17] ASGE guideline: Guidelines for endoscopy in pregnant and lactating women. Gastrointest Endosc 2005;61(5):357–62.

[18] ASA. Practice guidelines for sedation and analgesia for non-anesthesiologists. Anesthesiology 2002;96:1000–17.

[19] Koren G, Pastuszak A, Ito S. Drugs in pregnancy. N Engl J Med 1998;338(16):1128–37.

[20] General considerations and maternal evaluation. In: Cunningham FG, Leveno LK, Bloom SL, Hauth JC, et al, editors. Williams obstetrics. 22nd editon. New York: Lippincott McGraw-Hill; 2005. p. 973–86.

[21] American College of Obstetricians and Gynecologists. Nonobstetric surgery in pregnancy. Committee opinion no. 284. Obstet Gynecol 2003;102(2):431.

[22] Loughrey J, Genç M. Orthopedic problems and maternal trauma. In: Datta S, Hepner D, editors. Anesthetic and obstetric management of high-risk pregnancy. 3rd edition. New York: Springer-Verlag; 2004. p. 233–44.

[23] Birnbach D, Browne I. Anesthesia for obstetrics. In: Miller R, editor. Anesthesia. vol 2. 6th edition. Philadelphia: Elsevier Churchill Livingstone; 2005.

[24] Levinson G. Anesthesia for surgery during pregnancy. In: Hughes S, Levinson G, Rosen M, editors. Anesthesia for obstetrics. 4th edition. Philadelphia: Lippincott Williams & Wilkins; 2002. p. 249–65.

[25] Macarthur A. Craniotomy for suprasellar meningioma during pregnancy: role of fetal monitoring. Can J Anaesth 2004;51(6):535–8.

[26] Ong BY, Baron K, Stearns EL, et al. Severe fetal bradycardia in a pregnant surgical patient despite normal oxygenation and blood pressure. Can J Anesth 2003;50(9):922–5.

[27] Seagard JL, Elegbe EO, Hopp FA, et al. Effects of isoflurane on the baroreceptor reflex. Anesthesiology 1983;59(6):511–20.

[28] Horrigan TJ, Villarreal R, Weinstein L. Are obstetrical personnel required for intraoperative fetal monitoring during nonobstetric surgery? J Perinatol 1999;19(2):124–6.

[29] Mazze RI, Kallen B. Reproductive outcome after anesthesia and operation during pregnancy: a registry study of 5405 cases. Am J Obstet Gynecol 1989;161(5):1178–85.

[30] Williams KP, Galerneau F. Intrapartum fetal heart rate patterns in the prediction of neonatal acidemia. Am J Obstet Gynecol 2003;188(3):820–3.

[31] Intrapartum assessment. In: Cunningham FG, Leveno KL, Bloom SL, et al, editors. Williams obstetrics. 22nd edition. New York: McGraw-Hill Companies, Inc.; 2005. p. 443–71.

[32] Immer-Bansi A, Immer FF, Henle S, et al. Unnecessary emergency caesarean section due to silent CTG during anaesthesia? Br J Anaesth 2001;87(5):791–3.

[33] Kawkabani N, Kawas N, Baraka A, et al. Severe fetal bradycardia in a pregnant woman undergoing hypothermic cardiopulmonary bypass. Journal of Cardiovascular and Vascular Anesthesia 1999;13(3):346–9.

[34] Thurlow JA, Kinsella SM. Intrauterine resuscitation: active management of fetal distress. Int J Obstet Anesth 2002;11(2):105–16.

[35] Dodson BA, Rosen MA. Anesthesia for neurosurgery during pregnancy. In: Hughes S, Levinson G, Rosen M, editors. Anesthesia for obstetrics. 4th edition. Philadelphia: Lippincott Williams & Wilkins; 2002. p. 509–27.

[36] Anderson G. Pregnancy-induced changes in pharmacokinetics: a mechanistic-based approach. Clin Pharmacokinet 2005;44(10):969–1008.

[37] Chavkin W, Kessler DA, Merkatz RB, et al. FDA policy on women in drug trials. N Engl J Med 1993;329(24):1815–6.

[38] Chang NS, Simone AF, Schultheis LW. From the FDA: what's in a label? A guide for the anesthesia practitioner. Anesthesiology 2005;103(1):179–85.

[39] Greene MF. Teratogenicity of SSRIs—serious concern or much ado about little? N Engl J Med 2007;356(26):2732–3.

[40] Ginsberg JS, Chan WS, Bates SM, et al. Anticoagulation of pregnant women with mechanical heart valves. Arch Intern Med 2003;163(6):694–8.

[41] American College of Obstetricians and Gynecologists. Safety of Lovenox in pregnancy. Committee opinion no. 276. Obstet Gynecol 2002;100(4):845–6.

[42] American College of Obstetricians and Gynecologists. Guidelines for diagnostic imaging during pregnancy. Committee opinion no. 299. Obstet Gynecol 2004;104(3):647–51.

[43] McCollough CH, Schueler BA, Atwell TD, et al. Radiation exposure and pregnancy: when should we be concerned? Radiographics 2007;27(4):909–17.

[44] Ratnapalan S, Bona N, Chandra K, et al. Physicians' perceptions of teratogenic risk associated with radiography and CT during early pregnancy. Am J Roentgenol 2004;182(5): 1107–9.

[45] Zajicek A, Giacoia GP. Obstetric clinical pharmacology: coming of age. Clin Pharmacol Ther 2007;81(4):481–2.

[46] U.S. Food and Drug Administration. General information about pregnancy exposure registries. Available at: http://www.fda.gov/womens/registries/registries.html. Accessed November 12, 2007.

[47] Black RS, Brocklehurst P. A systematic review of training in acute obstetric emergencies. Br J Obstet Gynaecol 2003;110(9):837–41.

[48] Grady K, Howell C, Cox C, editors. Managing obstetric emergencies and trauma: the MOET course manual. 2nd edition. London: RCOG Press; 2007.

ELSEVIER
SAUNDERS

Anesthesiology Clin
26 (2008) 109–125

ANESTHESIOLOGY
CLINICS

Principles and Practices of Obstetric Airway Management

Eric Goldszmidt, MD, FRCPC[a,b,*]

[a]University of Toronto, Toronto, Ontario, Canada
[b]Department of Anesthesia and Pain Management, Mount Sinai Hospital,
600 University Avenue #1514, Toronto, Ontario, Canada M5G 1X5

Management of the pregnant airway requires constant vigilance among anesthesiologists. This partially may result from the fact that airway deaths continue to be a significant cause of anesthesia-related maternal mortality. It also is widely accepted that the maternal airway is more difficult to manage, largely as a result of the physiologic changes of pregnancy.

The aim of this article is to appraise key concepts relating to the principles and the practice of obstetric airway management. The literature underlying the assumptions about maternal mortality and the increased difficulties in managing maternal airways are reviewed critically. The physiologic and nonphysiologic factors that may contribute to maternal airway difficulties are discussed as are effects of labor on the airway. Management strategies and useful airway adjuncts also are presented.

Principles

Epidemiology and maternal mortality data

Large population studies of maternal mortality reveal the relative importance of problems related to maternal airway management. These can be compared with observations made in similar studies of general populations.

Although the total number of maternal deaths had been decreasing steadily in the United Kingdom between 1968 and 1984, anesthetic deaths consistently accounted for approximately 10% of the total direct maternal deaths [1]. During the triennium, 1982 to 1984, anesthesia was the third

This work was supported by institutional sources.
* Department of Anesthesia and Pain Management, Mount Sinai Hospital, 600 University Avenue #1514, Toronto, Ontario, Canada M5G 1X5.
E-mail address: e.goldszmidt@utoronto.ca

leading cause of death resulting in 19 of 243 deaths, 15 of which resulted from airway difficulties [2]. During the enquiry spanning 1994 to 1996, anesthesia was responsible for only one of the 268 deaths [3]. Most recently, during the triennium 2000 to 2002, there were six direct deaths resulting from anesthesia (of a total of 261 direct and indirect deaths) of which three were airway deaths [4]. The details are disturbing. All were associated with trainee-grade anesthesiologists who had inadequate senior backup. Two of the cases involved unrecognized esophageal intubations where capnometry was not used. The third case was an aspiration death related to difficulty intubating the esophagus of a morbidly obese parturient.

United States data reveal a similar trend. Hawkins and colleagues [5] looked at all anesthesia-related deaths in obstetrics in the United States from 1979 to 1990 using the Centers for Disease Control and Prevention Pregnancy-Related Mortality Surveillance System. They found that 49% of all anesthesia-related deaths were secondary to airway or respiratory causes. This increased to 73% when only deaths resulting from general anesthesia were considered. The number of deaths per million general anesthetics increased from 20 (1979–1984) to 32.3 (1985–1990). This was associated with a concomitant decrease in the death rate from regional anesthesia. The relative risk (RR) of mortality from general versus regional anesthesia was 16.7. This study was updated to cover the period 1991 to 1996 [6]. During this subsequent time period, the RR fell to 6.7. This decrease may be related to increased usage of pulse oximetry and capnometry and to a more structured approach to difficult intubation. Berg and coworkers [7] used the same database to examine pregnancy-related deaths from 1987 to 1990. Anesthesia accounted for 2.5% of all maternal deaths. Of these, 58% were classified as airway related; the remainder were unspecified.

Panchal and colleagues [8] used data collected by the state of Maryland between 1984 and 1997. Their team examined all hospital admissions to short-stay nonfederal institutions. All maternal deaths were collected for study. There were 135 deaths of which anesthesia-related complications accounted for 7 (5.2%). A Dutch national confidential enquiry [9] studied 113 cases of direct maternal death in the Netherlands between 1983 and 1992. Anesthesia-related complications accounted for only four of these (3%). A smaller study [10] using death certificates in the state of Tennessee between 1989 and 1992 identified 129 women who died within 1 year of delivery. Of these deaths, none was attributable to anesthetic complications. In North Carolina, from 1981 to 1985, May and Greiss [11] showed that 10% of all maternal deaths were secondary to general anesthesia. Endler and colleagues [12] looked at anesthesia-related maternal mortality in Michigan from 1972 to 1984. They found that anesthesia accounted for 6.9% of all maternal deaths and that airway problems were responsible for 40% of those deaths. When this study was updated for the period from 1985 to 2003 [13], some interesting observations were made. During this time, there were eight (2.3%) anesthesia-related deaths. Half of these were related to general anesthesia or deep sedation but none was the result of difficulty intubating. All were postoperative deaths related to airway obstruction or hypoventilation during emergence or recovery.

These results are in contrast with population studies looking at anesthetic mortality in general populations.

In Western Australia, from 1990 to 1995 [14], there were only 26 deaths directly related to anesthesia; none of these related to airway. In a study of 325,585 anesthetics in Finland in 1986 [15], only five deaths were caused by anesthesia and 15 deaths implicated anesthesia as a minor factor. Of those, 20 deaths only 5 (25%) were related to airway issues (aspiration) and all were judged to have been a minor factor. Finally, in New South Wales, Australia, from 1984 to 1990 [16], only 2.3% of anesthetic-related deaths were the result of airway problems.

There are no studies that explicitly compare the incidence of airway morbidity and mortality for obstetric and nonobstetric patients. From the available data, it can be concluded that anesthetic-related deaths are rare and the incidence in the obstetric and nonobstetric populations seems to be declining over time. In the obstetric population, however, airway problems seem to remain the predominant cause of anesthesia-related death. This is not surprising given the usually young, healthy nature of the obstetric population compared with the surgical population as a whole. The introduction of pulse oximetry and end-tidal carbon dioxide monitoring came into common use over the span of some of these studies as did practice guidelines related to difficult intubation. These may have contributed to some of the declining rates. Also, the increasing use of regional anesthesia for obstetrics exposes fewer and fewer women to airway management in general. This same change in practice, however, also might imply that the patients receiving general anesthesia for caesarean section represent a sicker and more urgent group in more recent studies compared with older cohorts.

Physiologic factors relating to obstetric airway management

Multiple physiologic changes of pregnancy may interact to add anatomic and situational difficulties to the management of the maternal airway, particularly with respect to intubation by direct laryngoscopy. There is much interpersonal variation with respect to how each of these interacts with individual underlying anatomy.

The principal changes contributing to anatomic difficulties relate to the upper airway. Pregnancy is a state of fluid retention. Within the upper airway, this may manifest as edema. This edema may be exacerbated by iatrogenic fluid administration and by pathologies, such as preeclampsia. Maternal weight gain also may result in increased fat deposition within the upper airways. These factors may contribute to increasing tongue size and decreased soft tissue mobility. The oral mucosa also may be more friable than usual resulting in bleeding from minimal trauma that may obscure attempts at laryngoscopy.

Changes in pulmonary physiology [17] result in rapid desaturation post induction. These changes include increased oxygen consumption and decreased functional residual capacity. These do not add anatomic difficulties but rather shorten the allowable time from induction to intubation while limiting how long intubation may be attempted.

A major physiologic factor that adds complexity to the situation is gastrointestinal changes [17], which increase the risk for reflux of gastric contents and aspiration. Anatomic changes related to relaxation of the lower esophageal sphincter and displacement of the stomach increase risk for reflux as early as the first trimester. Gastric emptying, however, is unaffected until labor or opioid analgesics supervene. During this time, delayed gastric emptying may be observed, further increasing the risks for aspiration.

Finally, during pregnancy, as the breasts engorge, they may interfere with placement of the laryngoscope, necessitating use of a short handle.

Nonphysiologic factors relating to obstetric airway management

In addition to the physiologic factors, several situational issues arise during airway management of pregnant patients that also contribute to difficulties.

Firstly, given current practice patterns, the majority of intubations are for emergent cases. This creates haste and anxiety for operators. This is a set-up for lapses in judgment that may contribute to making a situation more difficult than it would be otherwise. Many of these cases occur outside of usual hours when minimal backup is available.

Intubations usually are accomplished by rapid sequence intubation with application of cricoid pressure. The rapid sequence aspect, although completely appropriate, adds further haste to the situation, possibly contributing to difficulties. The cricoid pressure, if applied improperly, may obscure airway anatomy. Although the usefulness of this maneuver is questioned [18], it still is considered by most practitioners to be the standard of care. Furthermore, in an attempt to minimize fetal exposure to induction and maintenance agents, induction is held until the last possible moment with a patient draped and surgical team ready to make an incision. This is suboptimal from an airway management point of view and subjects anesthesiologists to further pressure.

Finally, depending on local circumstances, the assistance received at induction may be substandard. This may be because of the diminishing incidence of general anesthetics on the labor floor. As a result, assistants are less familiar with airway management. Although most anesthesiologists continue to manage airways routinely in other aspects of their practice, the labor floor assistants usually do not.

Is the pregnant airway truly more difficult to intubate?

To answer this question ideally, a prospective study would be required, comparing intubation of pregnant and nonpregnant patients under standardized conditions using predetermined criteria while controlling for other predictors of difficult intubation, including experience of the operators and anatomic characteristics. If the incidence of difficult intubation in pregnancy were 2%, the study would require more than 4600 patients to demonstrate a 50% difference compared with the nonpregnant state. In the absence of this type of evidence, the existing airway literature can be a guide. This has been addressed recently in a systematic review of the topic [19].

The existing literature covers many different types of studies. Few of these include pregnant and nonpregnant patients. Some of these studies were designed to assess various methods of airway evaluation whereas others were retrospective audits from quality assurance data or other databases. Definitions for difficult and failed intubations and operators and conditions tend to vary from study to study, making comparison difficult.

Four studies compare obstetric and nonobstetric airways. Wong and Hung [20] prospectively studied 151 pregnant and 260 nonpregnant Chinese patients, looking for predictors of difficult intubation in that population. They defined difficult intubation as a Cormack and Lehane [21] grade 3 or 4 view at laryngoscopy. In this small study, there was no difference between the groups, with incidences of 1.99% and 1.54%, respectively. Yeo and colleagues [22] similarly compared 283 gynecologic patients with 277 obstetric patients. They found the incidence of difficult intubation to be 2.2% and 1.8%, respectively. Dhaliwal and coworkers [23] compared 15,150 main operating room (OR) anesthetics to 466 obstetric suite anesthetics using prospectively collected quality assurance data. The incidences of difficult intubation (1.16% versus 0.86%) and failed intubation (0.28% versus 0%) were similar. They did report that 1.5% of the maternity cases required ventilation by facemask during the rapid sequence induction compared with 0.1% of the OR cases; however, the denominator for the OR rapid sequence cases is unknown. Samsoon and Young [24] retrospectively recalled known failed intubations patients from an obstetric registry. The aim of their study was to assess their modification of the Mallampati score [25] (the addition of the fourth class). The study was extended to nonobstetric patients to increase the number of cases. They identified 7 of 1980 obstetric patients (0.35%) and 6 of 13,380 OR patients (0.04%). There is no way to be sure all cases were identified. Furthermore, failures and circumstances were unknown. All of these patients, when recalled at later dates, demonstrated class 4 oropharyngeal views even when no longer pregnant (except for one previous obstetric patient who had tracheal stenosis). This begs the question whether or not they would be difficult in the nonpregnant state or if pregnancy exacerbated the situation.

Six cohort studies of obstetric airways have been published. Barnardo and Jenkins [26] published the results of a prospective audit of obstetric anesthesia activities in the South Thames region of the United Kingdom during the years 1993 to 1998. They defined failed intubation as an intubation not accomplished with a single dose of succinylcholine. They documented an incidence of 36 of 8970 (0.4%). They were able to review 26 of these cases. Twenty-three of these were cesarean sections, of which only four were elective. Sixteen of these cases occurred after hours. Only five of these were cases with a grade 4 view and only one of the operators was a consultant. More than half of the charts failed to demonstrate evidence of an airway assessment. Fortunately, there were no adverse maternal outcomes. Al Rhamadhani and colleagues [27] prospectively studied sternomental distance as a predictor of difficult laryngoscopy in 523 cesarean section patients. The incidence of difficult intubation as defined by a grade 3 or 4 view was 18 of 523 (3.5%). Of these, only one was grade 4. Intubation failed in three of these patients (0.57%). Tsen and coworkers [28] retrospectively reviewed the charts of 536 parturients who had general anesthesia for cesarean sections. The incidence of difficult intubation was 5.8% and failure was 0.19%. During the course of the study (1990–1995), it was observed that the incidence of general anesthesia decreased; however, those receiving it suffered from more systemic disease. Hawthorne and colleagues [29] prospectively audited the incidence of failure to intubate (defined as intubation not accomplished with a single dose of succinylcholine) over a 17-year period (1978–1994). He included data published previously [30]. All patients were visited postoperatively and had an airway assessment. The overall incidence of failure was 23 of 5802 (0.4%). A majority of the cases were emergencies that took place after hours and involved house officers. On postoperative examination, all patients had at least one airway abnormality and more than half had multiple abnormalities. Two of these patients had known previous difficult intubations; two others subsequently were shown to have Klippel-Feil syndrome; one had masseter muscle spasm; and one was intubated easily after being turned to the lateral position. Thus, at least six of the 23 patients could be argued to have had intubation difficulties unrelated to pregnancy. Six patients were reported as having pharyngeal edema; two were preeclamptic; and two generally were edematous—all changes that could be related to pregnancy. Fourteen of these cases were previously or subsequently intubated easily under other circumstances while the patients were no longer pregnant. Rocke and coworkers [31] prospectively assessed the airways of 1500 patients undergoing general anesthesia for cesarean section to correlate the airway examination with subsequent intubation results. There were only two failed intubations, one of which was intubated easily by the consultant resulting in an incidence of 1 of 1500 (0.07%). The incidence of difficulty was 2%. The multivariate analysis showed that only Mallampati score, short neck, retrognathia, and overbite correlated with difficult intubation. Facial and tongue edema, the only factor they assessed that could be attributable to pregnancy itself, did not correlate.

Glassenberg and coworkers [32] reviewed the intubation results of 2266 parturients who had general anesthetics during two time periods (1980–1984 and 1985–1989). The change in practice that occurred during the second time period was that 127 patients who had anticipated difficult airways were intubated awake. During these two time periods, the incidence of difficulty as defined by requiring multiple attempts increased from 2.2% to 2.6%. The failure rate dropped from 0.37% to 0.2%. Neither of these differences was statistically significant. The investigators also report that half of the failed intubations occurred in patients whose airway examinations appeared normal. The question they ask is whether or not there is an irreducible minimum incidence of failure to intubate, which is inherent in the inability to predict accurately all patients who should be intubated awake. This concept is reinforced by a study of 5379 general surgical patients [33] that looked for predictors of difficult intubation. This study found that 40% of the difficult or failed intubations had not been predicted preoperatively by experienced practitioners who filled out questionnaires after encountering the problem. This issue seems to apply equally outside the labor and delivery suite.

Despite all their limitations, the obstetric airway series suggest that the incidence of difficult intubation ranges from approximately 1% to 6% and the incidence of failed intubation from 0.1% to 0.6%. How does this compare with nonpregnant or general surgical patients? A contemporary review by the Canadian Airway Focus Group [34] suggests that the incidence of difficult intubation in the general population is in the range of 1.5% to 8.5%, whereas the incidence of failed intubation ranges from 0.13% to 0.3%. These are similar to the results found in pregnant patients. The intubation results from large cohorts [35–37] (6184–18,500 patients) of nonpregnant patients also fall within this range.

Airway changes during pregnancy

Airway changes during pregnancy, labor, and delivery are described. Many case reports describe patients who have developed airway edema during labor and delivery [38,39], secondary to preeclampsia [39–41] and post massive fluid and blood transfusion for postpartum hemorrhage [42]. Changes in Mallampati score and actual difficulties in intubation resulted.

These observations are supported by some evidence. One study [43] found that the inability to fully visualize the uvula during a Mallampati test at 36 weeks' gestation was more common in women who had preeclampsia. Another group [44] did a photographic study to look at the changes in Mallampati score during labor in 70 women. They were assessed in early labor, after delivery, and at 48 hours. Thirty-three percent changed their airway one grade higher whereas 5% went up two grades. Eighty-two percent reverted to their admission grade by 48 hours. This same group did an airway study [45] using acoustic reflectometry, which measures pharyngeal volume and area, which may be surrogate markers for ease of intubation. They looked at only five patients and found that their mean pharyngeal volumes were significantly lower after delivery.

Pilkington and colleagues [46] studied the effect of pregnancy itself on the airway. He submitted 242 pregnant women to photographic Mallampati tests that were performed in a standardized manner at 12 and 38 weeks' gestation. Two photographs were taken each time and all were graded by three blinded assessors. At 12 weeks, 36% were grade 3 and 42% grade 4, but by 38 weeks, 29% were grade 3 and 56% were grade 4. The increased Mallampati scores correlated with gains in body weight, implying that oropharyngeal edema was responsible for the observed changes. The significance of these findings with respect to airway management is unknown. The most striking issue is that the original study by Mallampati documented only 7% of patients in these categories. The investigators attributed this lower incidence to the lack of standardization in how the test was done in the original study. If the high baseline rates of class 3 and 4 airways in this study are accurate, the usefulness of this test is questionable.

Practices

Prevention

Planning for and preventing airway problems in obstetric anesthesia is the cornerstone of practice. Although not all difficult situations are predictable, having safe practices and strategies in place before these events may help lessen the consequences and provide for better outcomes.

The first principal in the prevention of airway misadventure is an attempt to predict which patients may be at risk. Although the ability to predict difficult intubation is poor, no obstetric patient should have an induction of general anesthesia without an airway assessment. In their audit, Barnardo and Jenkins [26] noted that on reviewing the charts, evidence of an airway assessment could be found in less than half of them. In a separate audit [29], Hawthorne and colleagues did retrospective airway assessments on all difficult and failed intubations. They noted that one third were predicted to be difficult and that two out of 23 cases had medical records documenting prior difficulties with intubation. Although no single test has good predictive value, Rocke and coworkers' [31] multivariate analysis of risk factors for difficult intubation in obstetrics demonstrates that risk increases dramatically as the number of abnormal airway findings increases. This is confirmed in a recent meta-analysis of general patients [47].

One strategy to avoid being caught with a potentially difficult airway requiring an urgent general anesthetic is to attempt to avoid the situation completely. Routine assessment of all patients in the labor and delivery area, or at least all high-risk patients, might allow for proper patient counseling and insertion of "prophylactic" epidurals, which could be used in the unlikely event that patients identified as being at risk for difficulties with airway management present for emergent cesarean section. This includes morbidly obese parturients who may represent a particularly at-risk group [48]. In busy units where assessment of all patients is not realistic, education of the nursing and obstetric staff as to warning signs might be possible, thus allowing them to function as first-line screeners.

Active obstetric management also may be of benefit by reducing the need for urgent cesarean sections. Dysfunctional labors, typically associated with emergent operations, might be identified earlier, thus avoiding this endpoint.

Given that not all difficulties are completely avoidable, it is advisable to have experienced operators immediately available when general anesthesia is administered for cesarean section. This message is reinforced by the Confidential Enquiries into Maternal Deaths in the United Kingdom, where trainees were found to be involved in several direct deaths [4]. This also was the case as described by Barnardo and Jenkins [26] and Hawthorne and colleagues [29] in their audits. Whether or not the presence of consultants would affect the incidence of difficult or failed intubation remains unknown; however, it is reasonable to expect that the management of these cases might be more optimal, resulting in less morbidity.

The final concept regarding prevention relates not to preventing a difficult intubation but to preventing one of its potential consequences, that is aspiration. The ultimate prophylactic regimen is the avoidance of general in favor of regional anesthesia. Where this is not possible, a variety of strategies are widely advocated as prophylaxis. Nonparticulate antacids, H_2 receptor antagonists, or proton-pump inhibitors and prokinetics (eg, metoclopramide) are used widely (described elsewhere) [49,50]. Oral intake of solids usually is restricted [51] and when general anesthesia is induced, a rapid-sequence induction with cricoid pressure is used. Although intuitive, none of these strategies ever has been demonstrated to reduce maternal morbidity [49,52]. Also, the risk for aspiration applies equally to parturients emerging from anesthesia and adequate care also must be taken at this time.

Management

A simple algorithm for management of the difficult maternal airway is shown in Fig. 1.

As discussed previously, all candidates for general anesthesia must have an airway assessment. In cases where airway difficulties are anticipated, general anesthesia should not be induced. Options in this situation include awake intubation or regional or local anesthesia. Although most practitioners likely could institute regional anesthesia more rapidly than they could secure an awake airway, this may not be the best solution for all situations. It is in this setting that a "prophylactic" epidural would be useful if

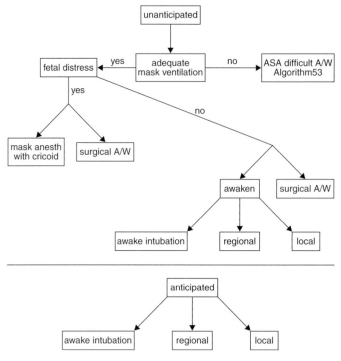

Fig. 1. Algorithm for management of the difficult maternal airway (A/W).

a patient had been laboring. In settings where regional is contraindicated or has failed, skilled help is essential for rapidly securing an awake airway in an emergent situation. Techniques for awake intubation are well described [53]. The most efficient strategy is to begin topicalization of the maternal airway while preparations simultaneously are made for the intubation. There are many options and none is superior to the other but individual practitioners should do what they can do best and most efficiently. The simplest strategy is known as an "awake look" [53,54]. Here, direct laryngoscopy is attempted after topicalization of the airway. During this maneuver, a practitioner may intubate directly or assess the true difficulty of intubation and reconsider the diagnosis. Not all practitioners are comfortable with this strategy. Other techniques for securing the airway of an awake patient include fiberoptic intubation or the intubating laryngeal mask both of which can be performed on a topicalized airway [53,55].

In the setting of the unanticipated difficult airway (which may represent up to 50% of all difficult intubations), practitioners must assure themselves that the intubation attempt has been optimal (most qualified operator, good positioning, and optimal laryngoscope blade). Pregnant patients tend to desaturate quickly; thus, there may not be much time for multiple attempts. The important variables include whether or not there is adequate mask ventilation and the presence of ongoing fetal distress. In situations where there is inadequate mask ventilation, the American Society of Anesthesiologists difficult airway algorithm applies [56]. In situations with adequate mask ventilation, which may include any type of laryngeal mask, it may be reasonable to proceed, particularly in the presence of ongoing fetal distress. In doing so, consideration must be given to whether or not to allow spontaneous mask ventilation or to institute neuromuscular blockade and manually or mechanically ventilate the patient. It also is recommended that cricoid pressure be maintained in situations where it does not interfere with ventilation. The obstetric team should be warned that fundal pressure and head-down positioning should be avoided so as not to potentiate any possible regurgitation of gastric contents. This may necessitate a forceps- or vacuum-assisted delivery. A surgical airway still is an option but the risks for and delay in doing this must be balanced against the risk for proceeding with a mask airway. In the absence of fetal distress, the most prudent course of action is to awaken the patient and proceed per the anticipated difficult airway algorithm. Again, although it is an option, a surgical airway in this setting is unnecessary.

Rescue devices and alternative airways in obstetrics

The most popular rescue device for failed intubation situations is the laryngeal mask airway (LMA). This device can be used as a ventilatory device or a conduit for intubation. In a study of 1097 healthy, selected women having elective cesarean sections under general anesthesia [57], the LMA was 99% effective on the first attempt and 1% effective on the second or third attempt as a ventilatory device. In a survey of 209 obstetric units in the United Kingdom [58], 21 of 24 anesthesiologists who had personal experience with LMAs in failed intubations were successful in using it for ventilation. Eight of these claimed that it was a "lifesaver." The remaining three were successful using a facemask. Bailey and Kitching [59] reported on an informal survey that described the successful use of the LMA as a rescue ventilatory device in nine cases in four departments in the United Kingdom. Brimacombe [60] suggests that the use of the LMA in the difficult obstetric airway is supported by a few studies and many case reports with an expected failure rate of approximately 12%.

The ProSeal LMA [61] is a new LMA that forms a seal and conduit with the respiratory tract and the gastrointestinal tract. The conduit to the gastrointestinal tract allows for gastric drainage and escape of regurgitated fluids whereas the newly designed airway cuff seals at higher pressures than a classic LMA allowing for higher ventilatory pressures, a finding constant across a wide range of body mass index scores. Compared to a classic LMA, these features may be advantageous in the pregnant population. Several case reports have demonstrated good success and no morbidities rescuing failed intubations [62–65] and failed intubation/failed ventilation

[64,66] scenarios with the ProSeal LMA. In several of these cases, the Pro-Seal was successful in women who had edematous upper airways [62,63,66]. Although these cases likely could have been salvaged just as easily with a classic LMA, the ProSeal allowed insertion of a gastric drainage tube. The value of gastric drainage in this situation and the value of a ProSeal (compared with a classic LMA) on maternal morbidity remain unknown.

The intubating LMA (ILMA) [67] is a rigid LMA designed to serve as a conduit for blind endotracheal intubation while allowing ventilation to take place between intubation attempts. The ILMA can be used for awake intubation after airway topicalization [55] (an alternative to awake fiberoptic intubation) or as a rescue device. Variations include using it as a conduit for a fiberscope or with the use of a lighted stylet. Although there is minimal published experience in the pregnant population, awake use and rescue are described [68,69].

Although the LMA is the best known of the alternative airway devices, another device that may be useful in obstetrics is the GlideScope. The GlideScope is a video laryngoscope with a camera embedded at the tip of the blade that precludes the requirement to obtain a direct view of the glottis. Three series evaluating the devices in almost 1000 unselected patients have shown that it consistently yields an equivalent or superior view to direct laryngoscopy [70–72]. In pregnant patients, Cormack and Lehane grade 3 views at laryngoscopy are a common problem among difficult intubations, and in the nonpregnant population, the GlideScope consistently provides improved glottic views in patients with poor views at direct laryngoscopy [72]. Although there are no publications documenting its use in obstetric patients this device has potential as a rescue device or as a primary tool in cases where difficult intubation is anticipated [73]. In the author's institution, it is used frequently in the main OR and has been used for several anticipated difficult intubations on the labor and delivery floor.

Alternative devices used successfully in pregnant patients include the Esophageal Tracheal Combitube [74] and the Laryngeal Tube S [75].

No single device can be recommended, as much of the data are based on case reports and series that are dependent on local availability and individual skills. Rather, individual practitioners should have a personal armamentarium of alternative airway management techniques (available to them) that they are proficient with and can use reliably in difficult situations.

Summary

Despite the concerns related to the physiologic changes of pregnancy, the best available evidence, from cohort studies, is not convincing regarding the premise that the pregnant population, as a whole, is more difficult to intubate. Studies seem to suggest that a subset of women may develop some oropharyngeal edema during pregnancy and during labor and delivery.

Superimposed preeclampsia and parenteral fluid administration also may contribute to this phenomenon. In certain cases, excessive edema may be present that might contribute to increasing difficulties at intubation. These may or may not be isolated cases. What probably is most important is the airway anatomy on which these changes are superimposed. Some women likely have more "airway reserve" for the accumulation of edema than others with respect to ease of intubation. Whether or not those patients at risk for difficult intubation by preoperative airway assessment can be detected is unknown. It is likely that this ability is limited and that there is an irreducible minimum incidence of difficult and failed intubation despite the best efforts at assessment and prediction.

What seems surer, however, is that induction of general anesthesia for cesarean section is a more complex situation than average, which may lend itself to an increased incidence of difficulty and complications. Given the prevalence of regional anesthesia for cesarean section, most teams have a declining experience at providing general anesthesia for cesarean section. This may contribute to increased problems. Pregnant women are at increased risk for aspiration and may be fasted inadequately. Consequently, all intubations require a rapid-sequence approach. They desaturate quickly allowing for less time to manage difficulties. Many women receiving general anesthesia have significant comorbidities and their operations often are more emergent and occur frequently outside of normal hours. Anesthesiologists may have substandard assistance and are under considerable pressure to proceed quickly. Assessment and judgment may be compromised. For all these reasons, even though the pregnant airway may not be more difficult anatomically, the circumstances are more challenging and must be respected.

Planning and prevention are fundamental to the management of the maternal airway. Patients must receive careful airway assessments, particularly when general anesthesia is contemplated. Prophylactic epidurals may help avoid difficult situations and gastrointestinal prophylaxis may decrease morbidity from aspiration. Experienced help always should be readily available. Anticipated difficult airways should be managed with regional techniques or awake intubation. Unanticipated cases are managed according to difficult airway algorithms. In cases where adequate mask ventilation is possible and fetal distress is ongoing, it may be reasonable to proceed carefully with the delivery. The laryngeal mask and its variations (ProSeal and ILMA) seem to be the most useful adjuncts to airway management in difficult situations. The much newer GlideScope holds some promise in this area based on preliminary studies in nonpregnant patients.

References

[1] De Swiet M. Maternal mortality: confidential enquiries into maternal deaths in the United Kingdom. Am J Obstet Gynecol 2000;182:760–6.

[2] Turnbull AC. Report on confidential enquiries into maternal deaths in England and Wales, 1982–1984. London: H.M.S.O.; 1989.

[3] Great Britain Department of Health. Why mothers die: report on confidential enquiries into maternal deaths in the United Kingdom. 1994–1996: executive summary and key recommendations. 1998.

[4] Cooper GM, McClure JH. Maternal deaths from anaesthesia. An extract from Why Mothers Die 2000–2002, the Confidential Enquiries into Maternal Deaths in the United Kingdom: Chapter 9: Anaesthesia. Br J Anaesth 2005;94:417–23.

[5] Hawkins JL, Koonin LM, Palmer SK, et al. Anesthesia-related deaths during obstetric delivery in the United States, 1979–1990. Anesthesiology 1997;86:277–84.

[6] Hawkins JL, Chang J, Callaghan W, et al. Anesthesia-related maternal mortality in the United States, 1991–1996. An update. Anesthesiology 2002;96:A1046.

[7] Berg CJ, Atrash HK, Koonin LM, et al. Pregnancy-related mortality in the United States, 1987–1990. Obstet Gynecol 1996;88:161–7.

[8] Panchal S, Arria AM, Labhsetwar SA. Maternal mortality during hospital admission for delivery: a retrospective analysis using a state-maintained database. Anesth Analg 2001; 93:134–41.

[9] Schuitemaker N, van RJ, Dekker G, et al. Confidential enquiry into maternal deaths in The Netherlands 1983–1992. Eur J Obstet Gynecol Reprod Biol 1998;79:57–62.

[10] Jocums SB, Berg CJ, Entman SS, et al. Postdelivery mortality in Tennessee, 1989–1991. Obstet Gynecol 1998;91:766–70.

[11] May WJ, Greiss FC Jr. Maternal mortality in North Carolina: a forty-year experience. Am J Obstet Gynecol 1989;161:555–60.

[12] Endler GC, Mariona FG, Sokol RJ, et al. Anesthesia-related maternal mortality in Michigan, 1972 to 1984. Am J Obstet Gynecol 1988;159:187–93.

[13] Mhyre JM, Riesner MN, Polley LS, et al. A series of anesthesia-related maternal deaths in Michigan, 1985–2003. Anesthesiology 2007;106:1096–104.

[14] Eagle CC, Davis NJ. Report of the Anaesthetic Mortality Committee of Western Australia 1990–1995. Anaesth Intensive Care 1997;25:51–9.

[15] Tikkanen J, Hovi-Viander M. Death associated with anaesthesia and surgery in Finland in 1986 compared to 1975. Acta Anaesthesiol Scand 1995;39:262–7.

[16] Warden JC, Horan BF. Deaths attributed to anaesthesia in New South Wales, 1984–1990. Anaesth Intensive Care 1996;24:66–73.

[17] Backus Chang A. Physiologic changes of pregnancy. In: Chestnut DH, editor. Obstetric anesthesia principles and practice. Philadelphia: Elsevier Mosby; 2004. p. 15–36.

[18] Brock-Utne JG. Is cricoid pressure necessary? Paediatr Anaesth 2002;12:1–4.

[19] Goldszmidt E. Is there a difference between the obstetric and non-obstetric airway? In: Halpern SH, Douglas MJ, editors. Evidence-based obstetric anesthesia. Oxford (UK): Blackwell Publishing; 2005. p. 225–36.

[20] Wong SH, Hung CT. Prevalence and prediction of difficult intubation in Chinese women. Anaesth Intensive Care 1999;27:49–52.

[21] Cormack RS, Lehane J. Difficult tracheal intubation in obstetrics. Anaesthesia 1984;39: 1105–11.

[22] Yeo SW, Chong JL, Thomas E. Difficult intubation: a prospective study. Singapore Med J 1992;33:362–4.

[23] Dhaliwal AS, Tinnell CA, Palmer SK. Difficulties encountered in airway management: a review of 15,616 general anesthetics at a university medical center. Anesth Analg 1996;82:S92.

[24] Samsoon GL, Young JR. Difficult tracheal intubation: a retrospective study. Anaesthesia 1987;42:487–90.

[25] Mallampati SR, Gatt SP, Gugino LD, et al. A clinical sign to predict difficult tracheal intubation: a prospective study. Can Anaesth Soc J 1985;32:429–34.

[26] Barnardo PD, Jenkins JG. Failed tracheal intubation in obstetrics: a 6-year review in a UK region. Anaesthesia 2000;55:690–4.

[27] Al Ramadhani S, Mohamed LA, Rocke DA, et al. Sternomental distance as the sole predictor of difficult laryngoscopy in obstetric anaesthesia. Br J Anaesth 1996;77:312–6.

[28] Tsen LC, Pitner R, Camann WR. General anesthesia for cesarean section at a tertiary care hospital 1990–1995: indications and implications. Int J Obstet Anesth 1998;7: 147–52.

[29] Hawthorne L, Wilson R, Lyons G, et al. Failed intubation revisited: 17-yr experience in a teaching maternity unit. Br J Anaesth 1996;76:680–4.

[30] Lyons G. Failed intubation. Six years' experience in a teaching maternity unit. Anaesthesia 1985;40:759–62.

[31] Rocke DA, Murray WB, Rout CC, et al. Relative risk analysis of factors associated with difficult intubation in obstetric anesthesia. Anesthesiology 1992;77:67–73.

[32] Glasssenberg R, Vaisrub N, Albright G. The incidence of failed intubation in obstetrics–is there an irreducible minimum? Anesthesiology 1990;73:A1062.

[33] Koay CK. Difficult tracheal intubation—analysis and management in 37 cases. Singapore Med J 1998;39:112–4.

[34] Crosby ET, Cooper RM, Douglas MJ, et al. The unanticipated difficult airway with recommendations for management. Can J Anaesth 1998;45:757–76.

[35] Yamamoto K, Tsubokawa T, Shibata K, et al. Predicting difficult intubation with indirect laryngoscopy. Anesthesiology 1997;86:316–21.

[36] El Ganzouri AR, McCarthy RJ, Tuman KJ, et al. Preoperative airway assessment: predictive value of a multivariate risk index. Anesth Analg 1996;82:1197–204.

[37] Rose DK, Cohen MM. The airway: problems and predictions in 18,500 patients. Can J Anaesth 1994;41:372–83.

[38] Farcon EL, Kim MH, Marx GF. Changing Mallampati score during labour. Can J Anaesth 1994;41:50–1.

[39] Jouppila R, Jouppila P, Hollmen A. Laryngeal oedema as an obstetric anaesthesia complication: case reports. Acta Anaesthesiol Scand 1980;24:97–8.

[40] Rocke DA, Scoones GP. Rapidly progressive laryngeal oedema associated with pregnancy-aggravated hypertension. Anaesthesia 1992;47:141–3.

[41] Heller PJ, Scheider EP, Marx GF. Pharyngolaryngeal edema as a presenting symptom in preeclampsia. Obstet Gynecol 1983;62:523–5.

[42] Bhavani-Shankar K, Lynch EP, Datta S. Airway changes during Cesarean hysterectomy. Can J Anaesth 2000;47:338–41.

[43] Dupont X, Hamza J, Jullien P, et al. Is pregnancy induced hypertension a risk factor for difficult intubation? Anesthesiology 1990;73:A985.

[44] Bhavani-Shankar K, Bulich LS, Kafiluddi R, et al. Does labor and delivery induce airway changes? Anesthesiology 2000;93:A1072.

[45] Chandrasekhar S, Topulus G, Bhavani-Shankar K. Upper airway study in pregnancy using acoustic reflectometry. Anesthesiology 2001;95:A1035.

[46] Pilkington S, Carli F, Dakin MJ, et al. Increase in Mallampati score during pregnancy. Br J Anaesth 1995;74:638–42.

[47] Shiga T, Wajima Z, Inoue T, et al. Predicting difficult intubation in apparently normal patients: a meta-analysis of bedside screening test performance. Anesthesiology 2005;103: 429–37.

[48] Hood DD, Dewan DM. Anesthetic and obstetric outcome in morbidly obese parturients. Anesthesiology 1993;79:1210–8.

[49] O'Sullivan GM, Guyton TS. Aspiration: risk, prophylaxis, and treatment. In: Chestnut DH, editor. Obstetric anesthesia principles and practice. Philadelphia: Elsevier Mosby; 2004. p. 523–34.

[50] Practice guidelines for preoperative fasting and the use of pharmacologic agents to reduce the risk of pulmonary aspiration: application to healthy patients undergoing elective procedures: a report by the American Society of Anesthesiologist Task Force on Preoperative Fasting. Anesthesiology 1999;90:896–905.

[51] Practice guidelines for obstetrical anesthesia: a report by the American Society of Anesthesiologists Task Force on Obstetrical Anesthesia. Anesthesiology 1999;90:600–11.

[52] Neilipovitz DT, Crosby ET. No evidence for decreased incidence of aspiration after rapid sequence induction. Can J Anaesth 2007;54:748–64.

[53] Benumof JL. Management of the difficult adult airway. With special emphasis on awake tracheal intubation. Anesthesiology 1991;75:1087–110.

[54] Johnson KB, Swenson JD, Egan TD, et al. Midazolam and remifentanil by bolus injection for intensely stimulating procedures of brief duration: experience with awake laryngoscopy. Anesth Analg 2002;94:1241–3.

[55] Dhar P, Osborn I, Brimacombe J, et al. Blind orotracheal intubation with the intubating laryngeal mask versus fibreoptic guided orotracheal intubation with the Ovassapian airway. A pilot study of awake patients. Anaesth Intensive Care 2001;29:252–4.

[56] Practice guidelines for management of the difficult airway: an updated report by the American Society of Anesthesiologists Task Force on Management of the Difficult Airway. Anesthesiology 2003;98:1269–77.

[57] Han TH, Brimacombe J, Lee EJ, et al. The laryngeal mask airway is effective (and probably safe) in selected healthy parturients for elective Cesarean section: a prospective study of 1067 cases. Can J Anaesth 2001;48:1117–21.

[58] Gataure PS, Hughes JA. The laryngeal mask airway in obstetrical anaesthesia. Can J Anaesth 1995;42:130–3.

[59] Bailey SG, Kitching AJ. The Laryngeal mask airway in failed obstetric tracheal intubation. Int J Obstet Anesth 2005;14:270–1.

[60] Brimacombe JR. Difficult airway. In: Brimacombe JR, editor. Laryngeal mask anesthesia principles and practice. Philadelphia: Saunders; 2005. p. 305–55.

[61] Brain AI, Verghese C, Strube PJ. The LMA 'ProSeal'—a laryngeal mask with an oesophageal vent. Br J Anaesth 2000;84:650–4.

[62] Cook TM, Brooks TS, Van der Westhuizen J, et al. The Proseal LMA is a useful rescue device during failed rapid sequence intubation: two additional cases. Can J Anaesth 2005;52:630–3.

[63] Awan R, Nolan JP, Cook TM. Use of a ProSeal laryngeal mask airway for airway maintenance during emergency Caesarean section after failed tracheal intubation. Br J Anaesth 2004;92:144–6.

[64] Sharma B, Sahai C, Sood J, et al. The ProSeal laryngeal mask airway in two failed obstetric tracheal intubation scenarios. Int J Obstet Anesth 2006;15:338–9.

[65] Vaida SJ, Gaitini LA. Another case of use of the ProSeal laryngeal mask airway in a difficult obstetric airway. Br J Anaesth 2004;92:905.

[66] Keller C, Brimacombe J, Lirk P, et al. Failed obstetric tracheal intubation and postoperative respiratory support with the ProSeal laryngeal mask airway. Anesth Analg 2004;98:1467–70, table.

[67] Brain AI, Verghese C, Addy EV, et al. The intubating laryngeal mask. II: a preliminary clinical report of a new means of intubating the trachea. Br J Anaesth 1997;79:704–9.

[68] Degler SM, Dowling RD, Sucherman DR, et al. Awake intubation using an intubating laryngeal mask airway in a parturient with spina bifida. Int J Obstet Anesth 2005;14:77–8.

[69] Minville V, N'guyen L, Coustet B, et al. Difficult airway in obstetric using Ilma-Fastrach. Anesth Analg 2004;99:1873.

[70] Cooper RM, Pacey JA, Bishop MJ, et al. Early clinical experience with a new videolaryngoscope (GlideScope) in 728 patients. Can J Anaesth 2005;52:191–8.

[71] Rai MR, Dering A, Verghese C. The Glidescope system: a clinical assessment of performance. Anaesthesia 2005;60:60–4.

[72] Sun DA, Warriner CB, Parsons DG, et al. The GlideScope Video Laryngoscope: randomized clinical trial in 200 patients. Br J Anaesth 2005;94:381–4.

[73] Cooper RM. Use of a new videolaryngoscope (GlideScope) in the management of a difficult airway. Can J Anaesth 2003;50:611–3.

[74] Munnur U, De Boisblanc B, Suresh MS. Airway problems in pregnancy. Crit Care Med 2005;33:S259–68.

[75] Zand F, Amini A. Use of the laryngeal tube-S for airway management and prevention of aspiration after a failed tracheal intubation in a parturient. Anesthesiology 2005;102: 481–3.

ELSEVIER
SAUNDERS

Anesthesiology Clin
26 (2008) 127–143

ANESTHESIOLOGY
CLINICS

Anesthesia for the Pregnant HIV Patient

Rachel Hignett, MA, MB BChir, MRCP, FRCA[a,*],
Roshan Fernando, MB BCh, FRCA[b]

[a]The Royal Infirmary of Edinburgh, Little France Crescent, Old Dalkeith Road,
Edinburgh, EH16 4SA, UK
[b]University College Hospital, 235 Euston Road, London, NW1 2BU, UK

Since the first cases of a new acquired immune deficiency syndrome were recognized in 1981 [1], the human immunodeficiency virus (HIV) has wreaked havoc, causing the greatest global health catastrophe of the late 20th century [2]. The HIV virus is a sophisticated and highly effective pathogen: over the past quarter century the acquired immunodeficiency syndrome (AIDS) has claimed more than 25 million lives world-wide. The most recent United Nations AIDS update from December 2006 estimates 39.5 million people living with HIV. Of these, an estimated 17.7 million are women, the majority of whom are of childbearing age [3]. Numbers of HIV infected individuals continue to increase, in part because of increasing numbers of infections. However, this rise is also attributed to increased longevity of those already infected, following the dramatic success of highly active antiretroviral therapy (HAART). For these reasons, the anesthesiologist is ever more likely to encounter HIV-infected parturients in the delivery suite as part of routine practice, and should be aware of the current trends in obstetric—as well as anesthetic—best practice and management. Management of HIV-infected parturients in resource-limited settings is beyond the scope of this article.

Pathophysiology of HIV

HIV is a lentiform virus, a subtype of the human retroviruses [4]. The HIV virus exists as HIV-1 and HIV-2, which produce similar clinical syndromes. However, HIV-2 is mostly confined to areas of West Africa and therefore will not be the subject of this article. HIV consists of single

---

* Corresponding author.
E-mail address: rachelhignett@doctors.org.uk (R. Hignett).

doi:10.1016/j.anclin.2007.11.002

stranded RNA. It binds to human cells that express the CD4 receptor: that is, CD4 T-helper lymphocytes, macrophages, mucosal langerhans dendritic cells, and brain microglial cells. On entering human cells, reverse transcriptase synthesizes double-stranded DNA, enabling integration of the virus into the host genome by viral integrase. Rapid viral replication occurs initially, with early infection of lymphoid and brain tissue. This includes early infection of CD4 T-lymphocytes. CD4 T-lymphocyte cell counts are subsequently used as a marker of disease progression, as cell numbers decline with advanced disease. This decline in CD4 T-lymphocytes leads to opportunistic infections and malignant disease, which is the hallmark of AIDS.

Transmission

Transmission of HIV occurs via human secretions and blood. The most common mode of transmission world-wide is heterosexual transmission via semen and vaginal secretions. Within the first 2 to 6 weeks of infection, an acute flu-like illness commonly occurs. Following this, viral levels decrease to, and equilibrate at, a viral set-point [4]. The level of this viral set-point is predictive of speed of disease progression: where the viral set-point is higher, rapid progression to AIDS is more likely. Most individuals will be asymptomatic for 6 to 12 years before declining CD4 T-lymphocyte counts and rising viral loads (ie, number of viral particles) herald the onset of advanced disease. Most opportunistic infections occur with CD4 T-lymphocyte counts below 200 cells per mm^3.

Seroconversion and diagnosis

Seroconversion may occur within 2 to 8 weeks after infection, and most occur by 3 months [4]. A few individuals do not seroconvert until 6 months. HIV diagnosis is by enzyme-linked immunoassay (EIA) and more specific Western blot techniques to detect antibodies generated to viral envelope glycoproteins or to the p24 core antigen. Direct detection of HIV RNA or proviral DNA by polymerase chain reaction is an alternative means of diagnosis, and may enable this to occur earlier, compared with antibody detection. In addition to these, there are rapid EIA tests using blood or oral fluids [4,5]. These enable screening of patients arriving on the labor ward who were not screened for HIV earlier in pregnancy.

Obstetric considerations

Effect of pregnancy on HIV prognosis

Pregnancy has not been shown to alter the viral load, progression to AIDS, or survival of women infected with HIV [6,7]; conversely in developed countries, maternal mortality is very rarely attributed to HIV. CD4 T-lymphocyte counts fall in pregnancy because of hemodilution and normally return to prepregnancy levels in the postpartum period [8]. Viral loads have been shown to increase in the 6-week postpartum period in some studies, both in women who were continued on HAART and in women who discontinued HAART at delivery [9,10]. Some of this elevation may be attributed to changes in pharmacokinetics in the postpartum period.

Mother to child transmission of HIV

The vast majority of childhood HIV infections are a result of mother-to-child transmission (MTCT). Without specific interventions and therapies, the risk of vertical transmission is up to 40% [11]. There are many maternal, fetal, obstetric, and viral risk factors that maybe targeted to reduce vertical transmission rates. In the United States, avoidance of breastfeeding lowers the risk to 15% to 25% [12], and therefore breastfeeding is not recommended for HIV-positive mothers in the United States. In developed countries, using combined strategies that focus on multiple risk factors, including antiretroviral therapy (ART), prelabor cesarean section (PLCS), and avoidance of breastfeeding, MTCT rates can be reduced to below 1% to 2%. The risk of MTCT occurring in utero is 4.4%, with 60% of infections occurring intrapartum and the remainder occurring postnatally because of breastfeeding [12].

The most significant risk factor for vertical transmission is the severity of maternal HIV disease, as demonstrated by low CD4 T-lymphocyte counts and high viral loads [13,14]. Suppression of viral loads to below 500 copies per milliliter minimizes this risk. The Pediatric AIDS Clinical Trials Group (PACTG) protocol 076 in 1994 demonstrated a reduction in MTCT of HIV of nearly 70% with the use of the nucleoside reverse transcriptase inhibitor zidovudine (ZDV) [11]. This protocol consists of administration of zidovudine to the mother and infant as part of a three-part regimen. It is given antenatally from 14 to 34 weeks gestation, intravenously in the intrapartum period, and orally to the neonate for 6-weeks. Following the incorporation of the PACTG protocol 076 into routine practice, epidemiologic studies in France [15] and the United States [16] have demonstrated a dramatic fall in perinatal infections. Many different combination antiretroviral drug regimes are now used in pregnancy to further suppress viral loads and to further reduce transmission risk. The efficacy of this combination drug approach has been the subject of a recent Cochrane Collaboration review [17]. However, cases of MTCT have been documented in women with very low or undetectable viral loads [18]. Genital tract viral loads are a risk factor for vertical transmission and levels do not always correlate with plasma viral loads [19]. Other maternal risk factors for vertical transmission include malnutrition, concomitant sexually transmitted diseases, and the use of recreational drugs.

The fetus may be put at increased risk of encountering HIV-RNA in maternal blood via obstetric risk factors, which include invasive fetal monitoring and fetal blood sampling, amniotomy, prolonged rupture of membranes, and use of instrumental deliveries. The fetus may be at increased risk because of low birth-weight, prematurity, and possible genetic susceptibility. The specific HIV genotype may also be a factor [20].

Antenatal HIV testing

Since publication of the PACTG protocol 076 in 1994 [11], it is recommended that all women are offered opt-out HIV antibody testing as early as possible in their antenatal care [21]. Even with routine antenatal screening, potentially avoidable neonatal HIV infections occur in babies of women presenting in labor with a negative or missing antenatal HIV test result. In the United States, a second HIV test in the third trimester is recommended for HIV-negative women considered at high-risk of HIV infection, and can be considered in all women with an initial negative test [21]. The Mother-Infant Rapid Intervention At Delivery study (MIRIAD), assessed rapid HIV testing on 17 United States delivery suites in women with negative or missing HIV test results, and found this approach to be both feasible and accurate [5]. Of 7,753 women who underwent rapid testing, 52 (0.7%) were found to be HIV positive. The American College of Obstetricians and Gynecologists recommends that all women arriving on delivery suite without an established HIV test result should have rapid HIV testing as part of an opt-out protocol [22].

Antiretroviral medications

Over the past two decades, new antiretroviral therapies have evolved rapidly, and have dramatically improved the outcome for HIV-infected patients. There are currently three commonly used classes of ART, including nucleoside analog reverse transcriptase inhibitors (NRTI), nonnucleoside analog reverse transcriptase inhibitors (NNRTI), and protease inhibitors (PI). NRTI inhibit completion of reverse transcription by binding to viral DNA, NNRTI directly inhibit the enzyme reverse transcriptase, and PI bind to and inhibit the protease enzyme. In addition to these, there are also newer fusion inhibitors, and integrase inhibitors. The Food and Drug Administration (FDA) approved the first integrase inhibitor, raltegravir, for treatment of HIV in October 2007. In the treatment of the nonpregnant population, combinations of drugs, usually three or more, are used to aggressively suppress HIV viraemia and disease progression by attacking different stages of the HIV virus life cycle. This is termed "highly active antiretroviral therapy" or HAART [23]. This combination drug approach also preserves immune function more effectively and reduces the incidence of drug resistance. The preferred HAART regimes in the United States for nonpregnant antiretroviral-naive adults are two NRTIs and one PI (with or without ritonavir boosting, as will be discussed later in this article) or two NRTIs and one NNRTI [24]. Efficacy of ART is judged by a reduction or suppression of viral load, increase in CD4 T-lymphocyte count, and on clinical grounds. Where response to treatment proves to be unsatisfactory, adjustments in drug regimens are made.

Antiretroviral medications in pregnancy

In pregnancy, ART is used to treat maternal HIV disease and to dramatically reduce vertical transmission. ART reduces perinatal transmission by suppressing viral load in the mother and by providing prophylaxis in the infant, both in utero via the placenta and after delivery. Women who warrant triple therapy for their own health should continue this or commence it de novo in pregnancy [24]. Drug regimes are adjusted and individualized from the nonpregnant standard regimes to take account of different pharmacokinetics in pregnancy, side effects in the mother and fetus, stage of disease, and previous antiretroviral treatment. ART drug resistance testing should be undertaken [24] both before starting de novo treatment and where viral suppression is inadequate, so that drug regimes can be optimized. Compliance with prescribed drugs is crucial, as subtherapeutic drug levels may lead to failure of viral suppression and the emergence of resistance.

Where therapy is not required for maternal health, triple therapy is advocated in the short term to reduce MTCT [24]. Combination ART is considered the gold standard for reducing the risk of MTCT. Antiretroviral-naive patients are usually commenced on two NRTIs and either a NNRTI or a PI [24]. Prophylaxis is more effective when given for a longer duration; therefore, recent recommendations advise starting treatment at 28 weeks [24]. All women should receive antiretroviral prophylaxis regardless of viral load or CD4 T-lymphocyte count [24]. An alternative to this is monotherapy in women who are willing to undergo a prelabor cesarean section. It is recommended that ZDV is incorporated into drug regimes in pregnancy, as per the PACTG protocol 076 [11]. Detailed and regularly updated guidelines on ART regimes for HIV-infected women in pregnancy can be accessed via http://www.aidsinfo.nih.gov. Even given the undeniable advantages of ART, the mother requires careful counseling about the relative risks and benefits of treatment in each individual case. There are well-documented side effects and drug interactions, both in the mother and fetus, and possible long-term side effects, as-yet unrecognized, in the fetus.

Teratogenicity

Teratogenic effects have not been observed with commonly used antiretroviral agents, but data regarding safety are limited, especially as new antiretroviral agents continue to evolve rapidly. All women who receive HAART in pregnancy should be enrolled into the Antiretroviral Pregnancy Registry (APR). Details can be found at http://www.APRegistry.com. This is a prospective epidemiologic database that aims to detect major teratogenicity resulting from ART. To date, the APR has failed to demonstrate an increase in overall birth defects in babies born to mothers on ART taken during the first trimester [25] (3.0 per every 100 live births, 95% confidence interval or CI 2.4–3.8), compared with women who have taken ART in the second and third trimesters (2.6 per every 100 live births) and compared with the Centers for Disease Control's (CDC) population-based birth defects surveillance system from 1968 to 2003 (Metropolitan Atlanta Congenital Defects Program) (2.67 per every 100 live births) [26]. Similar findings were reported from PACTG 076 [11].

There is limited evidence from animal data and case reports linking some antiretroviral drugs with birth defects. Efavirenz (Sustiva), a NNRTI, has been associated with neural tube defects in both primates and human beings and is classed as FDA pregnancy category D. There have been three reported cases of neural tube defects and one case of Dandy-Walker syndrome, all in babies exposed to efavirenz in the first trimester [27]. Following reports of birth defects in rodents, avoidance in the first trimester is also advised with zalcitabine, delavirdine, and tenofovir. The APR has reported an increase in birth defects in women who received first trimester didanosine, although no specific pattern of birth defects has so far emerged [25]. The use of this drug in pregnancy is currently under review.

It is recommended that all women who have taken HAART in the first trimester should undergo a detailed anomaly scan during the second trimester [24].

Complications of antiretroviral therapy in children

In the short term, neonates receiving ZDV may develop anemia [11]. In the longer term, there have been concerns raised by several conflicting reports in the medical literature regarding mitochondrial dysfunction in infants exposed in utero to NRTIs. If there is a true causal relationship between in utero exposure and infant severe mitochondrial dysfunction, then the incidence appears to be extremely low [24].

Follow-up from PACTG 076 has so far failed to demonstrate any increased immunologic dysfunction, neurodevelopment, or growth in children exposed to ZDV in utero and in the neonatal period [28]. Six-year follow-up from PACTG 076 has also failed to show an increase in childhood cancers. Long-term follow-up through adulthood is recommended for all children exposed to in utero ART [24].

Maternal complications of antiretroviral therapy

There are numerous side effects and possible drug interactions of ART (Table 1). Long-term use of NRTIs are known to cause mitochondrial toxicity, which may result in neuropathy, myopathy, cardiomyopathy, pancreatitis, hepatic steatosis, and lactic acidosis, which usually resolve on discontinuation of the drugs. Some of these clinical syndromes have

Table 1
Antiretroviral drugs and potential adverse effects

Class of antiretroviral drug	Generic and trade name	Potential adverse effects
Nucleoside reverse transcriptase inhibitors (NRTIs)	Abacavir (ABC, Ziagen) Adefovir (Hepsera) Didanosine (ddI, Videx) Lamivudine (3TC, Epivir) Stavudine (d4T, Zerit) Zidovudine (ZDV, Retrovir) Zidovudine and Lamivudine (Combivir)	Generally well tolerated Adverse side effects include peripheral neuropathy, anemia, gastrointestinal disturbance, pancreatitis, raised transaminases, skin rash Lactic acidosis with combined stavudine and didanosine
Nonnucleoside reverse transcriptase inhibitors (NNRTIs)	Delavirdine (Rescriptor) Nevirapine (Viramune) Efavirenz (Sustiva)	Gastrointestinal disturbance, hepatic impairment, rash
Protease inhibitors (PIs)	Amprenavir (Agenerase) Indinavir (Crixivan) Nelfinavir (Viracept)[a] Ritonavir (Norvir) Saquinavir (Invirase, Fortovase)	Gastrointestinal disturbance, hepatic impairment, hyperglycemia, new-onset diabetes mellitus, exacerbation of diabetes mellitus, diabetic ketoacidosis, lipodystrophy

[a] Potential fetal and maternal toxicity caused by impurity in Viracept, from animal data. Therefore, the FDA advises that women switch from nelfinavir regimes for the foreseeable future.

similarities to hepatic disorders in the third trimester, such as the syndrome of hemolysis, elevated liver enzymes and low platelets (HELLP), and acute fatty liver of pregnancy (AFLP), and should be born in mind as a differential diagnosis. Recent evidence suggests that HELLP syndrome and AFLP may be caused by disorders of fetal or maternal mitochondrial fatty acid oxidation [29]. The combination of stavudine (d4T) and didanosine (ddI) cause lactic acidosis in pregnancy and should be avoided [24].

Protease inhibitors taken for long durations are known to cause glucose intolerance, new-onset diabetes mellitus, worsening of diabetes mellitus, diabetic ketoacidosis, hyperlipidemia, fat redistribution, and raised aminotransferases, among many other side effects. To date, rates of gestational diabetes have not been shown increase with the use of PIs in pregnancy [24]. Recent recommendations advise a glucose tolerance test at 24 to 28 weeks for patients on ART during pregnancy [24].

Drug interactions with antiretroviral therapy

Protease inhibitors may be inhibitors or inducers of cytochrome P-450 (CYP) 3A4, which is involved in the metabolism of many drugs (see anesthetic considerations). Ritonavir is a potent inhibitor of this enzyme and is often used in ART regimes, termed "ritonavir-boosted," to enhance the efficacy of other ART drugs. The NNRTI efavirenz and delavirdine are also inhibitors of CYP 3A4.

Effect of antiretroviral therapy on pregnancy outcome

Concerns exist about the effect of HAART on the outcome of pregnancy, although data are conflicting. Townsend and colleagues 2007 [30], in a UK epidemiologic study of 4,445 women on ART, reported an incidence of delivery before 37 weeks of 13.1% (95% CI 12.1–14.2), even when CD4 T-lymphocyte counts and HIV-related symptoms were accounted for. The risk was highest for women on HAART (14.1%), and lower for dual or monotherapy (10.1%). Delivery before 35 weeks was more strongly associated with HAART. Similarly, the European Collaborative Study and the Swiss Mother and Child HIV Cohort Study [31], which looked at 3,920 mother-child pairs, found a 2.6-fold (95% CI 1.4–4.8) increased odds of preterm delivery for infants exposed to HAART, compared with no treatment or monotherapy, after adjustment for CD4 T-lymphocyte counts and intravenous drug use. However, a meta-analysis of seven studies conducted in the United States, of 2,123 women who received HAART in pregnancy, compared with 1,143 women who did not, failed to demonstrate a difference in preterm labor, low birth rate, or Apgar scores [32]. Another recent meta-analysis of 14 European and United States studies, found no overall evidence of preterm delivery in women taking ART in pregnancy, compared with those who did not [33]. Other data relating to risk of fetal death and severe growth restriction (lower than 1,500 grams) are also conflicting.

Management of delivery

A meta-analysis by the International Perinatal HIV Group in 1999 of 15 prospective cohort studies [34], a randomized controlled trial by the European Mode of Delivery Collaboration also published in 1999 [35], and a Cochrane Collaboration systematic review in 2005 by Read and Newell [36] strongly support the use of PLCS in the prevention of MTCT, which has become standard practice for the management of delivery in HIV-infected women. This management has dramatically reduced the incidence of MTCT. However, these studies were undertaken before viral loads were measured routinely in pregnancy, and when antiretroviral therapy consisted of using single agent zidovudine or no ART. As a result, the practice of PLCS for all women is now being called into question. The American College of Obstetricians and Gynecologists recommend an elective cesarean section at 38-weeks gestation in women with more than 1,000 viral copies per milliliter [37]. However, British HIV Association guidelines suggest that PLCS may be unnecessary in women with undetectable viral loads on HAART who are low risk for requiring surgical interventions during delivery [38]. The recent AmRo study [39], investigated the rate of MTCT in 143

HIV-infected women taking HAART by mode of delivery. Of the 89 women (62%) who delivered vaginally, there were no cases of MTCT. ZDV is commenced intravenously 3 hours before PLSC, or at the onset of labor, and stopped at delivery. With the exception of stavudine (d4T), which should be stopped during intravenous ZDV infusion [24], other antiretrovirals should be continued orally near to the time of delivery. The infant should receive 6 weeks of ZDV therapy. The impact of cesarean section after the onset of labor or rupture of membranes in reducing MTCT is not known.

Where possible, in laboring women, fetal blood sampling, invasive fetal monitoring, amniotomy, and instrumental deliveries should be avoided, as these may increase the risk of MTCT [24]. Prolonged rupture of membranes has been shown to be a risk factor for MTCT. A meta-analysis by the International Perinatal HIV group reported an increased risk of MTCT of 2% for every hour of ruptured membranes in patients who received ZDV or no ART and who had duration of ruptured membranes of less than 24 hours [34]. There is currently limited data assessing the risk of MTCT in women with ruptured membranes who are taking combination ART with effective viral suppression. In the 2007 AmRo study [39], there were no cases of MTCT in 143 HIV-infected women taking HAART. Of these, data regarding rupture of membranes was available in 93. Duration of membrane rupture was longer than 4 hours in 43% of women.

Complications of cesarean section in HIV-infected patients

Several studies have looked at the complication rates following cesarean births in HIV-infected women compared with uninfected controls. The majority show some increase in minor complications, such as fever, but not major complications [35]. Some of these studies have observed a higher complication rate in women with more advanced disease, as demonstrated by CD4 T-lymphocyte counts less than 200 cells per mm^3. This has been confirmed by a Cochrane Collaboration systematic review by Read and Newell [36] in 2005. As in the non-HIV infected population, complications following PLCS are less than those following emergency cesarean section, but higher than those following vaginal delivery [36]. No randomized controlled trials have been undertaken to assess the effect of prophylactic antibiotics given to HIV-infected women during cesarean section, but recent guidelines recommend their use [24].

Anesthetic considerations

Assessment of HIV-infected patients

The majority of pregnant HIV-infected women whom the anesthesiologist is likely to encounter, are healthy and can be treated as normal. However, women with advanced disease, especially with CD4 T-lymphocyte counts below 200 cells per mm^3 and high viral loads, are susceptible to opportunistic infections, malignancies, and pathology directly attributed to the HIV virus itself. No organ system in the body is exempt from the effects of HIV. The anesthesiologist needs to carefully review each patient, looking at the patient's functional status, clinical manifestations of HIV, side effects of drug treatment, and results from laboratory tests. All patients should have full blood count analysis, coagulation screen, glucose measurement, and hepatic and renal function tests. Markers for disease severity (ie, CD4 T-lymphocyte count and viral load) should be performed within 3 months of the estimated date of delivery. Routine electrocardiograms and chest radiographs should be considered. Those with cardio-respiratory symptoms and signs warrant a more thorough cardiac and respiratory workup.

Respiratory system

Opportunistic infections, such as mycobacterium tuberculosis (MTB), bacterial pneumonias, and aspergillosis cause respiratory distress and hypoxemia. Pneumocystis carinii pneumonia (PCP) is encountered less frequently than in the past because of routine use of PCP prophylactic drug regimes for patients with advanced HIV disease, and more effective treatment of HIV per se. Neuraxial anesthesia may be preferable in these patients, although a high motor block with intercostal muscle weakness may not be tolerated in severe cases.

Cardiovascular system

HIV is known to cause, and is associated with cardiomyopathies, pulmonary hypertension, right and left ventricular dysfunction, myocarditis, pericardial effusions, and coronary artery disease. Studies have estimated the incidence of HIV-related cardiomyopathy to be between 2.7% [40] and 40% [41]. Pulmonary hypertension is rare and has a grave prognosis, as in the non-HIV population [42]. Myocarditis may occur commonly in the later stages of disease [40] and may be caused by opportunistic infections, such as MTB, cryptococcus, and toxoplasmosis, but the cause is usually not found in up to 80% of cases. Side effects of antiretroviral drugs include hyperglycemia, hyperlipidemia, lipodystrophy, and accelerated coronary arteriosclerosis. Of the antiretroviral therapies, PIs are most commonly associated with accelerated atherosclerosis. All patients need to have cardiovascular assessment, and some may warrant a detailed cardiac work-up. As longevity of patients continues to increase on ART, such side effects and their consequences are expected to increase.

Central nervous system

The central nervous system (CNS) is infected within the initial weeks following systemic HIV infection [43]. There may be many varied signs and symptoms of CNS involvement during the acute stage of infection, which include headaches, photophobia, meningitis, encephalitis, Guillain-Barré syndromes, peripheral and central neuropathies, and depression.

Autoimmune based demyelinating syndromes may develop in the latent phase. In advanced disease, patients may present with space occupying lesions because of toxoplasmosis, MTB, and lymphomas. Patients may also develop meningitis for example, because of cryptococcus, MTB and syphilis, encephalopathy, myelopathy, myopathy, and neuropathies. Autonomic neuropathy has also been described in HIV infected individuals [44]. Patients presenting with an altered mental state, headaches, and neurologic signs should be investigated with neuro-imaging, as space occupying lesions with raised intracranial pressure and CNS infections would contraindicate neuraxial blockade. Peripheral neuropathy is the most common neurologic manifestation of HIV disease, with 35% of AIDS patients affected [45]. A thorough neurologic examination should be conducted and abnormalities carefully documented before regional techniques are used.

Hematologic abnormalities

Anemia, leucopenia, lymphopenia, and thrombocytopenia may result from HIV infection, antiretroviral drugs, and bone marrow infiltration by opportunistic infection or neoplastic disease. Infection of CD4 T-lymphocytes occurs in the earliest stages of the disease, and falling CD4 T-lymphocyte counts are used as a marker of disease severity. Thrombocytopenia has been attributed to HIV-related immune thrombocytopenia, HIV infection of megakaryocytes, and reversible bone marrow suppression because of drugs such as ZDV and ganciclovir. The medical literature contains reports of thrombotic episodes in advanced HIV disease [46], which may be of particular significance to pregnant patients. Careful assessment of bleeding and coagulation parameters should be sought to guide the choice of technique, and consideration given to the management of postdelivery venous thromboembolism risk.

Renal abnormalities

HIV-infected patients are at risk of renal disease from multifactorial causes. HIV nephropathy presents as nephritic syndrome. Antiretroviral drugs may cause renal insults, for example acute tubular necrosis (adefovir) and nephrolithiasis (indinavir).

Gastrointestinal system

Patients with advanced disease may develop dysphagia, most frequently because of *Candida albicans*. Gastroesophageal reflux is also common in the later stages and may compound the significant risk of pulmonary aspiration in pregnant women.

Choice of anesthetic technique

Concerns have been expressed in the past over the use of both general and neuraxial anesthesia in HIV-infected patients. However, both techniques appear to be safe, bearing in mind the usual caveats and contra-indications relating to non-HIV infected patients.

General anesthesia can lead to transient immune depression, but this does not appear to be of clinical significance in HIV-positive patients. Gershon and Manning-Williams [47] studied 11 subjects undergoing general anesthesias in the peripartum period. There was no increase in complications or worsening of HIV disease in this group at 24 to 48 hours and 4 to 6 weeks postpartum, compared with patients receiving neuraxial blocks, local anesthesia or seda-tion, and no anesthesia. Concerns have also been expressed over the use of succinylcholine in patients with neuropathies and myopathies, but reports of adverse events, such as hyperkalemia, are lacking. Patients with AIDS-re-lated dementia are sensitive to opioids and benzodiazepines, but this group of patients is unlikely to be encountered in the obstetric population.

Neuraxial techniques have also been areas for concern in HIV-infected individuals. It has been postulated that extradural and spinal blocks might cause primary CNS HIV infection, that they might worsen pre-existing CNS disease, or that they might introduce other pathogens into the CNS. It is now known that HIV is a neurotropic virus and infects the CNS during the earliest stages of infection [43]. HIV virions and antibodies have been isolated from the CNS at the time of initial diagnosis. There is no evidence in the medical literature to suggest that neuraxial blockade is detrimental to HIV-infected patients.

In 1995, Hughes and colleagues prospectively studied 30 HIV-infected parturients [48]. Of these, 18 received neuraxial blocks for labor analgesia, or anesthesia. After extensive follow-up for 4 to 6 months postpartum, there were no adverse neurologic or immune sequelae. Gershon and Manning-Williams [47] studied 96 asymptomatic HIV-infected parturients retro-spectively to determine the effect of anesthetic technique on the stability of immune function. Comparison of 36 patients receiving neuraxial blocks, with 11 receiving general anesthesias, 22 receiving local anesthesia or sedation, and 27 patients receiving no anesthesia failed to reveal differences in compli-cation rates at 24 to 48 hours and 4 to 6 weeks postpartum, and there were no neurologic sequelae at 2-year follow-up. Second trimester CD4/CD8 ratios from 31 women subsequently receiving neuraxial blocks, local anesthesia, or no anesthesia, did not alter significantly at 24 to 48 hours postpartum. A third study by Avidan and colleagues (2002) [49], compared spinal an-esthesia in 44 HIV-infected parturients receiving ART, with 45 HIV-negative controls undergoing cesarean section. There was no difference in intraoper-ative hemodynamic stability or postoperative complications between the two groups. CD4 T-lymphocyte counts showed a significant increase in the immediate postpartum period in the HIV group, but CD4/CD8 ratios and viral loads remained stable.

The results from these studies are reassuring, but it should be born in mind that all of these studies were conducted on relatively healthy HIV-in-fected individuals. The effect of regional anesthesia on patients with advanced disease is not yet known. In addition to the usual advantages of neuraxial blockade in parturients, these techniques avoid potential drug interactions between drugs used for general anesthesia and antiretroviral agents.

Epidural blood patch

Concerns have also been expressed over the use of epidural blood patches used to treat postdural puncture headache (PDPH) in HIV-infected individuals. Despite the theoretical risks, there have been no reports of serious complications related to this technique in HIV-infected patients. Tom and colleagues [50], in a study of six HIV-infected patients who received an epidural blood patch to treat PDPH, reported no adverse sequelae over a 2-year follow-up period. Conversely, not treating a severe PDPH with an epidural blood patch may lead to debilitating neurologic sequelae [51].

Drug interactions

Some antiretroviral drugs are inhibitors of CYP 3A4, which is necessary for the metabolism of many drugs. Ritonavir is a potent inhibitor of this enzyme and has been shown to significantly reduce the rate of metabolism of fentanyl, midazolam, amiodarone, and quinidine. In a study using volunteers, fentanyl clearance was shown to be reduced by 67% in patients taking ritonavir [52]. Caution should be used when using fentanyl in patients taking ritonavir, and other CYP 3A4 inhibitors, especially in high dose. Conversely, nevaripine is a cytochrome P-450 inducer and increased doses of the above drugs maybe required.

Caution should also be used in the choice of drugs used to treat postpartum hemorrhage [24] because of uterine atony in patients taking CYP 3A4 inhibitors such as ritonavir, and the NNRTI efavirenz and delavirdine. Ergotamines, for example methergine, may result in an exaggerated vasoconstrictive response when these drugs are concomitantly administered. Alternatives should be used in the first instance, such as oxytocin, prostaglandin F2 alpha, and misoprostol. Should these drugs prove to be inadequate, the risk and benefits of methergine should be considered, and if given should be titrated slowly in small doses.

Patients infected with HIV may also be taking many other drugs for the prophylaxis and treatment of opportunistic infections. There is great potential for drug interactions with these drugs, antiretrovirals, and drugs used in anesthesia, and advice from HIV specialists should be sought if these pose a concern.

Universal precautions and occupational exposure to HIV

It is recommended that all health care workers who may come into contact with blood, blood products, body tissues, and secretions, use universal precautions in all patients to reduce the risk of occupational exposure to organisms such as HIV. This should include gloves, eye protection, and face-masks, gowns, and appropriate footwear. Risk of seroconversion varies with type of exposure. A needlestick injury involving HIV-infected blood is associated with a 0.3% risk of seroconversion [53], compared with a 0.09% risk in mucous membrane exposure [54]. Percutaneous injuries at higher risk include hollow needle injury, deep injuries into muscle or blood vessels, and injuries from infected patients with advanced disease [55]. CDC guidelines from 2005 [56] state that exposure sites should be washed with soap and water, or mucous membranes irrigated with water. The situation should be assessed for risk of seroconversion and experts contacted for advice about postexposure prophylaxis, which is normally taken over a 4-week period.

Summary

Numbers of HIV-infected individuals across the globe are increasing, as is the proportion of women infected with HIV. However, better understanding of the HIV virus and rapidly evolving treatments has provided hope for millions of people world-wide. With the evolution of ART, HIV infection has changed from a fatal condition to a chronic disease. In the pregnant population, recent understanding of factors influencing vertical transmission has enabled dramatic reductions in MTCT to below 2%. HIV-infected parturients should be cared for by a multidisciplinary team in which the anesthetist plays an important role. Most patients whom the anesthetist encounters will be healthy, but all warrant thorough assessment to tailor appropriate analgesic and anesthetic techniques.

References

[1] Gottlieb M. Pneumocystis carinii pneumonia and mucosal candidiasis in previously healthy homosexual men: evidence of a new acquired cellular immunodeficiency. N Engl J Med 1981; 305:1425–30.

[2] Fauci AS. The AIDS epidemic: considerations for the 21st century. N Engl J Med 1999;341: 1046–50.

[3] UNAIDS/WHO. AIDS epidemic update: December 2006. Available at: http://www.unaids. org/en/HIV_data/epi2006/. Accessed November 18, 2007.

[4] Luzzi GA, Peto TEA, Weiss RA, et al. HIV and AIDS. In: Warrell DA, David DJ, Cox TM, et al, editors. Oxford textbook of medicine. 4th edition. Oxford (UK): Oxford University Press; 2004.

[5] Jamieson DJ, Cohan MH, Maupin R, et al. Rapid human immunodeficiency virus-1 testing on labor and delivery in 17 US hospitals: the MIRIAD experience. Am J Obstet Gynecol 2007;197:S72–82.

[6] French R, Brocklehurst P. The effect of pregnancy on survival in women infected with HIV: a systematic review of the literature and meta-analysis. Br J Obstet Gynaecol 1998;105: 827–35.

[7] Minkoff H, Hershow R, Watts DH, et al. The relationship of pregnancy to human immuno-deficiency virus disease progression. Am J Obstet Gynecol 2003;189:552–9.

[8] Burns DN, Nourjah P, Minkoff H, et al. Changes in CD4+ and CD8+ cell levels during pregnancy and post partum in women seropositive and seronegative for human immunodeficiency virus-1. Am J Obstet Gynecol 1996;174:1461–8.

[9] Cao Y, Krogstad P, Korber BT, et al. Maternal HIV-1 viral load and vertical transmission of infection: the Ariel Project for the prevention of HIV transmission from mother to infant. Nat Med 1997;3:549–52.

[10] Watts DH, Lambert J, Stiehm ER, et al. Progression of HIV disease among women following delivery. J Acquir Immune Defic Syndr 2003;33(5):585–93.

[11] Connor EM, Sperling RS, Gelber R, et al. Reduction of maternal-infant transmission of human immunodeficiency virus type 1 with zidovudine treatment. Pediatric AIDS Clinical Trials Group Protocol 076 Study Group. N Engl J Med 1994;331:1173–80.

[12] Hughes SC. HIV and pregnancy: twenty-five years into the epidemic. Int Anesthesiol Clin 2007;45:29–49.

[13] Mofenson LM, Lambert JS, Stiehm ER, et al. Risk factors for perinatal transmission of human immunodeficiency virus type 1 in women treated with zidovudine. Pediatric AIDS Clinical Trials Group Study 185 team. N Engl J Med 1999;341:385–93.

[14] Garcia PM, Kalish LA, Pitt J, et al. Maternal levels of plasma human immunodeficiency virus type 1 RNA and the risk of perinatal transmission. N Engl J Med 1999;341:394–402.

[15] Mayaux MJ, Teglas JP, Mandelbrot L, et al. Acceptability and impact of zidovudine for prevention of mother-to-child human immunodeficiency virus-1 transmission in France. J Pediatr 1997;131(6):857–62.

[16] Harris NH, Thompson SJ, Ball R, et al. Zidovudine and perinatal human immunodeficiency virus type 1 transmission: a population-based approach. Pediatrics 2002;109:60.

[17] Volmink J, Siegfried NL, van der Merwe L, et al. Antiretrovirals for reducing the risk of mother-to-child transmission of HIV infection. Cochrane Database Syst Rev 2007, Issue 1. Art. No.:CD003510. DOI:10.1002/14651858.CD003510.pub2.

[18] Ioannidis JPA, Abrams EJ, Ammann A, et al. Perinatal transmission of human immunodeficiency virus type 1 by pregnant women with RNA virus loads < 1000 copies/ml. J Infect Dis 2001;183:539–45.

[19] Kovacs A, Wasserman SS, Burns D, et al. Determinants of HIV-1 shedding in the genital tract of women. Lancet 2001;358:1593–601.

[20] Reinhardt PP, Reinhardt B, Lathey JL, et al. Human cord blood mononuclear cells are preferentially infected by non-syncytium-inducing, macrophage-tropic human immunodeficiency virus type 1 isolates. J Clin Microbiol 1995;33:292–7.

[21] Branson BM, Handsfield HH, Lampe MA. Revised recommendations for HIV testing of adults, adolescents, and pregnant women in health-care settings. Morbidity and Mortality Weekly 2006;55(RR-14):1–17.

[22] ACOG. ACOG committee opinion number 304, November 2004. Prenatal and perinatal human immunodeficiency virus testing: expanded recommendations. Obstet Gynecol 2004; 104(5 Pt 1):1119–24.

[23] AIDSinfo. Glossary of HIV/AIDS-related terms. 5th edition. 2005. Available at: http://aidsinfo.nih.gov/contentfiles/GlossaryHIV-relatedTerms_FifthEdition_en.pdf. Accessed 19 November, 2007.

[24] Perinatal HIV Guidelines Working Group. Public health service task force recommendations for use of antiretroviral drugs in pregnant HIV-infected women for maternal health and interventions to reduce perinatal HIV transmission in the United States. 2007. 1–96. Available at: http://aidsinfo.nih.gov/ContentFiles/PerinatalGL.pdf. Accessed November 6, 2007.

[25] Antiretroviral Pregnancy Registry Steering Committee. Antiretroviral Pregnancy Registry international interim report for 1 Jan 1989–31 January 2007. Wilmington (NC): Registry Coordinating Center; 2004. Available at: http://www.APRegistry.com. Accessed 19th November 2007.

[26] Correa A, Cragan J, Kucik J, et al. Metropolitan Atlanta Congenital Defects Program 40th Anniversary Edition Surveillance Report: reporting birth defects surveillance data 1968–2003. Birth Defects Research (Part A) 2007;79:65–93.

[27] News Item: Bristol-Myers Squibb has issued a 'Dear Health Care Provider' letter advising of a change in the pregnancy category for sustiva [efavirenz]. Reactions Weekly 2005;1056:2.

[28] Culnane M, Fowler M, Lee SS, et al. Lack of long-term effects of in utero exposure to zidovudine among uninfected children born to HIV-infected women. Pediatric AIDS Clinical Trials Group Protocol 219/076 Teams. JAMA 1999;281(2):151–7.

[29] Ibdah JA, Yang Z, Bennett MJ. Liver disease in pregnancy and fetal fatty acid oxidation defects. Mol Genet Metab 2000;71:182–9.

[30] Townsend CL, Cortina-Borja M, Peckham CS, et al, International Perinatal HIV Group European Mode of Delivery Collaboration. Antiretroviral therapy and premature delivery in diagnosed HIV-infected women in the United Kingdom and Ireland. AIDS 2007;21: 1019–26.

[31] European Collaborative Study, Study SMaCHC. Combination antiretroviral therapy and duration of pregnancy. AIDS 2000;14(18):2913–20.

[32] Tuomala RE, Shapiro DE, Mofenson LM, et al. Antiretroviral therapy during pregnancy and the risk of an adverse outcome. N Engl J Med 2002;346:1863–70.

[33] Kourtis AP, Schmid CH, Jamieson DJ, et al. Use of antiretroviral therapy in pregnant HIV-infected women and the risk of premature delivery: a meta-analysis. AIDS 2007;21: 607–15.

[34] International Perinatal HIV Group. The mode of delivery and the risk of vertical transmission of human immunodeficiency virus type 1- a meta-analysis of 15 prospective cohort studies. N Engl J Med 1999;340:977–87.

[35] European Mode of Delivery Collaboration. Elective caesarean-section versus vaginal delivery in prevention of vertical HIV-1 transmission: a randomized clinical trial. Lancet 1999; 353:1035–9.

[36] Read JS, Newell ML. Efficacy and safety of cesarean delivery for prevention of mother-to-child transmission of HIV-1. Cochrane Database Syst Rev 2005, Issue 4. Art. No.: CD005479. DOI:10.1002/14651858.CD005479.

[37] ACOG. ACOG committee opinion number 234, May 2000. Scheduled cesarean delivery and the prevention of vertical transmission of HIV infection. Int J Gynaecol Obstet 2001;73: 279–81.

[38] BHIVA. British HIV Association (BHIVA) Guidelines for the Management of HIV infection in Pregnant Women and the Prevention of Mother-to-Child Transmission of HIV. 2005. p. 1–104. Available at: http://www.bhiva.org/cms1191558.asp. Accessed November 19, 2007.

[39] Boer K, Nellen J, Patel D, et al. The AmRo study: pregnancy outcome in HIV-1 infected women under effective highly active antiretroviral therapy and a policy of vaginal delivery. Br J Obstet Gynaecol 2007;114:148–55.

[40] Barbaro G, Di Lorenzo G, Grisorio B, et al. Cardiac involvement in the acquired immunodeficiency syndrome: a multicenter clinical-pathological study. AIDS Res Hum Retroviruses 1998;14:1071–7.

[41] Barbaro G. Cardiovascular manifestations of HIV infection. Circulation 2002;106:1420–5.

[42] Pellicelli AM, Barbaro G, Palmieri F, et al. Primary pulmonary hypertension in HIV patients: a systematic review. Angiology 2001;52:31–41.

[43] Spector SA, Hsia K, Pratt D, et al. Virologic markers of human immunodeficiency virus type 1 in cerebrospinal fluid. The HIV Neurobehavioral Research Center Group. J Infect Dis 1993;168:68–74.

[44] Villa A, Foresti V, Confalonieri F. Autonomic nervous system dysfunction associated with HIV infection in intravenous heroin users. AIDS 1992;6:85–9.

[45] Wulff EA, Wang AK, Simpson DM. HIV-associated peripheral neuropathy, epidemiology, pathophysiology and treatment. Drugs 2000;59:1251–60.

[46] Saif MW, Greenberg B. HIV and thrombosis: a review. AIDS Patient Care STDS 2001;15: 15–24.

[47] Gershon RY, Manning-Williams D. Anaesthesia and the HIV-infected parturient: a retrospective study. Int J Obstet Anesth 1997;6:76–81.

[48] Hughes SC, Dailey PA, Landers D, et al. Parturients infected with human immunodeficiency virus and regional anesthesia: clinical and immunologic response. Anesthesiology 1995;82: 32–7.

[49] Avidan MS, Groves P, Blott M, et al. Low complication rate associated with cesarean section under spinal anesthesia for HIV-1 infected women on antiretroviral therapy. Anesthesiology 2002;97:320–4.

[50] Tom DJ, Gulevich SJ, Shapiro HM, et al. Epidural blood patch in the HIV-1 positive patient. Anesthesiology 1992;76:943–7.

[51] Loo CC, Dahlgreen G, Irestedt L. Neurological complications in obstetric regional anaesthesia. Int J Obstet Anesth 2000;9:99–124.

[52] Olkkola KT, Palkama VJ, Neuvonen PJ. Ritonavir's role in reducing fentanyl clearance and prolonging its half-life. Anesthesiology 1999;91:681–5.

[53] Bell DM. Occupational risk of human immunodeficiency virus infection in health-care workers: an overview. Am J Med 1997;102(5B):9–15.

[54] Ippolito G, Puro V, De Carli G. Italian Study Group on Occupational Risk of HIV Infection. The risk of occupational human immunodeficiency virus in health care workers. Arch Intern Med 1993;153:1451–8.

[55] Cardo DM, Culver DH, Ciesielski CA, et al. A case-control study of HIV seroconversion in health care workers after percutaneous exposure. N Engl J Med 1997;337:1485–90.

[56] CDC. Updated U.S. Public Health Service guidelines for the management of occupational exposures to HBV, HCV, and HIV and recommendations for postexposure prophylaxis. MMWR 2005;50(no.RR-11):1–42.

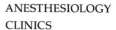

ANESTHESIOLOGY
CLINICS

ELSEVIER
SAUNDERS

Anesthesiology Clin
26 (2008) 145–158

Ultrasound-Facilitated Epidurals and Spinals in Obstetrics

Jose Carlos Almeida Carvalho, MD, PhD, FANZCA, FRCPC

Department of Anesthesia and Pain Management, Mount Sinai Hospital, 600 University Avenue, Room 781, Toronto, Ontario, M5G 1X5, Canada

Regional anesthesia is currently the gold standard of practice for pain control in obstetrics, and it is unlikely that this will change soon. The search for improvements in the quality and safety of epidurals and spinals in obstetrics deserves therefore our closest attention.

Failures and complications of regional anesthesia can be related to many causes, one of the most important being the blind nature of such techniques. The practice of epidurals and spinals relies primarily on the palpation of anatomic landmarks that are not always easy to find. A good assessment of the spine includes a careful examination to be sure that the vertebrae are aligned, and to locate the iliac crests (Tuffier's line), lumbar posterior spinous processes, and interspaces. These landmarks identify the level of the spine at which the puncture will be performed and the optimal puncture site. Other important aspects of the spinal or epidural puncture, such as the angle of the needle during its insertion and the distance from the skin to the ligamentum flavum, cannot be assessed based on inspection and palpation. If a patient is overweight, has a curvature of the spine, or has any abnormal anatomy that is not visible or palpable, the spinal or epidural technique becomes not only blind, but also unpredictable. The somewhat unreliable nature of the technique can lead to complications, such as patient discomfort, trauma to various structures (nerves, vessels, ligaments, and bones), potential infectious risk from multiple attempts, failure, and accidental dural puncture with subsequent postdural puncture headache.

Failures and complications in spinals and epidurals can be minimized by optimal positioning of the patient, meticulous assessment of the anatomic landmarks, and refined technique. However, limitations still apply, notably

E-mail address: jose.carvalho@uhn.on.ca

1932-2275/08/$ - see front matter © 2008 Elsevier Inc. All rights reserved.
doi:10.1016/j.anclin.2007.11.007 *anesthesiology.theclinics.com*

the failure of clinicians to accurately determine the puncture level. When the accuracy of the puncture level determined by palpation is compared with that determined by MRI, clinicians are correct in their assessment only 30% of the time. Although they are only out by one space most of the time, this error in assessment can be as much as four spaces. The implications of such imprecision for the safety of the procedure are obvious, especially in case of spinal anesthesia [1,2].

Despite considerable improvement in the quality of needles, catheters, drugs, and delivery systems for epidurals and spinals, the technical aspects of the procedures have not evolved in the past 70 years. The techniques for identifying the epidural space currently in use were proposed by Dogliotti (loss of resistance) and Gutierrez (hanging drop) in the 1930s. The most common complication in labor epidurals, the accidental dural puncture, still occurs in up to 1.6% of cases, causing significant morbidity for the obstetric patient in the postpartum period [3].

Similar to the experience with peripheral nerve blocks, the ultimate advance in spinal and epidural techniques will only occur when we are able to have image-guided procedures. This will enhance precision and reduce complications, therefore improving patient outcomes and satisfaction. Ultrasound has recently been introduced into clinical anesthesia to facilitate lumbar spinals and epidurals [4,5]. The use of preprocedure ultrasound imaging or, eventually, real-time ultrasound guidance should improve not only clinical practice, but also teaching.

Spinal ultrasound is particularly challenging because the structures to be imaged are protected by a very complex, articulated encasement of bones, which affords a very narrow acoustic window for the ultrasound beam. In addition, the structures are located deeper than those we image when we use ultrasound for peripheral nerve blocks or the placement of central lines. There are, however, two useful acoustic windows for the assessment of lumbar spine sonoanatomy: One is accessed by using a transverse midline approach, the other by using a paramedian longitudinal approach [6,7]. The information from each of these two scanning planes complements the other. The ultrasound probe used for spinals and epidurals must be a low-frequency (2–5 MHz) curved probe. When compared with the high–frequency (10–15 MHz) linear probe, the low-frequency ultrasound penetrates deeper, which is more appropriate for this purpose. On the other hand, the image resolution is lower, which limits the precision of the assessment.

A thorough knowledge of the lumbar spine anatomy is necessary for the understanding of the sonoanatomy information being generated. The key elements visualized in the longitudinal and transverse approaches include boney structures and ligaments.

Anatomical elements identifiable by the longitudinal approach include:

- Sacrum
- Articular process

- Ligamentum flavum and posterior dura mater
- Anterior dura mater, posterior longitudinal ligament, and vertebral body

Anatomical elements identifiable by the transverse approach include:

- Spinous process
- Articular process
- Transverse process
- Ligamentum flavum and posterior dura mater
- Anterior dura mater, posterior longitudinal ligament, and vertebral body

With spinal ultrasound, only two patterns have to be recognized: one for the longitudinal paramedian approach, and the other for the transverse approach. This makes spinal ultrasound simpler to use than ultrasound for peripheral nerve blocks where different sonographic patterns have to be recognized. When using the longitudinal paramedian approach, a pattern appears that is commonly described in the literature as the "saw sign" (Fig. 1). As for the pattern of the transverse approach, I usually describe it as the "flying bat" (Fig. 2).

An accurate assessment of the sonoanatomy of the lumbar spine requires a systematic technique. For the longitudinal paramedian approach, the paramedian longitudinal scan is performed by positioning the ultrasound probe vertically, perpendicular to the long axis of the spine. The probe is initially placed over the sacral area, 3 cm to the left of the midline and slightly angled to target the center of the spinal canal. From this point, a continuous hyperechoic (bright) line representing the ultrasound image of the sacrum is visualized. The probe is then slowly moved cephalad until a hyperechoic sawlike image is seen (Fig. 3). The "saw" represents the articular processes (teeth of the saw) and the interspaces (spaces between the teeth), the latter consisting of the ligamentum flavum and posterior dura mater and, deeper in, the anterior dura mater, the posterior longitudinal ligament, and the vertebral

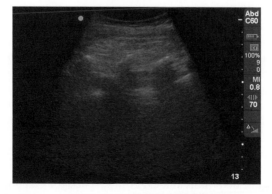

Fig. 1. Longitudinal paramedian view of the lumbar spine with the typical saw sign.

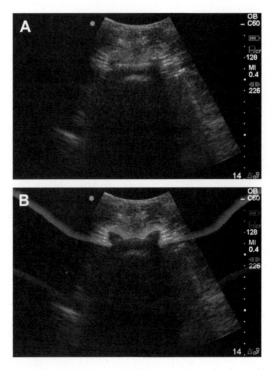

Fig. 2. Transverse view of a lumbar interspace shows a pattern that resembles a flying bat. (*A*) Actual image. (*B*) Artistic concept of the "flying bat."

body (Fig. 4). The exact level of each of the interspaces, L5-S1 to L1-L2, can then be marked on the skin to facilitate the rest of the examination.

For the transverse approach, a transverse scanning of each individual space can be performed once the interspaces are determined. This is accomplished by positioning the probe horizontally, perpendicular to the long axis of the spine, at the marked levels. With this approach, the midline of the spine corresponding to the spinous process is identified as a small hyperechoic signal immediately underneath the skin, which continues as a long triangular hypoechoic (dark) acoustic shadow (Fig. 5). The probe is then moved slightly cephalad or caudad to capture a view of an acoustic window (interspace). Within the interspace, on the midline, a hyperechoic band corresponding to the ligamentum flavum and the dorsal dura is visualized. A second hyperechoic band, parallel to the first band, corresponds to the anterior dura, the posterior longitudinal ligament, and the vertebral body. In addition, paramedian hyperechoic structures, corresponding to the articular and transverse processes, are also visualized via the acoustic window (Fig. 6).

The ultrasonographic assessment of the lumbar spine as described above helps the clinician determine the exact interspace for the puncture and the optimal insertion point. The determination of the optimal insertion point is

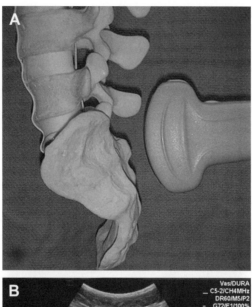

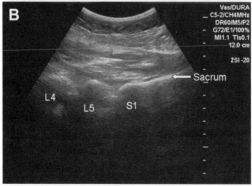

Fig. 3. Longitudinal approach, whether midline or paramedian, identifies the sacrum and the lumbar interspaces. (*A*) Orientation of the ultrasound probe. (*B*) Hyperechoic image of the sacrum and of the saw sign, which represents the articular processes of the lumbar vertebrae and the interspaces.

easily made with the transverse approach. Once the clear image of the interspace is obtained, the image is frozen. At that moment, with the probe kept steady, two marks are drawn on the skin, one coinciding with the center of the upper horizontal surface of the probe (midline) and the other coinciding with the middle point of the right lateral surface of the probe (interspace). The puncture site is determined by the intersection of the extensions of the two marks on the skin in the vertical and horizontal planes (Fig. 7). It is not easy to predict the angle at which the epidural needle should be advanced during placement. In the author's experience, a reliable technique is to ensure that the needle should follow the same angle at which the best image of the "flying bat" was captured. This technique is based on the premise that,

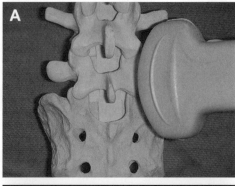

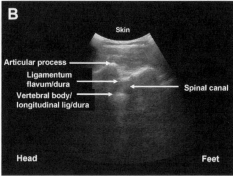

Fig. 4. Longitudinal paramedian approach with the typical saw sign. (*A*) Orientation of the ultrasound probe. (*B*) Hyperechoic image of the articular processes, the ligamentum flavum–posterior dura mater unit, and the anterior dura mater–posterior longitudinal ligament–vertebral body unit. The spinal canal can be seen between the anterior and posterior dura mater.

because the ultrasound beam penetrates without being distorted, it provides a good path for the needle to follow.

With the aid of a built-in caliper, the distance from the skin to the epidural space can be measured. This is helpful in determining the distance from skin to dura and assists the regionalist in needle placement and depth perception. With the current resolution offered by portable ultrasound machines, the captured image of the ligamentum flavum and posterior dura mater appears as a single unit. At present, the distance from the skin to the inner side (ie, the deepest border of this ligamentum flavum–posterior dura mater unit) is standardized to represent the actual needle depth (Fig. 8). The built-in caliper can also be used to measure the antero-posterior diameter of the dural sac, which might be useful information in the practice of techniques, such as spinal and combined spinal-epidural anesthesia.

Although it has been suggested that the paramedian longitudinal approach is the best acoustic window in spinal ultrasonography [6], the transverse approach is more useful in clinical practice, especially if the midline approach is to be used for the puncture, which is the norm. the author's experience,

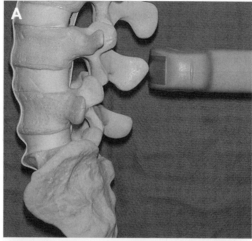

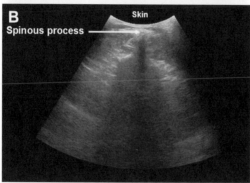

Fig. 5. Transverse approach at the tip of the spinous process easily identifies the midline of the spine. (*A*) Orientation of the ultrasound probe. (*B*) The tip of the spinous process appears as a small hyperechoic structure immediately beneath the skin, and determines a long vertical black hypoechoic shadow.

the paramedian longitudinal approach has been used to determine the level of the puncture. In some cases, especially where the quality of imaging is compromised or where there is a need of confirmation of a certain structure, the paramedian longitudinal approach is beneficial. It is therefore advisable that the anesthesiologist should be familiar with both approaches.

Based on the information provided by the ultrasound, anesthesiologists can determine the optimal insertion point, the estimation of the angle to be used, and the calculation of the distance from the skin to the epidural space. In addition to the loss of resistance, these are key factors in performing an uneventful puncture.

In a previous study done at Mount Sinai Hospital, the accuracy of the insertion point has been shown to be very high. When the preprocedural scanning is done with the above technique, there is no need to reinsert the

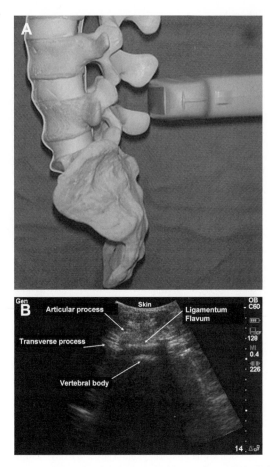

Fig. 6. Transverse approach at a lumbar interspace shows the typical "flying bat" sign. (*A*) Orientation of the ultrasound probe. Arrow indicates (*B*) Ligamentum flavum–posterior dura mater unit and anterior dura mater–posterior longitudinal ligament–vertebral body unit are seen as hyperechoic structures on the midline. Articular processes and transverse processes are seen as paramedian hyperechoic structures and determine corresponding acoustic shadows.

epidural needle in 91.8% of the patients, and no need to even redirect the needle in 73.7%. In our experience, the successful identification of the epidural space is accomplished with two or fewer redirections in 96.7% of the cases [7]. The precision of the estimation of the distance to the epidural space is also remarkable. In our series of 60 obstetric patients, we found that the mean difference between the distance estimated by the ultrasound and the actual needle depth was 0.01 (±0.345) cm, with a 95% limit of agreement for the difference between the two measurements being −0.666 to +0.687 cm. The epidural space depth determined by ultrasound was 4.66 (±0.68) cm (range 3.43–6.91 cm), whereas the one determined by the actual needle was 4.65 (±0.72) cm (range 3.5–6.5 cm) [7].

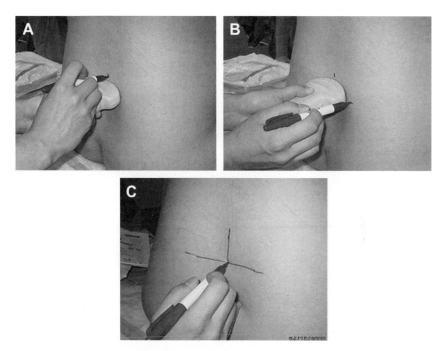

Fig. 7. The insertion point is determined by the intersection of the extensions of the two marks on the skin in the vertical and horizontal planes, one for the midline, the other for the interspace.

The sonoanatomy described above represents the normal findings with this new technology. Ultrasound technology has major benefits when it comes to dealing with parturients with altered anatomy. Two of these conditions are worth highlighting: obesity and scoliosis.

Obese patients can introduce some degree of difficulty to the use of spinal ultrasound. Image quality depends on how much fat tissue exists between the skin and the tip of the spinous process. In addition, if the distance to the ligamentum flavum is too great, the sharpness of the image can be compromised, but appropriate visualization is still possible (Fig. 9). In some patients, the tip of the spinous process is located more than 5 cm from the skin. The ligamentum flavum can be as deep as 8 cm, with extremes of 11 to 12 cm. One important detail while scanning obese patients is to estimate the degree of compression that the subcutaneous tissue allows. This is easily demonstrated on the ultrasound screen by compressing and relieving the subcutaneous tissue with the ultrasound probe. If the distance from the skin to the epidural space is measured during the compression of the subcutaneous tissue, such measurement will considerably underestimate the actual needle depth. One should therefore relieve the pressure on the skin, freeze the image, and measure, thereby ensuring a much better correlation between the measurements determined by both ultrasound and

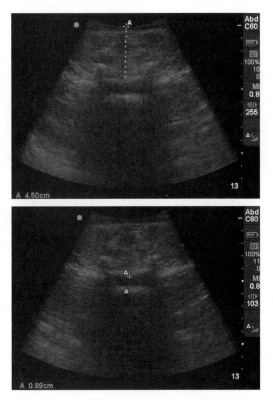

Fig. 8. Estimation of the needle depth (*dotted line*) by ultrasound with the aid of the built-in caliper. The author recommends positioning the caliper at the inner side (ie, the deepest border of the ligamentum flavum–posterior dura mater unit) (*top image*). The built-in caliper can also measure the antero-posterior diameter of the dural sac (*bottom image*). (*A*) Position of caliper.

needle. The vast majority of obese patients have the epidural space located at a maximum of 8 cm from the skin if the puncture is done at the optimal insertion point. The clinical implication of this information is that with the aid of ultrasound, an extra-long spinal or epidural needle is not likely necessary. Preprocedural scanning is helpful in determining the need for special needles. In some cases, the quality of the image obtained at 8 cm from the skin can be compromised in the transverse approach. In these cases, the distance from the skin to the ligamentum flavum can be double-checked with the longitudinal paramedian approach, which offers a sharper image of the ligamentum flavum and dura mater in this subset of patients. Measurements obtained with the midline approach and the paramedian approach are slightly different, either a few millimeters longer or shorter, depending on how much subcutaneous tissue fills the paraspinal groove. An additional advantage of ultrasound in these patients is its usefulness for positioning the patients appropriately. By viewing real-time ultrasound, minor changes in

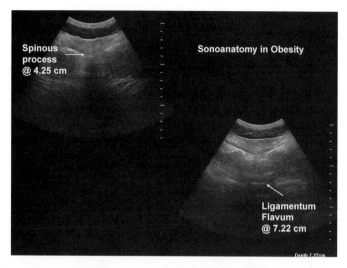

Fig. 9. Sonoanatomy of the lumbar spine of an obese patient. Note that the tip of the spinal process is 4.25 cm from the skin and 7.22 cm from the ligamentum flavum–posterior dura mater unit. If significant compression of the subcutaneous tissue is applied during the ultrasonographic assessment, a significant underestimation of the distance will occur.

patient position can make huge differences in opening up interspinous spaces and ensuring minimal spinal rotation or lateral flexion.

Patients who have scoliosis also present challenges. Scoliosis is not only associated with lateral curvatures of the spine on the longitudinal plane, but also with different degrees of rotation around the longitudinal axis. These abnormalities are frequent causes of difficult epidurals and spinals. In many cases, accurately determining the optimal puncture site is impossible without the use of the ultrasound. This is especially true in overweight patients in which the palpation is compromised. The abnormal interspace shows asymmetry of the bony structures, with asymmetric articular processes. In addition, one of the typical parallel hyperechoic lines corresponding to the ligamentum flavum and the vertebral body is either incomplete or missing (Fig. 10). When possible, these abnormal interspaces should be avoided and a space with preserved anatomy should be sought. In the past, a radiograph was needed to determine the optimal space in patients with scoliosis. Today, with the use of ultrasound, this can be avoided. Additionally, corrective surgery for scoliosis can obliterate potential spaces and the use of ultrasound can assist the anesthesiologist in optimal site selection.

Abnormal anatomy can be present in patients for reasons other than obesity and scoliosis. Patients with previous spine surgery may have extensive destruction of bony and soft tissue, with substitution by scar tissue. However, even in the presence of extensive spinal surgery, it is almost always possible to identify a space with preserved anatomy and therefore

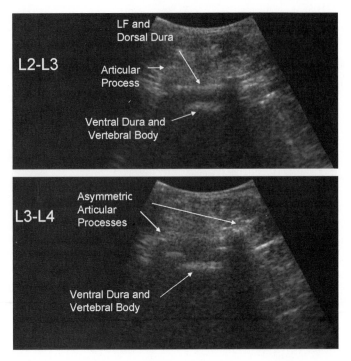

Fig. 10. Sonoanatomy in severe scoliosis. Sonoanatomy is typical and normal at L2-L3, while at L3-L4 articular processes are grossly asymmetric and the ligamentum flavum is not seen.

make regional anesthesia, such as a spinal, still possible. A promising application of ultrasound is for detecting abnormal sonoanatomy of the ligamentum flavum and thus to possibly avoid accidental dural puncture. In comparing patients with history of previous accidental dural puncture with patients who also had epidurals but without dural puncture, investigators at Mt. Sinai Hospital have found a much higher than normal incidence of abnormal ligamentum flavum on ultrasonography in the group with dural puncture. Although no clear explanation can be offered for these findings at present, it has been the author's practice to avoid the puncture of spaces in which the ligamentum flavum is either not seen or appears abnormal on ultrasound. The author hypothesizes that widespread use of ultrasonography may decrease the number of accidental dural punctures.

The advantages of ultrasound in assisting the placement of epidurals and spinals have been discussed in a few publications. Grau and colleagues [8] have determined that, compared with the epidurals done with the conventional palpatory method, ultrasound-assisted blocks are associated with fewer attempts during the procedure, greater efficacy, and higher patient satisfaction. This has been shown to be true not only in patients with spines that are considered easy for placement, but also in subgroups of patients with spines considered difficult for placement, such as patients with scoliosis, accentuated lordosis or kyphosis, or obesity [9].

The limitations of ultrasound use are confined to time, cost, and technical limitation. However as experience develops, many of these can be overcome with the promise of improved reliability.

The advantages of the use of ultrasound-assisted epidurals and spinals go far beyond routine clinical practice. Ultrasound is an accurate and extremely helpful teaching tool. Grau and colleagues [10] have shown that the learning curve for administering epidurals can be significantly improved when these procedures are done under ultrasound. As compared with the standard palpatory method, the ultrasound-assisted technique is associated with a higher success rate at all stages of the learning curve.

The use of sonoanatomy of the spine may well be a breakthrough in the practice of regional anesthesia. Research possibilities with this new tool are phenomenal. The author recently attempted to correlate the antero-posterior diameter of the dural sac with the spread of spinal anesthesia in cesarean deliveries [11]. Although not successful on the first attempt, it is believed that preprocedural scanning will allow for a better understanding of the physiology and pharmacology of epidural and spinal anesthesia.

Another fascinating possibility is the development of a "difficult spine score," similar to what has been developed for difficult intubation. Preprocedural assessment of the patient's spine will allow better planning and will, it is hoped, lead to better outcomes and greater patient satisfaction.

Finally, despite the obvious technical difficulties, it has been suggested that real-time spinal ultrasound can actually be used to guide the needle insertion [12] and even to detect position of vessels in the needle trajectory with the aid of Doppler [13]. Although these possibilities are fascinating, they do face important limitations. In the case of real-time ultrasound, an assistant is needed to capture the image of the interspace with a paramedian longitudinal approach while the primary anesthetist performs the needle insertion via midline approach. In the case of detection of vessels, the limiting factor is the extremely low blood flow in the epidural vessels, which makes imaging more difficult.

In summary, the preprocedural ultrasonographic assessment of the lumbar spine provides valuable information for the placement of spinals and epidurals, by determining:

The exact interspace (level) at which the puncture will be performed, which is especially important in spinal anesthesia
The best interspace (the clearest sonoanatomy)
The ideal insertion point
The angle of the puncture
The depth of the epidural space
Any abnormalities of the anatomy (eg, scoliosis)

This fascinating new tool will considerably improve the technical aspects of spinal and epidural techniques, with the following possible benefits:

When used as a teaching tool, it facilitates the learning curve and increases safety.

It shortens the duration of the procedure.

It increases the comfort of the procedure.

It decreases the number of attempts and the subsequent trauma.

It decreases the number of accidental dural punctures.

It forecasts difficult epidurals (similar to difficult intubations).

It transforms difficult epidurals into easy epidurals.

It helps the clinician in choosing the best equipment for the spinal/ epidural.

References

[1] Broadbent CR, Maxwell WB, Ferrie R, et al. Ability of anaesthetists to identify a marked lumbar interspace. Anaesthesia 2000;55:1122–6.

[2] Furness G, Reilly MP, Kuchi S. An evaluation of ultrasound imaging for identification of lumbar intervertebral level. Anaesthesia 2002;57:277–83.

[3] MacArthur C, Lewis M, Knox EG. Accidental dural puncture in obstetric patients and long term symptoms. BMJ 1993;306:883–5.

[4] Grau T, Leipold RW, Conradi R, et al. Ultrasound imaging facilitated localization of the epidural space during combined spinal and epidural anesthesia. Reg Anesth Pain Med 2001;26:64–7.

[5] Grau T, Leipold RW, Horter J, et al. The lumbar epidural space in pregnancy: visualization by ultrasonography. Br J Anaesth 2001;86:798–804.

[6] Grau T, Leipold RW, Horter J, et al. Paramedian access to the epidural space: the optimum window for ultrasound imaging. J Clin Anesth 2001;13:213–7.

[7] Arzola C, Davies S, Rofaeel A, et al. Ultrasound using the transverse approach to the lumbar spine provides reliable landmarks for labor epidurals. Anesth Analg 2007;104:1188–92.

[8] Grau T, Leipold RW, Conradi R, et al. Efficacy of ultrasound imaging in obstetric epidural anesthesia. J Clin Anesth 2002;14:169–75.

[9] Grau T, Leipold RW, Conradi R, et al. Ultrasound control for presumed difficult epidural puncture. Acta Anaesthesiol Scand 2001;45:766–71.

[10] Grau T, Bartusseck E, Conradi R, et al. Ultrasound imaging improves learning curves in obsteric epidural anesthesia: a preliminary study. Can J Anaesth 2003;50:1047–50.

[11] Arzola C, Balki M, Carvalho JCA. The antero-posterior diameter of the lumbar dural sac does not predict sensory levels of spinal anesthesia for cesarean delivery. Can J Anaesth 2007;54:620–5.

[12] Grau T, Leipold RW, Fatehi S, et al. Real-time ultrasonic observation of combined spinal-epidural anaesthesia. Eur J Anaesthesiol 2004;21:25–31.

[13] Grau T, Leipold RW, Horter J, et al. Colour doppler imaging of the interspinous and epidural space. Eur J Anaesthesiol 2001;18:706–12.

ANESTHESIOLOGY
CLINICS

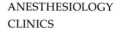

Anesthesiology Clin
26 (2008) 159–168

Can Medical Simulation and Team Training Reduce Errors in Labor and Delivery?

David J. Birnbach, MD, MPH[a],*, Eduardo Salas, PhD[b]

[a]*Univeristy of Miami-Jackson Memorial Hospital Center for Patient Safety,
Miller School of Medicine, University of Miami, 1611 North West 12th Avenue,
Miami, FL 33136, USA*
[b]*Department of Psychology, and Institute for Simulation and Training,
University of Central Florida, 4000 Central Florida, Orlando, FL 32816-0544, USA*

Open almost any magazine or newspaper and you will see a plethora of examples of what the public is learning about medical errors. Reports of medical mistakes causing patient suffering and death abound in the lay press. Patient safety is one of the most pressing challenges in health care today, and there is no question that medical errors occur and that patients are worried about them. How do we, as medical professionals, define "error"? The Institute of Medicine (IOM) has defined "medical error" as a "failure of a planned action to be completed as intended, or the use of a wrong plan to achieve an aim." Furthermore, communication problems are consistently identified as a leading cause of medical errors in obstetrics [1] and the Joint Commission on Accreditation of Healthcare Organizations (JCAHO) reports that lack of effective communication is the primary reason for sentinel events [2].

Traditional medical and nursing education has relied on the treatment of real patients in actual clinical settings. There is a belief now that the current availability of medical simulations and the knowledge gained from the science of team training may improve patient outcomes, and there is a paradigm shift occurring in many universities and training programs. Thus, most medical and nursing schools have purchased simulators and are attempting to use them in undergraduate and graduate education. The current popularity of medical simulation in the arena of patient safety is illustrated by the fact that a Google search for the phrases "patient safety"

---

* Corresponding author.
E-mail address: dbirnbach@med.miami.edu (D.J. Birnbach).

1932-2275/08/$ - see front matter © 2008 Elsevier Inc. All rights reserved.
doi:10.1016/j.anclin.2007.11.001   *anesthesiology.theclinics.com*

and "medical simulation" resulted in 1.8 million hits. This article discusses two strategies that, when combined, may reduce medical error in the labor and delivery suite: team training and medical simulation.

Teamwork, teams, and simulation-based training

Health care teams operate in an environment characterized by acute stress, heavy workload, and high stakes for decision and action errors [3]. The labor and delivery suite is no exception to this environment. In fact, the labor and delivery suite requires intense, error-free vigilance with effective communication and teamwork between many different clinical disciplines, including obstetricians, midwives, nurses, anesthesiologists, and pediatricians [4].

A recent American College of Obstetricians and Gynecologists Committee Opinion states that promoting safety requires that all those in the health care environment recognize that the potential for errors exists, and that teamwork and communication are the basis for fostering change and preventing errors. They further suggest that "a culture of safety should be the framework for any effort to reduce medical errors" [5]. Moreover, the JCAHO has recommended a risk-reduction strategy for decreasing perinatal death or injury. This strategy includes the implementation of team training and mock emergency drills for shoulder dystocia, emergency cesarean delivery, and maternal hemorrhage [6]. Similarly, the IOM has recommended that team training and implementation of team behaviors could improve patient safety [7,8]. Teamwork is a set of interrelated behaviors, cognitions and attitudes that bring about effective coordination, cooperation, and communication when these are conducted in a timely and adaptive fashion [3]. And team training promotes the acquisition of these adaptive behaviors, shared cognitions, and relevant attitudes. Team training is an instructional strategy that ideally combines practice-based delivery methods with realistic events guided by medical teamwork competencies (ie, the behaviors, cognitions, and attitudes).

Unfortunately, two of the fathers in the field of patient safety have suggested that the lack of progress following the release of the initial IOM report are a result of the "culture of medicine." They believe that this culture is deeply rooted, both by custom and training, in autonomous individual performance and a commitment to progress through research [9]. It is possible that the systemic and appropriate use of medical simulation, along with other important changes to the system, will facilitate the necessary cultural change and hence, improve patient safety. As Liang [10] has said, "a finger-pointing environment promotes fear and is counterproductive to promoting a collaborative, blame-free systems approach to reducing errors." It has recently been suggested that the concept of patient safety in obstetrics is "not as strong as desirable for the provision of reliable health care." The culture is one of a penalizing nature with suppressed error reporting, lack of proper communication, and feedback failure [11]. Obviously, this culture needs to change before health care practitioners can drastically improve patient safety in our country.

Patient safety is "predicated on trust, open communication, and effective interdisciplinary teamwork" [12]. But where do medical students, residents, attending physicians, nursing students, nurses, and midwives learn to work as teams?

Thomas and colleagues [13] conducted a qualitative assessment of teamwork and suggested that factors that influence working together could be divided into three categories: provider characteristics (personal attributes, reputation, expertise), workplace factors (staffing, work organization, work environment), and group influences (communication, relationships, and team). These categories can be addressed, at least in part, by working together in teams in a simulated environment and evaluating teamwork and human performance. Lyndon [14] has suggested that the application of human performance-based theory has demonstrated that "communication patterns, team function, workload, and coping mechanisms affect both individual and group ability to identify evolving problems and make appropriate management decisions in complex decision-making situations."

Why is teamwork training important for labor and delivery personnel? As noted, communication problems are consistently identified as a leading cause of medical error and can be well addressed during team training. The recent Confidential Enquiry in Maternal Deaths in the United Kingdom (2000-2002) has emphasized that "emergency drills for maternal resuscitation should be regularly practiced in clinical areas in all maternity units" [15]. As an example, a recent review of competence in managing cardiac arrest among obstetric trainees in the UK reported that there is a lack of knowledge about airway management and ventilation. These investigators suggest that to facilitate the retention of skills, regular short periods of practice on a manikin are essential [16]. Furthermore, we know from research that what works in simulation-based team training is when trainees have an opportunity to practice relevant competencies in a structured scenario and get diagnostic feedback on their individual and collective performance, clearly indicating the importance of guided practice (by scenario events) and measurement.

Simulation-based training in labor and delivery

What are "drills" and how do they work? According to Sorenson [17], "mock emergency training is an opportunity for staff to learn to identify risk factors and prepare for interventions in the event of an obstetric emergency." According to the Agency for Health Care Research and Quality, "drills that are carefully planned can decrease medical errors by addressing unintended events that may result in injury to a patient arising from unintentional actions, mistakes in judgment, or inadequate plans of action"

[18]. Simulation of labor and delivery events can range from high-fidelity human simulators (typically located off site) to low-tech simulations and drills that can often be done in the labor and delivery suite [17]. Labor and delivery events that are commonly addressed include maternal hemorrhage (antepartum as well as postpartum), failed intubation, failed neuraxial block, seizure, cardiac arrest, anaphylaxis, cord prolapse, and shoulder dystocia. In addition, Thomson and colleagues [19] reported that drills to practice management of eclampsia were successful at identifying deficiencies in team preparation.

Another area where simulation exercises may impact outcome is preparing individuals and teams in improved communication during transfer of patients care from one set of care-givers to another, termed "handovers." A recent survey from the UK found that handovers were rarely documented in writing and that 4% of units reported critical incidents following inadequate handovers in the past 12 months [20]. This interesting article describes the use of situation-background-assessment-recommendation (SBAR) and potential to practice sign-offs and handovers during practice drills.

These scenarios (guided by desired learning outcomes) can be designed so that they can be used to train nurses, obstetric residents, anesthesia residents, or midwives, either individually or, much more optimally, as teams. Team training is not only for those in training; attending physicians may also benefit from participation. Not only do these drills allow various team members to practice coming up with an appropriate plan during a crisis situation, but it also allows them to practice improved communication with their operating room team. They also provide an opportunity for the various team members, as well as administrators, to identify areas that need further preparation.

When an adverse perinatal outcome associated with an error occurs, it is likely that more than one individual will be involved and blamed [21]. Similarly, when an unexpected injury occurs to a mother or infant, there are usually several players involved and an issue with the "system" that allowed the error to occur. Obstetricians, anesthesiologists, pediatricians, labor nurses, midwives, and operating room staff all work together as part of a system and when an error occurs, it is usually associated with the system. Therefore, optimal simulation exercises involve all these key players and evaluate not only their behaviors and communication skills, but also problems within the system in which they work. Simulation allows the recreation of a labor and delivery room or operating room, where reality-based scenarios can be recreated allowing anesthesiologists, obstetricians, midwives, nurses, and pediatricians to practice their roles and communication skills.

Hunt and colleagues [22] have suggested that medical teams require practiced interaction and communication to be effective and efficient. According to these investigators, leadership, follower-ship, situational awareness, closed-loop communication, critical language and standardized responses, assertive communication, adaptive behaviors, workload management, and debriefing can be practiced to optimize the synergy of the team (Box 1).

Team training in obstetrics

While relatively new to obstetrics, drills have been successfully used in other areas of medicine, including anesthesia, intensive care, and emergency medicine, often using lessons learned from crew resource management (CRM) training. CRM began as a program to train pilots to "change what had been identified as human error in airplane crashes" [23]. CRM training has led to safety and performance improvements beyond those produced by improvements in equipment and technology [24,25].

Airlines use many tools to reduce human error; CRM training is just one. Others include the use of checklists, standardized maintenance, ability to report errors without disciplinary repercussions, and simulator training.

Box 1. Advantages of simulation for research, training, and performance assessment

- No risk to patients
- Many scenarios can be presented, including uncommon but critical situations in which a rapid response is needed
- Participants can see the results of their decisions and actions; errors can be allowed to occur and reach their conclusion (in real life a more capable clinician would have to intervene)
- Identical scenarios can be presented to different clinicians or teams
- The underlying causes of the situation are known
- With mannequin-based simulators, clinicians can use actual medical equipment, exposing limitations in the human-machine interface
- With full recreations of actual clinical environments, complete interpersonal interactions with other clinical staff can be explored and training on teamwork, leadership, and communication provided
- Intensive and intrusive recording of the simulation session is feasible, including audiotaping, videotaping, and even physiologic monitoring of participants; there are no issues of patient confidentiality; the recordings can be preserved for research, performance assessment, or accreditation

---

Data from Gaba DM. Anesthesiology as a model for patient safety in health care. BMJ 2000;320:785–8.

Not all of these, however, are easily adaptable to medicine. Helmreich [26] has identified several lessons learned from CRM that can be exported to medicine. He believes that errors in competence require technical training and that errors in decisions or communication require team training. Helmreich also suggests that the adaptation of CRM to medicine similarly requires the development of nonpunitive methods to collect information on errors that can be used to identify how teams perform. It has been suggested that elements of CRM that are useful in medical settings include briefings, conflict resolution procedures, and performance reviews [27]. There is evidence that operator attitudes about teamwork, hierarchy, errors, and stress affect performance among aviators working together in teams [28]. There is also evidence that there are problems with these attitudes in health care workers [29].

However, Salas and colleagues [30] have reported that CRM training will not be effective or achieve its desired outcomes in health care unless the following 12 prerequisites occur:

1. The physicians must be on board
2. The concept of teamwork becomes part of the "DNA" of the health care professional
3. CRM is supplemented by other teamwork-focused training strategies
4. The design, development, and delivery of CRM is scientifically rooted
5. CRM training is designed systematically
6. CRM is part of a learning organization's strategy to promote patient safety and quality care.
7. Teamwork is rewarded and reinforced by the health care provider
8. CRM training is evaluated at multiple levels of specific outcomes
9. CRM is supported by simulation or practice-based approaches
10. The health care provider is "ready" to receive training
11. The patient is part of the team
12. The team training is recurrent

As the health care system implements CRM training, these 12 issues must be addressed, resolved, and dealt with before benefits will be obtained.

While miscommunication is common in obstetrics, sometimes difficulties are caused not by problems with communication, but rather because of disruptive behavior on the part of a team member. In fact, it has been reported that disruptive and intimidating behavior occurs frequently in labor and delivery units. It has been estimated that 3% to 5% of physicians present a problem of disruptive behavior [31]. Although these behaviors are often demonstrated by physicians, they may also be manifested by other disciplines, such as nursing or administration, and must be considered when using simulation to improve team behaviors.

The disruptive behavior that occurs frequently in labor and delivery units has been defined to include angry outbursts, rudeness or verbal attacks, physical threats, intimidation, noncompliance with policies, and sexual harassment. It has contributed to the nursing shortage, near misses, and adverse occurrences, and was exhibited by a broad range of professionals. Disciplines demonstrating disruptive behavior included obstetricians, anesthesiologists, family practitioners, pediatricians, nurses, midwives, nurse anesthetists, and administrators. The behavior is not always effectively managed by the organization [32]. Disruptive behavior was actually reported in more than 60% of labor and delivery units that responded to the questionnaire. Bad behavior doesn't always involve physicians. It occurs between nurses as well, termed "horizontal hostility," and includes rudeness, verbal abuse, humiliating statements, unjustly critical statements, withholding information, and gossip [33].

Both high-tech and low-tech approaches to simulation have been used. Simulation centers often use high-fidelity simulation with interactive computerized manikins in a realistic environment. As described by Blackburn and Sadler [34], these simulations include a room set up as a normal working environment (eg, labor room or operating room) with a full complement of working equipment and staff. The manikin is quite realistic and has pulses, O_2 saturation, heart and breath sounds, ventilatory movements, and electrocardiogram tracing. All vital signs can be adjusted via computer control, as can the ability to intubate or ventilate. Not all simulation exercises and drills for obstetrics need to be performed in high-fidelity simulators and some investigators have advocated classroom training as superior [35]. Sorenson [17] has stated that simulation of labor and delivery events can range from high-fidelity human simulators (typically located off site) to low-tech simulations and drills that can often be done in the labor and delivery suite. The inability to arrange for staff of several disciplines to be off the labor and delivery floor simultaneously often precludes the use of high-tech simulation and may make on-site exercises advantageous.

As mentioned, some investigators believe that classroom training may be advantageous, and it has been suggested that high-fidelity simulation is too expensive [35,36]. Gaba [37], however, has countered that simulation need not be cost-prohibitive and that it provides the required "real-life" experience necessary for training of complex real-life scenarios. Morgan and colleagues [38] recently reported on an obstetric model that allowed for more realistic participation of real surgeons (rather than actors playing the role of surgeons) in a simulated scenario. This is the first published report of a high-fidelity simulation of obstetric team performance with anesthesiologists, nurses, and obstetricians involved in the hands-on management of obstetric crises.

There are several available options for teaching teamwork and crisis intervention in obstetrics. Multidisciplinary obstetric simulated emergency scenarios (MOSES) was first reported by the St. Bartholomew Hospital Group in 2002 [39]. Obstetricians, anesthesiologists, and midwives participated in team training on a high-fidelity simulator. MedTeams was developed by the United States Armed Forces and Dynamics Research

Corporation. Originally described in Emergency Departments [24,40,41], it has now been used for labor and delivery teams [4]. The course consists of "train the trainer" sessions that focus on seven different dimensions that are essential to teamwork. Behaviorally-anchored rating scales are used to assess various key behaviors [24]. A review of the program and challenges of implementation has recently been published [42]. Morey and colleagues [24] reported that the MedTeams Program reduced errors in the emergency room and observed a statistically significant improvement in behaviors. The clinical error rate in this study decreased in the MedTeams group from 31% to 4%. Other evidence-based programs have emerged recently, such as Team STEPPs [43], which has been developed by the Department of Defense and the Agency for Healthcare Research and Quality as a program to standardize team training, at least in the Department of Defense. The program is adaptable, medically relevant, is based on findings from the science of team performance, and is applicable to labor and delivery.

The most recent confidential enquiry into maternal deaths [15] has also recommended the managing obstetric emergencies and trauma course. This 3-day course, aimed at both anesthesiologists and obstetricians, includes lectures, skill stations, workshops, and simulations (www.alsg.org).

Summary

The authors believe that the data is very encouraging in support of the use of medical simulation and team training in labor and delivery. They improve teamwork and communication, as well as recognition of potential areas of weakness and, therefore, these are very viable strategies to mitigate medical errors. Despite an unproven track record for objective findings of improved patient safety, many investigators suggest that team training is useful in the health care arena and is "here to stay" [27,44,45].

Physicians and nurses who want to learn more about this field might consider attendance at the annual meeting of the Society for Simulation in Health Care, a society that was first established in 2004. This multidisciplinary society has grown exponentially and represents the rapidly growing group of educators and researchers who use a variety of simulation techniques for education, testing, and research in health care. According to the Society, the membership is now over 1,500 and united by its desire to improve performance and reduce errors in patient care, using all types of simulation including task trainers, human patient simulators, virtual reality, and standardized patients (http://www.ssih.org/public). Each year at their annual meeting there are numerous sessions relating to team training and patient safety in obstetrics.

Pearlman [46] stated it very eloquently when he wrote the following: "The effect of medical errors and unsafe systems of care has had a profound effect on the practice of obstetrics and gynecology. … We have the moral imperative as a specialty to fully engage in the identification of our own best practices, to advance safety research in obstetrics and gynecology, and to implement broadly those practices which are best." One of the steps that he proposed to initiate the required changes is to "incorporate patient safety education into all levels of training." The time is right, the technology is here, and the momentum has begun.

References

[1] Simpson KR, Knox GE. Adverse perinatal outcomes. Recognizing, understanding & preventing common accidents. AWHONN Lifelines 2003;7:224–35.

[2] Joint Commission. Root cause of sentinel events, all categories: 1995–2004. Available at: http://www.jointcommission.org. Accessed March 2006.

[3] Salas E, Rosen MA, King H. Managing teams managing crises: principles of teamwork to improve patient safety in the emergency room and beyond. Theoretical Issues in Ergonomics Science 2007;8:381–94.

[4] Nielsen PE, Goldman MB, Mann S, et al. Effects of teamwork training on adverse outcomes and process of care in labor and delivery: a randomized controlled trial. Obstet Gynecol 2007;109:48–55.

[5] ACOG. Committee opinion number 286. Int J Gynaecol Obstet 2004;86:121–3.

[6] Joint Commission on Accreditation of Healthcare Organizations. JCAHO sentinel event alert #30. 2004.

[7] Kohn LT, Corrigan JM, Donaldson MS, editors. To err is human: building a safer health system. Washington, DC: National Academy Press; 2000 [Institute of Medicine].

[8] Committee on Quality Health Care in America. Crossing the quality chasm: a new health system for the 21st century. Washington, DC: National Academy Press; 2001.

[9] Leape LL, Berwick DM. Five years after To Err Is Human: what have we learned? JAMA 2005;293:2384–90.

[10] Liang BA. The adverse event of unaddressed medical error: identifying and filling the holes in the health-care and legal systems. J Law Med Ethics 2001;29:346–68.

[11] Nabhan A, Ahmed-Tawfik MS. Understanding and attitudes towards patient safety concepts in obstetrics. Int J Gynaecol Obstet 2007;98:212–6.

[12] Simpson KR, James DC, Knox GE. Nurse-physician communication during labor and birth: implications for patient safety. J Obstet Gynecol Neonatal Nurs 2006;35:547–56.

[13] Thomas EJ, Sherwood GD, Mulhollem JL, et al. Working together in the neonatal intensive care unit: provider perspectives. J Perinatol 2004;24:552–9.

[14] Lyndon L. Communication and teamwork in patient care: how much can we learn from aviation? J Obstet Gynecol Neonatal Nurs 2006;35:538–46.

[15] RCOG. Why mothers die 2000–2002: the confidential enquiries into maternal deaths in the United Kingdom. London: RCOG Press; 2004. p. 96–101.

[16] Morris S, Stacey M. Resuscitation in pregnancy. BMJ 2003;327:1277–9.

[17] Sorensen SS. Emergency drills in obstetrics: reducing risk or perinatal death or permanent injury. JONAS Healthc Law Ethics Regul 2007;9:9–16.

[18] Agency for Healthcare Research and Quality. Guide to patient safety indicators. Available at: http://www.qualityindicators.ahrq.gov. Accessed Aug, 2007.

[19] Thompson S, Neal S, Clark V. Clinical risk management in obstetrics: eclampsia drills. BMJ 2004;328:269–71.

[20] Sabir N, Yentis SM, Holdcroft A. A national survey of obstetric anaesthetic handovers. Anaesthesia 2006;61:376–80.

[21] Furrow BR. Medical mistakes: tiptoeing toward safety. Houst J Health Law Policy 2003;3: 181–217.

[22] Hunt EA, Shilkofski NA, Stavroudis TA, et al. Simulation: translation to improved team performance. Anesthesiol Clin 2007;25:301–19.

[23] Helmreich RL, Merritt AC, Wilhelm JA. Evaluation of crew resource management training in commercial aviation. Int J Aviat Psychol 1999;9:19–32.

[24] Morey JC, Simon R, Jay GD, et al. Error reduction and performance improvement in the emergency department through formal teamwork training: evaluation results of the MedTeams project. Health Serv Res 2002;37:1553–81.

[25] Salas E, Wilson KA, Burke CS, et al. Using simulation-based training to improve patient safety: what does it take? Jt Comm J Qual Patient Saf 2005;31:363–71.

[26] Helmreich RL. On error management: lessons from aviation. BMJ 2000;320:781–5.

[27] Sundar E, Sundar S, Pawlowski J, et al. Crew resource management and team training. Anesthesiol Clin 2007;25:283–300.

[28] Bowers CA, Jentsch F, Salas E, et al. Analyzing communication sequences for team training needs assessment. Hum Factors 1998;40:672–80.

[29] Gaba DM, Singer SJ, Sinaiko AD, et al. Differences in safety climate between hospital personnel and naval aviators. Hum Factors 2003;45:173–85.

[30] Salas E, Wilson KA, Murphy CE, et al. What crew resource management training will not do for patient safety: unless.... Jt Comm J Qual Patient Saf 2007;3:62–4.

[31] Leape LL, Fromson JA. Problem doctors: is there a system-level solution? Ann Intern Med 2006;144:107–15.

[32] Veltman LL. Disruptive behavior in obstetrics: a hidden threat to patient safety. Am J Obstet Gynecol 2007;196:e1–4.

[33] Thomas SP. Horizontal hostility. Am J Nurs 2003;103:87–91.

[34] Blackburn T, Sadler C. The role of human patient simulators in health-care training. Hosp Med 2003;64:677–81.

[35] Pratt SD, Sachs BP. Team training: classroom training vs. high fidelity simulation. Point Counterpoint. AHRQ Web M&M. Available at: http://www.webmm.ahrq.gov/perspective. aspx?perspectiveID=21. Accessed March, 2006.

[36] Kurrek MM, Devitt JH. The cost for construction and operation of a simulation centre. Can J Anaesth 1997;44:1191–5.

[37] Gaba DM. Two examples of how to evaluate the impact of new approaches to teaching. Anesthesiology 2002;96:1–2.

[38] Morgan PJ, Pittini R, Regehr G, et al. Evaluating teamwork in a simulated obstetric environment. Anesthesiology 2007;106:907–15.

[39] Davis C, Gregg A, Thornley D. Initial feedback on MOSES (multidisciplinary obstetric simulated emergency scenarios): a course on team training, human behaviour and "fire drills". Anesthesiology 2002;96(Suppl 1):11.

[40] Simon R, Salisbury M, Wagner G. MedTeams: teamwork advances emergency department effectiveness and reduces medical errors. Ambul Outreach 2000:21–4.

[41] Risser DT, Rice MM, Salisbury ML, et al. The potential for improved teamwork to reduce medical errors in the emergency department. The MedTeams Research Consortium. Ann Emerg Med 1999;34:373–83.

[42] Harris KT, Treanor CM, Salisbury ML. Improving patient safety with team coordination: challenges and strategies of implementation. J Obstet Gynecol Neonatal Nurs 2006;35: 557–66.

[43] Alonso A, Baker DP, Holtzman A, et al. Reducing medical error in the Military Health system. How can team training help? Human Resource Management Review 2006;16: 396–415.

[44] Baker DP, Day R, Salas E. Teamwork as an essential component of high reliability organizations. Health Serv Res 2006;41:1576–98.

[45] Grogan EL, Stiles RA, France DJ, et al. The impact of aviation-based teamwork training on the attitudes of health-care professionals. J Am Coll Surg 2004;199:843–8.

[46] Pearlman MD. Patient safety in obstetrics and gynecology: an agenda for the future. Obstet Gynecol 2006;108:1266–71.

ELSEVIER
SAUNDERS

Anesthesiology Clin
26 (2008) 169–182

ANESTHESIOLOGY
CLINICS

The Use of Remifentanil in Obstetrics

David Hill, MD, FCARCSI, Dip Pain Med RCSI

Department of Anaesthesia, Ulster Hospital, Belfast, BT16 1RH, UK

Obstetric anesthesia has always had an uneasy relationship with systemic opioids. Sedation, nausea, delayed gastric emptying, and respiratory and neonatal depression combined with doubtful efficacy as a labor analgesic have limited their use [1,2]. Furthermore, the decline in the use of general anesthesia in obstetrics has made systemic opioids almost redundant. However, the introduction of remifentanil in the early 1990s heralded a growing interest among obstetric anesthesiologists. Because of its rapid onset and offset, remifentanil offers potential not only as a labor analgesic, but also as an adjunct to general anesthesia, particularly in high-risk women [3].

Fundamental to its use in obstetrics were data published as abstracts in 1996 and as papers in 1998 and 2001. The first study reported placental transfer of an intravenous remifentanil infusion during cesarean section under epidural anesthesia. Remifentanil readily crossed the placenta with an umbilical vein/maternal artery ratio of 0.82 and, if administered close to the delivery of the neonate, the umbilical artery/vein ratio was 0.29, suggesting rapid metabolism and redistribution in the neonate [4]. The second study reported the pharmacokinetics of remifentanil when used for postoperative pain relief in neonates. The pharmacokinetics were found to be similar to those for older children and adults [5].

Suitability of remifentanil as a labor analgesic

An effective alternative to regional analgesia for labor is needed. A growing number of women either do not want or cannot have an epidural for labor. An ideal intravenous opiate should have an onset and offset that can match the time course of uterine contractions, while preserving uterine contractility and a reassuring cardiotocograph (CTG). The analgesia experienced should be considered worthwhile. There should be little effect on maternal respiration. There should be minimal neonatal effects so that

---

E-mail address: davidhill@doctors.org.uk

1932-2275/08/$ - see front matter © 2008 Elsevier Inc. All rights reserved.
doi:10.1016/j.anclin.2007.11.004
anesthesiology.theclinics.com

administration can be continued up to and during delivery. Gastric emptying should not be delayed should (or in case general anesthesia is required.

Of the parental opiates used, meperidine (pethidine) fails on almost all
counts, despite being available as an option in 95% of United Kingdom
units [6]. Fentanyl has been reported to provide worthwhile analgesia with
peak effect at 3 to 4 minutes [7], but can cause measurable neonatal effects
with one study reporting naloxone administration to 37% of neonates at
birth with neurobehavioral effects lasting up to 7 days postdelivery [8].
Due to its low volume of distribution, alfentanil has a rapid onset of 1 minute. However, it provides inferior analgesia compared to that provided by
fentanyl and results in lower neurobehavioral scores than those parturient
who received meperidine [9].

Remifentanil exhibits rapid onset of effect of around 1 minute, rapid metabolism by tissue, and plasma esterase to inactive metabolites with a context
sensitive half-life of 3 minutes [3]. Consequently, there is no accumulation,
even after prolonged administration. These properties predict that intravenous remifentanil could be suitable for the cyclical pain of uterine contractions.

Computerized simulations of the effect site concentrations have predicted
that the half time for blood effect site equilibration was 1.3 to 1.6 minutes
[10]. Another study recording effects on ventilation in volunteers following
a 0.5-µg/kg bolus over 5 seconds reported onset of effect at 30 seconds and
peak effect at 2.5 minutes [11]. This suggests that it would be difficult, if not
impossible, to coincide peak effect with each uterine contraction. It is more
likely that peak effect would coincide with the second or subsequent
contraction.

This may explain why the first published attempt to use remifentanil for
labor analgesia fell short of expectations [12]. Its use in four women was reported. However, the bolus doses of remifentanil were manually administered by a third party, inevitably leading to delay in dosing. The
investigators concluded that remifentanil was ineffective. It is likely that
the peak effect occurred in the period between contractions.

Nevertheless, subsequent case reports [13–15] and studies [16–22] employing patient-controlled intravenous analgesia (PCIA) devices were more successful. Several investigators commented that timing of dosing was critical
[23]. They reported that "with tutoring, the patient can learn to anticipate
the next contraction and to make an early effective demand" [24].

Efficacy of analgesia

Doubts have been raised concerning the effectiveness of intravenous remifentanil for labor pain [25]. Initial case reports involved women who
could not have an epidural for one reason or another. These women, it
could be said, were willing to accept less than ideal analgesia.

To date, four observational studies have investigated remifentanil PCIA
for labor analgesia. Two have been dose-finding studies [16,17], one an

observational study employing a fixed PCIA dose [21], and one comparing two regimes of background infusion plus PCIA [26].

All four studies reported analgesia with remifentanil. In the feasibility study of Blair and colleagues [16], the median reduction in pain score was 30 mm compared with baseline with a bolus dose range of 0.25 to 0.5 µg/kg. The dose-finding study of Volmanen and colleagues [17] reported a median reduction in pain scores of 42 mm with a median dose of 0.4 µg/kg. The observational study of Volikas and colleagues [21] administered a fixed dose of 0.5 µg/kg and reported a mean reduction in pain scores from baseline of 26 mm. The remaining study compared a fixed background infusion dose and an escalating PCIA bolus dose with a fixed bolus dose and an escalating background infusion dose and reported a mean reduction in pain scores from baseline of 30 mm [26].

Three studies have evaluated PCIA remifentanil with meperidine. Only one compared with PCIA meperidine [19]. The others employed intramuscular [18] and an intravenous infusion of meperidine. The most relevant study where both drugs were administered by PCIA reported similar mean pain scores with both drugs.

It appears that the analgesia provided by intravenous PCIA remifentanil is not complete but achieves a reduction in pain scores of around 30 mm during the first stage of labor. Where pain scores were reported for the second stage of labor, they remained high at around 80 mm [16]. Nevertheless a common theme among all these studies was high maternal satisfaction, implying that this modest analgesia is worthwhile. Analgesia is only one component of a satisfactory birth experience and complete analgesia has not been reported as figuring high in the birthing process for the majority of women. In a review [27] of 137 reports involving the views of 14,000 women from nine countries, the important factors were:

- Personal expectations
- Support and coping skills
- Quality of the caregiver–parturient relationship
- Involvement in decisions

Several studies also report that dissatisfaction with analgesic care is more related to nonavailability and failed timing of pain relief [28,29]. This is where PCIA remifentanil has an advantage. It is easily set up, as the main skill required is intravenous cannula placement. It does not require the skills of an attending physician and, if managed by a trained nurse or midwife, it can become part of the caregiver support.

Optimal dosing regime

There is no consensus on the optimal dosing regime for remifentanil (Table 1). Each study has used its own dosing schedule with a bolus dose

Table 1
PCIA remifentanil analgesia and dosing details for labor analgesia

	Bolus dose	Lockout time	With Entonox?	Median or reduction in pain scores	Conversion to regional analgesia
Blair et al [16]	0.25–0.5 µg/kg/min	2 min	No	Median of 50 mm	2 of 21
Thurlow et al [18]	0.20 µg/kg/min	2 min	Yes	Median of 48 mm	7 of 18
Volmanen et al [20]	0.4 µg/kg/min	1 min		Reduction of 15 mm	Not reported
Blair et al [19]	40 µg	2 min	Yes	Median of 64 mm	2 of 20
Volmanen et al [17]	0.2–0.8 µg/kg/min	1 min	No	Reduction of 42 mm	Not reported
Evron et al [22]	0.27–0.93 µg/kg/min	3 min	No	Median of 35 mm	8 of 88
Volikas et al [21]	0.5 µg/kg/min	2 min	No	Median of 46 mm	5 of 50
Balki et al [26]	0.25 µg/kg/min plus intravenous infusion	2 min	No	Not reported	1 of 20

range of 0.2 to 0.93 µg/kg. The most popular dose is 0.5 µg/kg. Some investigators have commented on the wide individual variation of bolus dose required [17] to achieve effective analgesia. This would suggest a fixed-dose regime could underdose and lead to failure or could overdose and lead to maternal oxygen desaturation. Variable dosing regimes may improve matters, particularly during the second stage when reported pain scores are high. However, this would require physician attendance to ensure appropriate monitoring.

Reported lockout times have also varied, some described lockout times of 2 minutes while others describe a bolus dose delivered over 1 minute with a 1-minute lockout time. With an average uterine contraction time of 70 seconds [30], it would seem prudent to allow a dose every 2 minutes.

In the dose-finding study of Blair and colleagues [16], who recommend a PCIA bolus dose of 0.25 to 0.5µg/kg, the introduction of a background infusion of remifentanil did not improve analgesia, but caused excessive maternal sedation and oxygen desaturation. In contrast, a Canadian study has recommended a PCIA bolus of 0.25 µg/kg with a background infusion of 0.025 to 0.1 µg/kg/min [26]. The investigators claimed a conversion rate to regional analgesia of 5% compared with the 10% rate of other studies without a background infusion. More work needs done to define the optimal dosing regime before a background infusion can be recommended.

Maternal effects

Of major concern is the potential for maternal respiratory depression and oxygen desaturation. All studies report episodes of maternal oxygen desaturation but comment that they were transient and easily corrected with nasal oxygen or reduction in dose. When we look at the detail, Blair and colleagues [16] reported 4 out of 21 women with saturation of oxyhemoglobin below 90% for 15 seconds and the lowest respiratory rate was 8 breaths per minute. Balki and colleagues [26] reported a range of oxygen saturations, the lowest being 85%. Volmanen and colleagues [17] reported 10 out of 17 women with oxygen saturations below 94%.

The comparative studies help as Blair and colleagues [19] found that PCIA meperidine caused incidence of maternal oxygen desaturation similar to that for PCIA remifentanil. This helps to put maternal oxygen desaturation in context, as the findings are comparable to a study that included women with no analgesia where episodes of oxygen desaturation in labor occurred in 46% of women for between 30 seconds to 6 minutes per hour in the second stage of labor [31]. Nevertheless we cannot be complacent and, on balance, women receiving PCIA remifentanil should have one-to-one nursing care, availability of oxygen saturation monitoring, and oxygen supplementation.

Sedation was variously reported, but not excessive. Balki and colleagues [26] reported one excessively sedated women who also desaturated. It is for these rare but unexpected women that appropriate supervision and monitoring is needed.

Nausea and vomiting is endemic in childbirth and it is difficult to distinguish a true opioid effect. The highest incidence reported was 48% [16].

Fetal and neonatal effects

No studies identified an excess of non-reassuring CTG traces. The comparative study of PCIA remifentanil with PCIA meperidine found fewer non-reassuring CTGs and better neurobehavioral scores in the remifentanil group [19]. Volikas and colleagues [21] monitored CTG traces in all women. Fifteen traces out of 50 were reported as non-reassuring at some point. However, there was no association between commencement of PCIA and deterioration in the CTG requiring intervention or fetal blood gas sampling.

Apgar scores and cord blood gases, where reported, did not show any unexpected deviations from normal practice. No neonates required naloxone at birth, a result that seems to confirm remifentanil's rapid metabolism and redistribution in the neonate following placental transfer.

Concomitant use of Entonox

Opioid analgesia in labor, originally introduced as an alternative to inhalational analgesia, never came into common use because of the shortcomings of systemic opioids. As a result, Entonox (Linde, Munich, Germany), which is a 50:50 mixture of oxygen and nitrous oxide, and opioid analgesia together, became the norm when regional analgesia was not used. If remifentanil could provide worthwhile analgesia without the need for Entonox, this would be a considerable advantage. Entonox is not without problems, causing maternal hypoventilation between contractions [31] and health issues for staff who are chronically exposed to nitrous oxide [32].

There is evidence that remifentanil can provide superior analgesia to Entonox alone [20]. Remifentanil was compared with intermittently inhaled Entonox in a small crossover study of 15 women. The investigators reported a median reduction in pain scores of 1.5 mm with a 0.4-μg/kg bolus of remifentanil delivered over 1 minute with a lockout of 1 minute. The median reduction in pain scores was 0.5 mm with inhaled Entonox. Fourteen out of 15 women preferred remifentanil. No maternal oxygen desaturation was reported in either group.

In two studies from the United Kingdom comparing PCIA remifentanil with meperidine, women were allowed access to Entonox if desired. Thurlow and colleagues reported equal use of Entonox in both groups but did not specify the number of women using it [18]. Blair and colleagues reported that 19 of 19 women in the meperidine group and 18 of 20 in the remifentanil group used Entonox [19]. It appears that, if given the choice, women would opt for Entonox despite using remifentanil.

Supervision and monitoring

A recent audit of remifentanil PCIA use in 104 mothers reported overse-dation in 14% and oxygen desaturation below 90% in 6% [33]. This high-lights the need for appropriate monitoring, supervision, and training for the caregiver to manage likely adverse events. In this audit, maternal oxygen saturation was monitored for the first 30 minutes of use. If the parturient did not exhibit oxygen desaturation within this time, continuous oxygen satura-tion monitoring was discontinued.

Practical experience

In the author's institution, remifentanil PCIA is offered for routine use as a labor analgesic. The dosing regime is a fixed bolus of 40 µg delivered over 20 seconds with a 2-minute lockout. Supervision is by trained midwives who give one-to-one care. After initiation of analgesia, maternal oxygen satura-tion is measured continuously for 30 minutes. During this time, approxi-mately 10% of women exhibit oxygen desaturation and receive nasal oxygen supplementation. Hourly respiratory rate and oxygen saturation are measured during remainder of use. Other aspects of antepartum care are normal, with intermittent monitoring of CTG unless otherwise indicated.

Remifentanil analgesia for anesthesia interventions

Remifentanil has been reported to facilitate initiation of spinal anesthesia in a morbidly obese, needle-phobic parturient [34] and to facilitate epidural catheter placement in a parturient unable to keep still because of painful contractions [35].

In the former report, remifentanil was infused at 0.05 to 0.1 µg/kg/min and in the latter report it was infused at 0.1 to 0.25 µg/kg/min. In both cases, verbal contact was maintained and the intended procedure was performed with patient cooperation.

Remifentanil can offer sedation and analgesia for the anxious patient without the risk of persistent opioid effects. Its rapid offset was advanta-geous in the report of epidural placement when a second catheter had to be inserted after the first was placed intravenously. Remifentanil did not hinder or confuse the detection of an intravenous test dose.

Remifentanil supplementation of epidural anesthesia

Systemic opioids are the mainstay of managing discomfort during epidural anesthesia for cesarean section, yet there are few published reports of remifen-tanil for this purpose. While Kan and colleagues [4] infused 0.1 µg/kg/min to 19 women undergoing epidural anesthesia, the purpose of the study was to investigate placental transfer and neonatal effects. In this study, anesthesia was provided by 2% lidocaine with epinephrine (1:200,000). Episodes of discomfort were not reported, but 1 woman had a rescue bolus of remifentanil. The remifentanil infusion rates were decreased in 3 women before delivery because of hypotension. The infusion rates were decreased in 5 more women after delivery of the infant because of dizziness in 1 woman and excessive sedation in 4 women.

One study has investigated intravenous remifentanil as an adjunct to epidural anesthesia for cesarean section [36]. The investigators compared epidural bupivacaine 0.5% supplemented with either epidural fentanyl or intravenous remifentanil. The investigators found intravenous remifentanil as effective as epidural fentanyl.

Considering the adverse neonatal effects of alfentanil [9] and fentanyl [8], remifentanil seems a preferable choice for maternal discomfort during epidural anesthesia. The expected dose would be below 0.1 μg/kg/min with a low potential for neonatal effects. Further studies are needed.

General anesthesia with remifentanil for cesarean section

Although the use of general anesthesia is in decline in obstetric patients, there will always be a need in high-risk women where regional anesthesia is not appropriate. Opioids are generally withheld in obstetric general anesthesia until after the delivery of the neonate to avoid the potential for respiratory depression. However, the risk/benefit ratio can favor opioids in circumstances where maternal hemodynamic stability and blunting of responses to airway manipulation and surgical stimulation are deemed important.

Remifentanil could offer these benefits even in healthy obstetric patients without the disadvantage of neonatal depression associated with fentanyl [8] and alfentanil [37]. Furthermore, remifentanil has the potential to prevent maternal awareness and a low potential for uterine relaxation [38].

Remifentanil has been reported as an adjunct to general anesthesia in patients with coagulation factor and platelet deficits [39]; severe cardiac disease [40]; aortic disease [41]; intracranial disease [42]; hemolysis, elevated liver enzymes, and low platelets (HELLP) syndrome [43]; pre-eclampsia [44]; and succinylcholine apnea [45]. Remifentanil has also been combined with target controlled infusions of propofol for elective cesarean section [46].

Hemodynamic stability appears to be consistently achieved and, although various dose regimes have been reported, the incidence of hypotension appears reasonably low. Blunting of airway responses is also consistently reported. Ngan Kee and colleagues [47] compared a 1-μg/kg bolus of remifentanil with a saline injection at induction of general anesthesia for elective cesarean section. The remifentanil group had an improved hemodynamic response to laryngoscopy and intubation, confirming the findings of

previous uncontrolled case reports [39–45] and the findings of a study of remifentanil for rapid sequence induction in nonobstetric patients [48].

However, the neonatal effects do not appear to be as innocent as first predicted. Van de Velde and colleagues [46] reported a 50% incidence of respiratory depression at birth requiring intervention by a neonatologist,
although the incidences were brief and self-limiting. In this study, anesthesia
was maintained with target controlled infusions of propofol and remifentanil at an infusion dose of 0.2 µg/kg/min. The investigators concluded that
a physician experienced in newborn resuscitation should be present when using their technique. In six reports (Table 2), Apgar scores at 1 minute were
low and mask ventilation of the infant was required [40,47,50,52,53]. Two of
these infants required endotracheal intubation [44,52] and three were admitted to a neonatal intensive care unit [40,44,52]. In one report, Apgar scores
were not low at birth, but the infant received naloxone [51]. Neonatal chest-
wall rigidity was reported at birth in an infant whose mother had received
remifentanil at an infusion dose titrated between 0.1 and 1.5 µg/kg/min
[39]. This is the highest reported dose of remifentanil employed in an obstetric patient and highlights that opioid effects should be expected in neonates
of mothers exposed to high-dose remifentanil.

In general, it appears that the higher the maternal dose of remifentanil, the
more neonatal effects observed. Kan and colleagues [4] infused intravenous
remifentanil at a dose of 0.1 µg/kg/min to awake patients during epidural anesthesia for cesarean section. No adverse neonatal effects were reported. We
therefore can infer that doses above this, combined with general anesthesia,
make the need for neonatal resuscitation likely. However, mask ventilation
was usually brief before spontaneous respiration commenced.

It seems prudent to anticipate the need for neonatal resuscitation at delivery when remifentanil is used in high-risk women at high doses. If contemplating the use of remifentanil in healthy women, it would seem reasonable
to either avoid remifentanil until after delivery of the infant or restrict the
infusion dose to at or below 0.1 µg/kg/min until delivery of the infant. Richa
and colleagues [43] interrupted the remifentanil infusion immediately after
hysterotomy until delivery of the infant and reported no adverse neonatal
effects. Even after a single bolus dose, Ngan Kee and colleagues [47] found
that 7 out of 20 infants required mask ventilation and 2 received naloxone,
compared with 4 infants in the control group requiring mask ventilation and
none requiring naloxone. A physician experienced in neonatal resuscitation
should be available when remifentanil is used as an adjunct to general anesthesia in obstetric patients, even if the effects are short-lived.

Remifentanil for sedation in critically ill obstetric patients

Remifentanil has been advocated for sedation of the obstetric patient
where there is potential for emergency delivery of the fetus. In a case report

Table 2
Hemodynamic and neonatal effects and reported dose ranges for remifentanil during obstetric general anesthesia

	Remifentanil bolus at induction (μg/kg)	Maintenance remifentanil infusion dose range (μg/kg/min)	Response to laryngoscopy and intubation blunted?	Significant hypotension?	Neonatal effects
Carvalho et al [39]	2.5	0.1–1.5	Yes	No	M, C
McCarroll et al [49]	2.5 (over 5 min)	0.8	Yes	No	None
Alexander [50]	1.0	0.5	Yes	Yes for 3 of 6 patients	A, M (3 neonates)
Imarengiaye et al [51]	1.0	0.5–1.0	Yes	No	M, N
Johannsen and Munro [44]	1.17 (over 4 min)	0.37	Yes	No	A, M, E, I
Bedard et al [42]	2.0 (over 2 min)	0.2–1.0	Yes	Yes for 1 patient	I
Richa et al [43]	1.0	0.4–0.1	Yes	No	None
Wadsworth et al [52]	2.5	0.25	Yes	Yes for 1 of 2 patients	A, M, E, I (2 neonates)
Alexander and Fardell [45]	0.5	0.25	Yes	No	None
Brown and McAtamney [53]	2.5 (over 5 min)	0.25	Yes	No	M
Van de Velde et al [46]	0.5	0.2	Yes	Yes for 2 of 10 patients	A, M (6 of 13 neonates)
Johnston et al [54]	1.0	0.17	Yes	No	None
Orme et al [41]	2–4	0.05–0.15	Yes	Yes for 1 of 4 patients	None
Macfarlane et al [40]	1.5 (over 3 min)	0.05–0.15	Yes	No	A, M, I
Manullang et al [55]	1.0	0.05–0.1	Yes	No	None
Scott et al [56]	2.0	0.15–0.075	Yes	No	None
Ngan Kee et al [47]	1.0	None	Yes	No	A, M, N (2 neonates)

Abbreviations: A, low Apgar score; C, chest-wall rigidity; E, endotracheal intubation; I, admission to neonatal intensive care unit; M, mask ventilation; N, naloxone.

of varicella pneumonitis requiring respiratory support, remifentanil was employed for sedation [57]. The woman at 32 weeks' gestation had a high risk of delivery by emergency cesarean section and her sedation protocol was changed from morphine/midazolam/fentanyl/propofol to remifentanil and propofol. Continuous CTG recording did not detect a non-reassuring trace during the period of remifentanil-propofol sedation. The outcome was good, improvement led to extubation, and the pregnancy went to term.

It has been reported that between 0.1% and 0.9% of obstetric patients require critical care [58]. Mechanical ventilation and sedation was required in 40%. However, the minority 8% were antenatal [59]. It is in this group of women that the use of remifentanil may be justified in the sedation protocol.

Off-label use

Remifentanil is not licensed for use in obstetric patients. The administration of drugs outside their product license is common in obstetric anesthesia. Opioids by the spinal and epidural route, as well as all self-prepared mixtures of drugs, are not licensed. Propofol and doses above 250 mg of pentothal are not licensed either. Most of us are content to use drugs outside the product license. Almost all of the 169 members of the Obstetric Anaesthetists Association surveyed in 1997 [60] admitted to using drugs outside the product license in obstetric anesthesia. It is unlikely that the manufacturers of remifentanil would invest in the cost of obtaining a license for obstetric use. The onus remains on each clinician to assess the risk/benefit ratio. Currently, remifentanil is more suited than any other systemic opioid to obstetric anesthesia. Time will tell whether its use will become routine. In the meantime, we should continue to appraise and study its unique properties, bearing in mind that it is an opioid with all the attendant problems that opioids can bring.

Summary

Remifentanil is currently the most suitable systemic opioid for obstetric use. While it has a rapid onset and offset, the timing of onset and offset cannot be matched to that of a single uterine contraction. Nevertheless, remifentanil has been shown to provide effective analgesia, especially during the first stage of labor. An appropriate PCIA dose regime is a 40-μg bolus with a 2-minute lockout. Systems should be in place to ensure one-to-one monitoring with trained caregivers. Maternal desaturation occurs in approximately 10% of women. PCIA remifentanil is a viable alternative for those who do not want or are unable to have regional analgesia. It is only with experience in this group of women that it could be rolled out for routine use.

In high-risk obstetric patients requiring general anesthesia, remifentanil is successful in providing hemodynamic stability at intubation and during surgery. High doses of remifentanil with general anesthesia have unpredictable neonatal effects, making attendance by a physician trained in neonatal resuscitation mandatory. Remifentanil at induction alone or restricted to an infusion dose less than 0.1 μg/kg/min before delivery, is likely to cause neonatal respiratory depression at birth.

Remifentanil has a place in obstetric anesthesia and analgesia. With experience and training, this must be a safe place.

> Nothing is intrinsically good or evil, but its manner of usage may make it so.
> St Thomas Aquinas, *Disputed Questions on Evil*, 1272

References

[1] Olofsson C, Ekblom A, Ekman-Ordeberg G, et al. Lack of analgesic effect of systemically administered morphine or pethidine on labour pain. Br J Obstet Gynaecol 1996;103(10): 968–72. PMID: 8863693.

[2] Elbourne T, Wiseman RA. WITHDRAWN: types of intra-muscular opioids for maternal pain relief in labour. Cochrane Database Syst Rev 2007;(3):CD001237. PMID: 17636658.

[3] Egan TD. Pharmacokinetics and pharmacodynamics of remifentanil: an update in the year 2000. Curr Opin Anaesthesiol 2000;13(4):449–55. PMID: 17016340.

[4] Kan RE, Hughes SC, Rosen MA, et al. Intravenous remifentanil: placental transfer, maternal and neonatal effects. Anesthesiology 1998;88(6):1467–74. PMID: 9637638.

[5] Ross AK, Davis PJ, Dear GL, et al. Pharmacokinetics of remifentanil in anesthetized pediatric patients undergoing elective surgery or diagnostic procedures. Anesth Analg 2001; 93(6):1393–401. PMID: 11726413.

[6] Saravanakumar K, Garstang JS, Hasan K. Intravenous patient-controlled analgesia for labour: a survey of UK practice. Int J Obstet Anesth 2007;16(3):221–5. Epub 2007 Apr 24. PMID: 17459691.

[7] Shafer SL, Varvel JR. Pharmacokinetic, pharmacodynamics and rational opioid selection. Anaesthesiology 1991;74:53–63.

[8] Morley-Forster PK, Weberpals J. Neonatal effects of patient-controlled analgesia using fentanyl in labor. Int J Obstet Anesth 1998;7(2):103–7. PMID: 15321226.

[9] Morley-Forster PK, Reid DW, Vandeberghe H. A comparison of patient-controlled analgesia fentanyl and alfentanil for labour analgesia. Can J Anaesth 2000;47(2):113–9. PMID: 10674503.

[10] Egan TD, Minto CF, Hermann DJ, et al. Remifentanil versus alfentanil: comparative pharmacokinetics and pharmacodynamics in healthy adult male volunteers. Anesthesiology 1996;84(4):821–33 [Erratum in: Anesthesiology 1996 Sep;85(3):695]. PMID: 8638836.

[11] Babenco HD, Conard PF, Gross JB. The pharmacodynamic effect of a remifentanil bolus on ventilatory control. Anesthesiology 2000;92(2):393–8. PMID: 10691225.

[12] Olufolabi AJ, Booth JV, Wakeling HG, et al. A preliminary investigation of remifentanil as a labor analgesic. Anesth Analg 2000;91(3):606–8. PMID: 10960385.

[13] Thurlow JA, Waterhouse P. Patient-controlled analgesia in labour using remifentanil in two parturients with platelet abnormalities. Br J Anaesth 2000;84(3):411–3. PMID: 10793609.

[14] Jones R, Pegrum A, Stacey RG. Patient-controlled analgesia using remifentanil in the parturient with thrombocytopaenia. Anaesthesia 1999;54(5):461–5. PMID: 10995144.

[15] Owen MD, Poss MJ, Dean LS, et al. Prolonged intravenous remifentanil infusion for labor analgesia. Anesth Analg 2002;94(4):918–9 [table of contents]. PMID: 11916797.

[16] Blair JM, Hill DA, Fee JP. Patient-controlled analgesia for labour using remifentanil: a feasibility study. Br J Anaesth 2001;87(3):415–20. PMID: 11517125.

[17] Volmanen P, Akural EI, Raudaskoski T, et al. Remifentanil in obstetric analgesia: a dose-finding study. Anesth Analg 2002;94(4):913–7. PMID: 11916796.

[18] Thurlow JA, Laxton CH, Dick A, et al. Remifentanil by patient-controlled analgesia compared with intramuscular meperidine for pain relief in labour. Br J Anaesth 2002;88(3): 374–8. PMID: 11990269.

[19] Blair JM, Dobson GT, Hill DA, et al. Patient controlled analgesia for labour: a comparison of remifentanil with pethidine. Anaesthesia 2005;60(1):22–7. PMID: 15601268.

[20] Volmanen P, Akural E, Raudaskoski T, et al. Comparison of remifentanil and nitrous oxide in labour analgesia. Acta Anaesthesiol Scand 2005;49(4):453–8. PMID: 15777291.

[21] Volikas I, Butwick A, Wilkinson C, et al. Maternal and neonatal side-effects of remifentanil patient-controlled analgesia in labour. Br J Anaesth 2005;95(4):504–9. PMID: 16113038.

[22] Evron S, Glezerman M, Sadan O, et al. Remifentanil: a novel systemic analgesic for labor pain. Anesth Analg 2005;100(1):233–8. PMID: 15616083.

[23] Volmanen P, Alahuhta S. Will remifentanil be a labour analgesic? Int J Obstet Anesth 2004; 13(1):1–4. PMID: 15321431.

[24] Dhileepan S, Stacey RG. A preliminary investigation of remifentanil as a labor analgesic. Anesth Analg 2001;92(5):1358–9. PMID: 11323383.

[25] Lacassie HJ, Olufolabi AJ. Remifentanil for labor pain: Is the drug or the method the problem? Anesth Analg 2005;101(4):1242–3 [author reply 1243]. PMID: 16192558.

[26] Balki M, Kasodekar S, Dhumne S, et al. Remifentanil patient-controlled analgesia for labour: optimizing drug delivery regimens. Can J Anaesth 2007;54(8):626–33. PMID: 17666715.

[27] Hodnett ED. Pain and women's satisfaction with the experience of childbirth: a systematic review. Am J Obstet Gynecol 2002;186(5 Suppl Nature):S160–72 [Review]. PMID: 12011880.

[28] Robinson PN, Salmon P, Yentis SM. Maternal satisfaction. Int J Obstet Anesth 1998;7(1): 32–7. PMID: 15321244.

[29] Ranta PO. Obstetric epidural analgesia. Curr Opin Anaesthesiol 2002;15(5):525–31. PMID: 17019249.

[30] Caldero-Barcia, Poseiro JJ. Physiology of the uterine contraction. Clin Obstet Gynecol 1960; 3:386–408.

[31] Griffin RP, Reynolds F. Maternal hypoxaemia during labour and delivery: the influence of analgesia and effect on neonatal outcome. Anaesthesia 1995;50(2):151–6. PMID: 7710029.

[32] Krajewski W, Kucharska M, Wesolowski W, et al. Occupational exposure to nitrous oxide— the role of scavenging and ventilation systems in reducing the exposure level in operating rooms. Int J Hyg Environ Health 2007;210(2):133–8. PMID: 17045524.

[33] Laird R, Hughes D, Hill D. Audit of remifentanil patient-controlled analgesia for labour. Abstracts of free papers presented at the annual meeting of the Obstetric Anaesthetists Association, Sheffield, 7–8 June, 2007. Int J Obstet Anesth 2007;16:S43.

[34] Mastan M, Mukherjee S, Sirag A. Role of remifentanil for elective CS in a morbidly obese, needle-phobic parturient. Int J Obstet Anesth 2006;15(2):176.

[35] Brada SA, Egan TD, Viscomi CM. The use of remifentanil infusion to facilitate epidural catheter placement in a parturient: a case report with pharmacokinetic simulations. Int J Obstet Anesth 1998;7(2):124–7.

[36] Blair JM, Wallace N, Dobson G, et al. Remifentanil infusion as an adjunct to epidural anaesthesia for CS. Int J Obstet Anesth 2002;11:19.

[37] Gin T, Ngan-Kee WD, Siu YK, et al. Alfentanil given immediately before the induction of anesthesia for elective cesarean delivery. Anesth Analg 2000;90(5):1167–72. PMID: 10781473.

[38] Kayacan N, Ertugrul F, Arici G, et al. In vitro effects of opioids on pregnant uterine muscle. Adv Ther 2007;24(2):368–75. PMID: 17565928.

[39] Carvalho B, Mirikitani EJ, Lyell D, et al. Neonatal chest wall rigidity following the use of remifentanil for caesarean delivery in a patient with autoimmune hepatitis and thrombocytopenia. Int J Obstet Anesth 2004;13:53–6.

[40] Macfarlane AJR, Moise S, Smith D. Caesarean section using total intravenous anaesthesia in a patient with Ebstein's anomaly complicated by supraventricular tachycardia. Int J Obstet Anesth 2007;16(2):155–9.

[41] Orme RM, Grange CS, Ainsworth QP, et al. General anaesthesia using remifentanil for CS in parturients with critical aortic stenosis: a series of four cases. Int J Obstet Anesth 2004; 13(3):183–7. PMID 1532139.

[42] Bedard JM, Richardson MG, Wissler RN. General anesthesia with remifentanil for Cesarean section in a parturient with an acoustic neuroma. Can J Anaesth 1999;46:576–80.

[43] Richa F, Yazigi A, Nasser E, et al. General anesthesia with remifentanil for Cesarean section in a patient with HELLP syndrome. Acta Anaesthesiol Scand 2005;49(3):418–20.

[44] Johannsen EK, Munro AJ. Remifentanil in emergency CS in pre-eclampsia complicated by thrombocytopenia and abnormal liver function. Anaesth Intensive Care 1999;27:527–9.

[45] Alexander R, Fardell S. Use of remifentanil for tracheal intubation for CS in a patient with suxamethonium apnoea. Anaesthesia 2005;60(10):1036–8. [Erratum in: Anaesthesia. 2006 Feb;61(2):208]. PMID: 16179051.

[46] Van de Velde M, Teunkens A, Kuypers M. General anaesthesia with target controlled infusion of propofol for planned CS: maternal and neonatal effects of a remifentanil-based technique. Int J Obstet Anesth 2004;13(3):153–8.

[47] Ngan Kee WD, Khaw KS, Ma KC, et al. Maternal and neonatal effects of remifentanil at induction of general anesthesia for cesarean delivery: a randomized, double-blind, controlled trial. Anesthesiology 2006;104(1):14–20. PMID: 16394684.

[48] O'Hare R, McAtamney D, Mirakhur RK, et al. Bolus dose remifentanil for control of haemodynamic response to tracheal intubation during rapid sequence induction of anaesthesia. Br J Anaesth 1999;82:283–5.

[49] McCarroll CP, Paxton LD, Elliott P, et al. Use of remifentanil in a patient with peripartum cardiomyopathy requiring CS. Br J Anaesth 2001;86:135–8.

[50] Alexander R. Haemodynamic changes with administration of remifentanil following intubation for CS [abstract]. Eur J Anaesthesiol 2002;19(Suppl 24):A571.

[51] Imarengiaye C, Littleford J, Davies S, et al. Goal oriented general anesthesia for cesarean section in a parturient with a large intracranial epidermoid cyst. Can J Anaesth 2001;48: 884–9.

[52] Wadsworth R, Greer R, MacDonald J, et al. The use of remifentanil during general anaesthesia for caesarean delivery in two patients with severe heart dysfunction. Int J Obstet Anesth 2002;11(1):38–43.

[53] Brown J, McAtamney D. Remifentanil infusion for high-risk CS. Int J Obstet Anesth 2003; 12(1):63–4. PMID: 15321524.

[54] Johnston AJ, Hall JM, Levy DM. Anaesthesia with remifentanil and rocuronium for CS in a patient with long-QT syndrome and an automatic implantable cardioverter-defibrillator. Int J Obstet Anesth 2000;9(2):133–6. PMID: 15321099.

[55] Manullang TR, Chun K, Egan TD. The use of remifentanil for cesarean section in a parturient with recurrent aortic coarctation. Can J Anaesth 2000;47(5):454–9. PMID: 10831203.

[56] Scott H, Bateman C, Price M. The use of remifentanil in general anaesthesia for CS in a patient with mitral valve disease. Anaesthesia 1998;53:695–7.

[57] Thomas GL, Banerjee A. Remifentanil sedation in a critically ill obstetric patient. Anaesthesia 2005;60(11):1151–2. PMID: 16229707.

[58] Raman S, Cheng C. Intensive care use by critically ill obstetric patients: a five-year review. Int J Obstet Anesth 2003;12(2):89–92.

[59] Wheatley E, Farkas A, Watson D. Obstetric admissions to an intensive therapy unit. Int J Obstet Anesth 1996;5(4):221–4. PMID: 15321319.

[60] Howell PR, Madej TH. Administration of drugs outside of product licence: awareness and current practice. Int J Obstet Anesth 1999;8(1):30–6.

ANESTHESIOLOGY
CLINICS

Anesthesiology Clin
26 (2008) 183–195

Pharmacogenetics and Obstetric Anesthesia

Ruth Landau, MD, PD

Service d'Anesthésiologie, Département APSI, Hôpitaux Universitaires de Genève,
Rue Micheli-du-Crest 24, 1211 Genève 14, Switzerland

Pharmacogenetics is the study of the variability in drug response resulting from genetic variability. The first observations that genetic factors may have an impact on the response to various pharmacologic agents occurred in the mid-1950s, with Kalow and Gunn's [1] report of prolonged postoperative muscle relaxation after the administration of succinylcholine attributed to an inherited variation of drug metabolism involving the enzyme butyrylcholinesterase.

Recent developments in technology and genomic information have opened vast opportunities to expand and improve understanding of pharmacogenetics that promote targeted personalized medicine. Within the National Institutes of Health Pharmacogenetics Research Network, several research groups are concentrating on drugs used to treat specific medical disorders (asthma, depression, cardiovascular disease, nicotine addiction, and cancer), whereas others are focused on proteins that interact with drugs (membrane transporters and phase II drug-metabolizing enzymes) [2]. Comprehensive scientific information is stored and annotated in a publicly accessible database, the Pharmacogenetics and Pharmacogenomics Knowledge Base [3,4].

The ultimate goal of pharmacogenetics research is to help doctors tailor doses of medicines to a person's unique genetic make-up. This paradigm shift should make medicines safer and more effective for everyone. Although there still are no guidelines and immediate clinical implications for practitioners providing analgesia or anesthesia, it is essential to realize that trial-and-error pharmacotherapy and one-size-fits-all dogmas are bound to die. This review briefly outlines the genetic variability of pharmacokinetics

Presented in large part at the 39th Annual Meeting of SOAP research hour, Banff, Alberta, Canada, 2007.

E-mail address: ruth.landau@hcuge.ch

and pharmacodynamics and discusses selected fields relevant to obstetric anesthesiologists for whom the challenges of translating pharmacogenetics to clinical practice hopefully are on their way.

Pharmacology and polymorphisms

Most drug effects are determined by the interaction of several polymorphisms that influence the pharmacokinetics and pharmacodynamics of medications, including inherited differences in drug targets (eg, receptors) and drug disposition (eg, drug-metabolizing enzymes and transporters). This interplay may result in polygenic determinants that involve many potential combinations of drug metabolism, drug transporters, and drug-receptor genotypes with corresponding drug-response phenotypes yielding a wide range of therapeutic indexes (efficacy/toxicity ratios) for a given drug (Fig. 1) [5].

Drug-metabolizing enzymes

Polymorphisms of the cytochrome P450 (CYP) family are typical examples of single nucleotide polymorphisms (SNPs), affecting the response to many drugs metabolized into an active compound or inactivated by this metabolic pathway. A SNP in the catechol-*O*-methyltransferase (COMT) gene, associated with three- to fourfold reduction in the activity of the COMT enzyme, represents an interesting polymorphism that may have clinical effects on pain perception and analgesia [6].

Drug-transporting proteins

P-glycoprotein, one of the major drug transporter proteins, is polymorphic and could contribute to creating resistance to certain drugs, such as a decreased CD4 response in HIV-infected patients treated with HIV protease inhibitors or a decreased digoxin bioavailability.

Drug targets

Genes coding for receptors present at the cellular surface can be polymorphic and modify the effect of endogenous or exogenous molecules that bind and activate or inactivate the receptor. This is the case for many receptors, such as adrenergic receptors, the μ-opioid receptor (μOR), and the melanocortin-1 receptor associated with the redhead phenotype and involved with an unexpected analgesia-modulating effect.

Clinically relevant polymorphisms

Many drugs used in daily anesthetic practice may display important interindividual variability in their effects (reduced effect, unpredictable

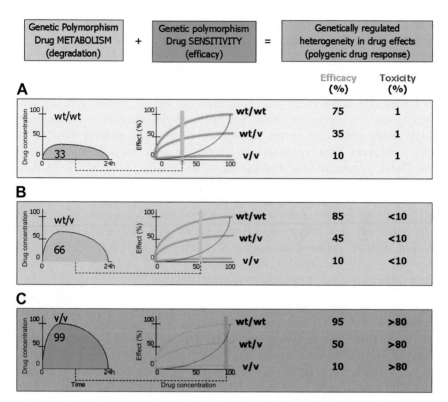

Fig. 1. Illustration of the polygenic determinants of drug response. The possible combined effects of two genetic polymorphisms are illustrated, one involving a drug-metabolizing enzyme (*left*) and the second involving a drug receptor (*middle*), demonstrating differences in drug clearance (area under the plasma concentration time curve) and receptor sensitivity in patients homozygous for the wild-type allele (wt/wt), heterozygous for one wild-type and one variant allele (wt/v), or who have two variant alleles (v/v) for the two polymorphisms. On the right, the nine potential combinations of drug-metabolism and drug-receptor genotypes are shown and the corresponding drug-response phenotypes calculated, yielding therapeutic indexes (efficacy/toxicity ratios). (*From* Landau R. Pharmacogenetics and obstetric anesthesia. Int Anesthesiol Clin 2007;45[1]:1–15; with permission.)

duration of action, side effects, and toxicity) because of polymorphisms. An exhaustive catalog of all alterations in efficacy and toxicity profiles is beyond the scope of this review; however, the following examples may serve to illustrate some implications of pharmacogenetics on clinical anesthesia and pain therapies.

The β₁-adrenergic receptor

The β_1-adrenergic receptor (β1AR, ADRB1) mediates chronotropic and inotropic responses to catecholamines, which are of particular interest to anesthesiologists. The Arg389 variant of a common polymorphism, Arg389-Gly, in vitro has a greater response to agonist stimulation, and individuals who have the Gly389 allele have a decreased response to β-blockade [7]. This polymorphism also is associated with differences in initial tolerability of β-blocker therapy in patients who have heart failure [8] and greater improvements in left ventricular remodeling in response to β-blockade [9]. The greater frequency of the Gly389 allele in African Americans (42%) than in Caucasians (28%) [10] may contribute to the decreased sensitivity to β-blockade reported in African Americans. Most recently, a multicentric Swiss study conducted in the perioperative period to address whether or not β-blockers improve long-term mortality after surgery under spinal anesthesia in patients who had known cardiovascular risks (the Swiss Beta Blocker in Spinal Anesthesia [BBSA] study) showed that individuals homozygous for Arg389 had better outcomes [11].

To date, there is no study addressing the potential association of this SNP and preeclampsia or any clinical trial examining the response to β-blockers in preeclamptic women according to genotype of β_1AR, which could provide an explanation for the observed ineffectiveness of labetalol in some hypertensive or preeclamptic women.

The β_2-adrenergic receptor

The β_2-adrenergic receptor ($\beta2AR$, ADRB2) is expressed at the surface of many cells, such as smooth muscle cells (bronchial, uterine, vascular, and so forth), with a relaxation of cells in response to endogenous catecholamines and synthetic β_2-agonists. Several SNPs are identified on the ADRB2, with at least three SNPs (Arg16Gly, Gln27Glu, and Thr164Ile) associated specifically with altered phenotypes [12].

Polymorphism of the ADRB2 has been studied regarding the following clinical situations: asthma, preterm labor and pregnancy outcome, and hemodynamic regulation and cardiovascular conditions.

Asthma

There are many studies assessing the association between asthma phenotypes and genetic variability of β_2AR. A recent meta-analysis concluded that neither the Gly16 nor the Glu27 allele contributes to asthma susceptibility overall or to bronchial hyperresponsiveness [13]. Gly16 homozygotes had a much higher risk for nocturnal asthma and asthma severity than Arg16 homozygotes. Therefore, SNPs of β_2AR gene are not major risk factors for the development of asthma; they are important, however, in determining drug response (pharmacogenetic effect).

Initial studies described an enhanced response to β_2-agonist bronchodilators in asthmatic subjects homozygous for the wild-type allele (Arg16) compared with patients homozygous for Gly16 [14], which seems consistent with the prediction of the in vitro findings that demonstrate increased receptor down-regulation in presence of the Gly16 variant. Recent genotype-stratified studies on treatment outcome in patients who had mild asthma, however, determined that patients homozygous for Gly16 improved in the long term with albuterol [15] or long-acting β_2-agonists [16], whereas those homozygous for Arg16 did not. With several studies showing that asthmatic patients who are Arg16 homozygous do not benefit from short-acting β-agonists in the absence or presence of concurrent inhaled cortico-steroid use, investigation of alternate treatment strategies that may help this group is on its way. Pharmacogenetics should influence the clinical management of asthma in the near future [17–20].

Preterm labor and delivery

Arg16 homozygosity of β_2AR genotype seems to confer a protective effect against preterm delivery [21,22], whereas the Glu27 variant might increase the risk for preterm delivery [23]. Furthermore, my colleagues and I have shown a pharmacogenetic effect, with a better response to β_2-agonist therapy (hexoprenaline) for tocolysis in women Arg16 homozygous who had idiopathic preterm labor between 24 and 34 weeks' gestation [24]. This had a significant impact on neonatal outcomes, with higher birthweights and less neonatal ICU admissions for respiratory or other complications re-sulting from prematurity in babies born to mothers who had that genotype.

It remains to be determined whether or not β_2AR genotype influences the severity of the disease (ie, that Arg16 homozygote women present with a milder disease than women who have other genotypes) or directly affects the response to therapy.

Hemodynamic regulation and cardiovascular conditions

Vascular tone and reactivity to β_2-agonists varies according to the genetic profile of β_2AR at positions 16 and 27. A large prospective cohort study in patients receiving β-blockers after an acute coronary event showed a differ-ential survival at 3 years according to β_2AR genotype, with a striking risk stratification when both genotypes were taken into account (mortality ranging from 6% in Gly16/Glu27 homozygotes to 20% in Arg16/Gln27 homozygotes) [25].

Although rare, the Thr164Ile variant is associated with a poor prognosis with congestive heart failure [26], resulting from an uncoupling of the β_2-agonist in the presence of the Ile164 variant, resulting in a decreased affinity for the receptor.

Within the field of anesthesia, there is less than a handful of studies assessing hemodynamic responses according to β_2AR genotype [11,27–29]. The pressor response to laryngoscopy and tracheal intubation is suggested as greater after intubation among Asian patients homozygous for Glu27 compared with those who have the other two genotypes [28]. In a similar study conducted in Turkey, however, Gln27 homozygous individuals were reported to respond to laryngoscopy and tracheal intubation with greater increases of heart rate than those carrying the Glu27 variant [27]. Interethnic variability is described for the β_2AR genotype [30]; along with different methodologies, this should be taken into account when interpreting such results.

A recent study in the obstetric population showed that the incidence and severity of maternal hypotension after spinal anesthesia for cesarean delivery and the response to treatment clearly are affected by β_2AR genotype. Women who are Gly16 homozygous, carrying one or two Glu at position 27 (heterozygous or homozygous for the Glu27 variant), were found to require significantly lower vasopressors (ephedrine) for treatment of hypotension during spinal anesthesia (Table 1) [29]. Again, this is a true pharmacogenetic effect of ADRB2 polymorphisms on the response to β_2-adrenoceptors stimulation. This pharmacogenetic effect explains in part why the many studies trying to prevent or treat hypotension during spinal anesthesia for caesarean section failed to define one single optimal strategy (fluid loading, ephedrine, or phenylephrine) for all patients.

Surprisingly, the BBSA study did not find any association between SNPs of β_2AR and the short- or long-term response to bisoprolol in patients who have known cardiovascular risks receiving spinal anesthesia for surgery [11].

Altogether, however, one should be cautious when extrapolating results from studies that report only one allele frequency at a single locus, because there are multiple allelic associations (linkage disequilibrium) between the three well-described SNPs. This may explain why several studies have reported ex vivo findings inconsistent with what is expected from in vitro work [31]. Future studies should focus on reporting the in vivo effects of naturally occurring haplotypes, so that further insights into the functional effects of β_2AR polymorphisms can be provided and translated effectively into clinical practice.

Table 1
Vasopressor use by β_2-adrenoceptor haplotype

	n	EPH 15	PE 15	Vasopressor units 15
Arg16Arg Gln16Gln	26	28 ± 13	78 ± 98	6.9 ± 2.6
Arg16Gly Gln27Gln	47	33 ± 23	82 ± 135	8.0 ± 5.2
Arg16Gly Gln27Glu	47	26 ± 16	122 ± 126	7.2 ± 3.9
Arg16Gly Glu27Glu	1	20	40	4.6
Gly16Gly Gln27Gln	15	23 ± 15	71 ± 89	5.8 ± 3.7
Gly16Gly Gln27Glu	22	16 ± 13[a]	44 ± 72	3.9 ± 3.0[b,c]
Gly16Gly Glu27Glu	12	13 ± 14[a]	59 ± 92	3.6 ± 3.4[d]

One-way analysis of variance with Bonferroni post hoc test. *P* values for analysis of variance: .001 for ephedrine dose, not significant for phenylephrine dose, and .0007 for vasopressor.

[a] Different from Arg16Gly Gln27Gln, *P* < .005.

[b] Different from Arg16Gly Gln27Gln, *P* < .01.

[c] Different from Arg16Gly Gln27Glu, *P* < .05.

[d] Different from Arg16Gly Gln27Gln, *P* < .02.

From Smiley RM, Blouin JL, Negron M, et al. beta2-adrenoceptor genotype affects vasopressor requirements during spinal anesthesia for cesarean delivery. Anesthesiology 2006;104(4):644–50; with permission.

Analgesia and pain-related candidate genes

Interindividual variability in pain perception and sensitivity to analgesic therapy with a large unpredictability in efficacy, side effects, and tolerance profiles to opioids is well described. Many candidate genes have been considered as suitable targets for the study of the genetic basis of pain and or analgesia [32].

Recently, a rare phenotype characterized by a total absence of pain perception (congenital indifference to pain) with no associated neuropathy has been associated with the gene SCN9A [33,34], encoding the α-subunit of the voltage-gated sodium channel, $Na_v1.7$. Individuals who have loss-of-function mutations of the $Na_v1.7$ lack protective mechanisms that allow tissue damage detection and suffer severe injuries because they do not learn pain-avoiding behaviors. This discovery opens new directions for development of novel generations of drugs with blocking $Na_v1.7$-blocking proprieties that should provide more selective and safe analgesia.

Meanwhile, this still is the era of opioid therapy, and the analgesic effect may be influenced by alterations in the metabolism of analgesic drugs (CYP), alterations in the metabolism of dopaminergic and adrenergic neurotransmitters (COMT), and mutations coding for the μOR.

Cytochrome P450

CYP is a superfamily of liver enzymes that catalyze phase 1 drug metabolism. One member of this family, CYP2D6, is of particular interest because it is involved with the metabolism of more than 100 drugs. It originally was discovered as a result of striking differences in the pharmacokinetics and effectiveness of drugs metabolized by this enzyme, including codeine, dextromethorphan, metoprolol, nortriptyline, and many more. The gene coding for this enzyme was found highly polymorphic, with more than 75 different CYP2D6 alleles [35], resulting in a variable enzymatic activity ranging from 1% to 200%. As a result, individuals can be classified as having an ultrarapid metabolism, an extensive metabolism, a normal metabolism, or a poor metabolism. CYP2D6 activity is absent in approximately 7% to 10% of whites [36]; because codeine must be converted into morphine to elicit its analgesic effect, individuals who have poor metabolism do not achieve analgesia with codeine [37], whereas they encounter side effects, such as nausea and vomiting, from the drug [38]. Conversely, codeine intoxication can be anticipated with ultrarapid CYP2D6 metabolism [39].

There has been a recent Food and Drug Administration warning on codeine use in nursing mothers after the death of a breastfed 13-day-old neonate believed to have suffered a morphine overdose because his mother was taking codeine and was a CYP2D6 ultrarapid metabolizer [40]. Although codeine undoubtedly is not a wonder analgesic, it still is prescribed because of the belief that as a weak opioid, it is safe. This case exemplifies precisely the irrefutable input of diagnostic pharmacogenetic testing.

The effect of tramadol analgesia also is influenced by the CYP2D6 genotype [41] in the sense that poor metabolizers may be overdosed (ie, opposite effect to that encountered with codeine), and interactions with any other coadministered medication undergoing CYP2D6 metabolism should be anticipated [42].

Catechol-O-methyltransferase gene

The COMT gene encodes a major enzyme involved in the metabolism of dopamine and norepinephrine. The Val138Met variant of the COMT gene is associated with a three- to fourfold reduction in COMT enzyme activity. The μ-opioid neurotransmitter system typically is activated in response to prolonged pain and its function is influenced by the COMT activity. Individuals homozygous for the Met138 allele have the lowest COMT enzyme activity and show diminished regional μ-opioid system responses (lower neuronal content of enkephalin), which might lead to decreased endogenous analgesia with higher sensory and affective ratings of pain [6]. Alternatively, the demonstrated increase of μOR might lead to an increased effect from morphine administration in individuals who have the Met/Met genotype. This is of particular interest because the prevalence of this genotype is high (32%) [43]. In addition, a pharmacogenetic effect of this SNP has been demonstrated in the context of chronic oral morphine therapy in cancer patients, with patients carrying the Met138 variant requiring less morphine compared with patients who are Val138 homozygous [43]. This bidirectional effect of the Val138Met polymorphism probably is because in those who have a low COMT activity, such as in individuals who are Met138 homozygous, there is a compensatory increase in regional μOR density that may cause morphine to be more effective in individuals carrying this genotype.

Because of the high prevalence of the variant Met138 genotype and the key role of COMT activity in the experience of pain, this polymorphism currently is a major target for genetic studies of interindividual differences in the adaptation and responses to pain and other stressful stimuli. Some recent studies report conflicting results, one study assessing postoperative pain ratings that did not find an association with the COMT genotype [44].

Finally, there is a increasing body of evidence that COMT activity is involved in the development of chronic pain in susceptible individuals [45]; as a result, polymorphism of the COMT gene in part may provide the genetic basis for individual variations in pain perception and the development of chronic pain conditions. With a growing interest in determining predictive factors for postcesarean pain and analgesia requirements and prevention of chronic pain after cesarean sections, studies including COMT activity and genetic determinations are becoming indispensable.

μ-opioid receptor

The μOR, encoded by genetic locus *OPRM1*, has been the focus of several genetic studies because this receptor is the primary site of action for many endogenous opioid peptides, including β-endorphin and enkephalin, and the major target for opioid analgesics, such as morphine, heroin, fentanyl, and methadone. The μOR is a G protein–coupled receptor (GPCR), and several SNPs have been described for *OPRM1*. At nucleotide position 118, an adenine substitution by a guanine (A118G), resulting in the asparagine residue at amino acid position 40 changed into an aspartate residue, has been reported to occur with an allelic frequency of 10% to 30% among whites [46,47] and a higher prevalence among Asians [48]. The major interest in this particular SNP is its pharmacologic [49] and physiologic consequences [50]. In vitro, the presence of at least one G118 allele is shown to increase the binding affinity and potency of β-endorphin [49]. Thus, individuals carrying the variant receptor gene could show differences in some of the functions mediated by β-endorphin action at the altered μOR, such as higher thresholds to pain. Consistent with this laboratory finding, one in vivo study of a human experimental pain model demonstrated that volunteers carrying a G118 allele exhibited lower sensitivity to pressure pain compared with A118 homozygotes [51]. The exact relationship of this polymorphism with the response to oral opioids for treatment of chronic pain, postoperative requirements of intravenous morphine, or the adverse effects and toxicity profiles has not been elucidated fully [52]. To date, only small series are available, with some evidence that individuals carrying the variant G118 allele may require higher doses of morphine [53,54], in contrast to what is expected if the variant μOR is associated with an increased endogenous opioid activity. Further studies to elucidate the impact of this genetic variant on labor pain and neuraxial opioid requirements for labor analgesia are ongoing; the A118G polymorphism has an impact on the median effective dose (produces desired effect in 50% of population) of intrathecal fentanyl in labor, with nulliparous women carrying the variant G118 allele requiring substantially lower doses of intrathecal fentanyl to achieve adequate analgesia early in labor (with a 1.5- to 2-fold difference between genetic groups) [55].

Undeniably, many candidate genes and elaborate models have been suggested for the study of the genetic component of pain [32,56], and several excellent reviews on the pharmacogenetics of opiods and analgesia recently were published [57–59]. In addition, a genetic database of knockout mice allowing the study of genetic variations in the context of specific pain phenotypes was made public in 2007 [60]. Nonetheless, because of the inherent complexity of studying pain (different nociceptive modalities, gender differences, limitations in extrapolating data from animal models to the response in humans, and interethnic and environmental differences) in addition to the obvious polygenic nature, it is the design and execution of large clinical studies analyzing multiple haplotypes simultaneously that remain the true challenges to date. Meanwhile, some groups already actively are working on gene therapies for pain, and the first results in animal models are starting to appear in journals [61–63]. It will be of interest to see the new insights and developments brought by more research on the SCN9A gene in the near future.

Future applications

To date, the choice of one medication over another does not take into account interindividual genetic variability. Some drugs have the potential for serious side effects or are ineffective in subsets of the population because of an unfavorable efficacy/toxicity ratio; therefore, pharmacogenetics has the potential to improve the clinical outcome of drug therapy. Targeting therapy to genotype implies that the efficacy/toxicity profile for each product according to genotype is determined and recommendations for drug use per genotype established; this has been done for some psychotropic drugs and is on its way for the management of asthma.

Considering the rapid decrease in the cost of genotyping, it is unlikely that technology will limit the widespread introduction of pharmacogenomics in clinical practice. The design and execution of large clinical trials in multiple populations, however, looking at multiple loci simultaneously, most likely will be the limiting factor. Pharmacogenetic tests have to be cost effective: typically, if a drug has a narrow therapeutic index (ie, high risk for toxicity), the pharmacokinetic/dynamic relationship is consistent, the response is difficult to predict, there is large interindividual variability in response, and the treatment is long term, diagnostic tests are cost-effective [64]. The pharmacogenetics of warfarin therapy have been studied extensively to the extent that prospectively validated algorithms taking into account metabolism of CYP2C9 and variability of the gene coding for the vitamin K epoxide reductase subunit 1 (VKORC1) soon should be available [65]. A Web-based report on the cost-effectiveness of warfarin pharmacogenetics estimated that testing for variants in the CYP2C9 and VKORC1 genes to guide initial dosing of warfarin therapy could provide $1,100,000,000 in cost savings to the United States health care system annually [66]. This report also estimates that 85,000 serious bleeding events and 17,000 strokes could be avoided annually. It remains to be seen whether or not these projections are overly optimistic, as suggested by some experts [67].

From a clinician's point of view, although it still is too early to foresee immediate implications of pharmacogenetics in general and pharmacogenetic diagnostic tests specifically in the daily practice of anesthesiologists, advances in the field of genomics certainly will identify which SNPs or haplotypes will have an impact on drug responses. These discoveries should allow targeting anesthetic drugs, hypertensive therapies, and acute and chronic pain therapies and personalizing strategies aimed at improving perioperative outcomes according to patients' genetic profiles, because "one size does not fit all" anymore.

References

[1] Kalow W, Gunn DR. The relation between dose of succinylcholine and duration of apnea in man. J Pharmacol Exp Ther 1957;120(2):203–14.

[2] Giacomini KM, Brett CM, Altman RB, et al. The pharmacogenetics research network: from SNP discovery to clinical drug response. Clin Pharmacol Ther 2007;81(3):328–45.

[3] Department of Genetics, Stanford University Medical Center. Pharmacogenetics and pharmacogenomics knowledge base. Available at: http://www.PharmGKb.org.

[4] Hodge AE, Altman RB, Klein TE. The PharmGKB: integration, aggregation, and annotation of pharmacogenomic data and knowledge. Clin Pharmacol Ther 2007;81(1):21–4.

[5] Evans WE, Relling MV. Moving towards individualized medicine with pharmacogenomics. Nature 2004;429(6990):464–8.

[6] Zubieta JK, Heitzeg MM, Smith YR, et al. COMT val158met genotype affects mu-opioid neurotransmitter responses to a pain stressor. Science 2003;299(5610):1240–3.

[7] Sofowora GG, Dishy V, Muszkat M, et al. A common beta1-adrenergic receptor polymorphism (Arg389Gly) affects blood pressure response to beta-blockade. Clin Pharmacol Ther 2003;73(4):366–71.

[8] Terra SG, Pauly DF, Lee CR, et al. beta-Adrenergic receptor polymorphisms and responses during titration of metoprolol controlled release/extended release in heart failure. Clin Pharmacol Ther 2005;77(3):127–37.

[9] Terra SG, Hamilton KK, Pauly DF, et al. Beta1-adrenergic receptor polymorphisms and left ventricular remodeling changes in response to beta-blocker therapy. Pharmacogenet Genomics 2005;15(4):227–34.

[10] Xie HG, Dishy V, Sofowora G, et al. Arg389Gly beta 1-adrenoceptor polymorphism varies in frequency among different ethnic groups but does not alter response in vivo. Pharmacogenetics 2001;11(3):191–7.

[11] Zaugg M, Bestmann L, Wacker J, et al. Adrenergic receptor genotype but not perioperative bisoprolol therapy may determine cardiovascular outcome in at-risk patients undergoing surgery with spinal block: the Swiss Beta Blocker in Spinal Anesthesia (BBSA) study: a double-blinded, placebo-controlled, multicenter trial with 1-year follow-up. Anesthesiology 2007;107(1):33–44.

[12] Liggett SB. Polymorphisms of the beta2-adrenergic receptor. N Engl J Med 2002;346(7): 536–8.

[13] Contopoulos-Ioannidis DG, Manoli EN, Ioannidis JP. Meta-analysis of the association of beta2-adrenergic receptor polymorphisms with asthma phenotypes. J Allergy Clin Immunol 2005;115(5):963–72.

[14] Lima JJ, Thomason DB, Mohamed MH, et al. Impact of genetic polymorphisms of the beta2-adrenergic receptor on albuterol bronchodilator pharmacodynamics. Clin Pharmacol Ther 1999;65(5):519–25.

[15] Israel E, Chinchilli VM, Ford JG, et al. Use of regularly scheduled albuterol treatment in asthma: genotype-stratified, randomised, placebo-controlled cross-over trial. Lancet 2004; 364(9444):1505–12.

[16] Wechsler ME, Lehman E, Lazarus SC, et al. beta-Adrenergic receptor polymorphisms and response to salmeterol. Am J Respir Crit Care Med 2006;173(5):519–26.

[17] Wechsler ME, Israel E. How pharmacogenomics will play a role in the management of asthma. Am J Respir Crit Care Med 2005;172(1):12–8.

[18] Israel E. Genetics and the variability of treatment response in asthma. J Allergy Clin Immunol 2005;115(Suppl 4):S532–8.

[19] Hall IP, Sayers I. Pharmacogenetics and asthma: false hope or new dawn? Eur Respir J 2007; 29(6):1239–45.

[20] Hall IP. Pharmacogenetics of asthma. Chest 2006;130(6):1873–8.

[21] Landau R, Xie HG, Dishy V, et al. beta2-Adrenergic receptor genotype and preterm delivery. Am J Obstet Gynecol 2002;187(5):1294–8.

[22] Doh K, Sziller I, Vardhana S, et al. Beta2-adrenergic receptor gene polymorphisms and pregnancy outcome. J Perinat Med 2004;32(5):413–7.

[23] Ozkur M, Dogulu F, Ozkur A, et al. Association of the Gln27Glu polymorphism of the beta-2-adrenergic receptor with preterm labor. Int J Gynaecol Obstet 2002;77(3):209–15.

[24] Landau R, Morales MA, Antonarakis SE, et al. Arg16 homozygosity of the beta2-adrenergic receptor improves the outcome after beta2-agonist tocolysis for preterm labor. Clin Pharmacol Ther 2005;78(6):656–63.

[25] Lanfear DE, Jones PG, Marsh S, et al. Beta2-adrenergic receptor genotype and survival among patients receiving beta-blocker therapy after an acute coronary syndrome. JAMA 2005;294(12):1526–33.

[26] Liggett SB, Wagoner LE, Craft LL, et al. The Ile164 beta2-adrenergic receptor polymorphism adversely affects the outcome of congestive heart failure. J Clin Invest 1998;102(8): 1534–9.

[27] Kaymak C, Kocabas NA, Durmaz E, et al. beta2 adrenoceptor (ADRB2) pharmacogenetics and cardiovascular phenotypes during laryngoscopy and tracheal intubation. Int J Toxicol 2006;25(6):443–9.

[28] Kim NS, Lee IO, Lee MK, et al. The effects of beta2 adrenoceptor gene polymorphisms on pressor response during laryngoscopy and tracheal intubation. Anaesthesia 2002;57(3): 227–32.

[29] Smiley RM, Blouin JL, Negron M, et al. beta2-adrenoceptor genotype affects vasopressor requirements during spinal anesthesia for cesarean delivery. Anesthesiology 2006;104(4): 644–50.

[30] Muszkat M. Interethnic differences in drug response: the contribution of genetic variability in beta adrenergic receptor and cytochrome P4502C9. Clin Pharmacol Ther 2007;82(2):215–8.

[31] Leineweber K, Brodde OE. Beta2-adrenoceptor polymorphisms: relation between in vitro and in vivo phenotypes. Life Sci 2004;74(23):2803–14.

[32] Belfer I, Wu T, Kingman A, et al. Candidate gene studies of human pain mechanisms: methods for optimizing choice of polymorphisms and sample size. Anesthesiology 2004; 100(6):1562–72.

[33] Cox JJ, Reimann F, Nicholas AK, et al. An SCN9A channelopathy causes congenital inability to experience pain. Nature 2006;444(7121):894–8.

[34] Goldberg YP, MacFarlane J, MacDonald ML, et al. Loss-of-function mutations in the Nav1.7 gene underlie congenital indifference to pain in multiple human populations. Clin Genet 2007;71(4):311–9.

[35] Allele Nomenclature Committee. Available at: http://www.imm.ki.se/cypalleles. Accessed August 13, 2007.

[36] Caraco Y. Genes and the response to drugs. N Engl J Med 2004;351(27):2867–9.

[37] Sindrup SH, Brosen K. The pharmacogenetics of codeine hypoalgesia. Pharmacogenetics 1995;5(6):335–46.

[38] Eckhardt K, Li S, Ammon S, et al. Same incidence of adverse drug events after codeine administration irrespective of the genetically determined differences in morphine formation. Pain 1998;76(1–2):27–33.

[39] Gasche Y, Daali Y, Fathi M, et al. Codeine intoxication associated with ultrarapid CYP2D6 metabolism. N Engl J Med 2004;351(27):2827–31.

[40] FDA News. Available at: http://www.fda.gov/bbs/topics/NEWS/2007/NEW01685.html. Accessed August 17, 2007.

[41] Enggaard TP, Poulsen L, Arendt-Nielsen L, et al. The analgesic effect of tramadol after intravenous injection in healthy volunteers in relation to CYP2D6. Anesth Analg 2006;102(1): 146–50.

[42] Stamer UM, Stuber F. Analgesic efficacy of tramadol if coadministered with ondansetron. Anesth Analg 2001;93(6):1626.

[43] Rakvag TT, Klepstad P, Baar C, et al. The Val158Met polymorphism of the human catechol-O-methyltransferase (COMT) gene may influence morphine requirements in cancer pain patients. Pain 2005;116(1–2):73–8.

[44] Kim H, Lee H, Rowan J, et al. Genetic polymorphisms in monoamine neurotransmitter systems show only weak association with acute post-surgical pain in humans. Mol Pain 2006;2:24–33.

[45] Diatchenko L, Slade GD, Nackley AG, et al. Genetic basis for individual variations in pain perception and the development of a chronic pain condition. Hum Mol Genet 2005;14(1):135–43.

[46] Landau R, Cahana A, Smiley RM, et al. Genetic variability of mu-opioid receptor in an obstetric population. Anesthesiology 2004;100(4):1030–3.

[47] Crowley JJ, Oslin DW, Patkar AA, et al. A genetic association study of the mu opioid receptor and severe opioid dependence. Psychiatr Genet 2003;13(3):169–73.

[48] Tan EC, Tan CH, Karupathivan U, et al. Mu opioid receptor gene polymorphisms and heroin dependence in Asian populations. Neuroreport 2003;14(4):569–72.

[49] Bond C, LaForge KS, Tian M, et al. Single-nucleotide polymorphism in the human mu opioid receptor gene alters beta-endorphin binding and activity: possible implications for opiate addiction. Proc Natl Acad Sci U S A 1998;95(16):9608–13.

[50] Chong RY, Oswald L, Yang X, et al. The mu-opioid receptor polymorphism A118G predicts cortisol responses to naloxone and stress. Neuropsychopharmacology 2006;31(1):204–11.

[51] Fillingim RB, Kaplan L, Staud R, et al. The A118G single nucleotide polymorphism of the mu-opioid receptor gene (OPRM1) is associated with pressure pain sensitivity in humans. J Pain 2005;6(3):159–67.

[52] Landau R. One size does not fit all: genetic variability of mu-opioid receptor and postoperative morphine consumption. Anesthesiology 2006;105(2):235–7.

[53] Chou WY, Wang CH, Liu PH, et al. Human opioid receptor A118G polymorphism affects intravenous patient-controlled analgesia morphine consumption after total abdominal hysterectomy. Anesthesiology 2006;105(2):334–7.

[54] Klepstad P, Rakvag TT, Kaasa S, et al. The 118 A > G polymorphism in the human microopioid receptor gene may increase morphine requirements in patients with pain caused by malignant disease. Acta Anaesthesiol Scand 2004;48(10):1232–9.

[55] Landau R, Kern C, Smiley R, et al. Polymorphism of mu-opioid receptor (A118G) affects intrathecal fentanyl ED50 for labor analgesia [abstract]. Anesthesiology 2005;(Suppl):A1469.

[56] Strong JA. Genetics of pain: lessons for future studies. Int Anesthesiol Clin 2007;45(2):13–25.

[57] Stamer UM, Bayerer B, Stuber F. Genetics and variability in opioid response. Eur J Pain 2005;9(2):101–4.

[58] Somogyi AA, Barratt DT, Coller JK. Pharmacogenetics of opioids. Clin Pharmacol Ther 2007;81(3):429–44.

[59] Lotsch J, Geisslinger G. Current evidence for a genetic modulation of the response to analgesics. Pain 2006;121(1–2):1–5.

[60] Lacroix-Fralish ML, Ledoux JB, Mogil JS. The Pain Genes Database: an interactive web browser of pain-related transgenic knockout studies. Pain 2007;131:3.e1–4.

[61] Hao S, Mata M, Fink DJ. Viral vector-based gene transfer for treatment of chronic pain. Int Anesthesiol Clin 2007;45(2):59–71.

[62] Tzabazis AZ, Pirc G, Votta-Velis E, et al. Antihyperalgesic effect of a recombinant herpes virus encoding antisense for calcitonin gene-related peptide. Anesthesiology 2007;106(6):1196–203.

[63] Mata M, Fink DJ. Gene therapy for pain. Anesthesiology 2007;106(6):1079–80.

[64] Swen JJ, Huizinga TW, Gelderblom H, et al. Translating pharmacogenomics: challenges on the road to the clinic. PLoS Med 2007;4(8):1317–24.

[65] Gage BF, Lesko LJ. Pharmacogenetics of warfarin: regulatory, scientific, and clinical issues. J Thromb Thrombolysis 2007;25:45–51.

[66] Reg-Markets.Org. Available at: http://www.aei-brookings.org/publications/abstract.php?pid=1127. Accessed November 2006.

[67] Veenstra DL. The cost-effectiveness of warfarin pharmacogenomics. J Thromb Haemost 2007;5(9):1974–5.

ELSEVIER
SAUNDERS

Anesthesiology Clin
26 (2008) 197–230

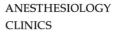

ANESTHESIOLOGY
CLINICS

Maternal Morbidity, Mortality, and Risk Assessment

Ashutosh Wali, MD, FFARCSI, Maya S. Suresh, MD*

*Department of Anesthesiology, Baylor College of Medicine, Faculty Center,
1709 Dryden Road, Suite 1700, MS: BCM 120, Houston, TX 77030, USA*

Maternal mortality is the tip of the maternal morbidity iceberg; several obstetric, anesthetic, and social challenges impact morbidity and mortality in women. Maternal mortality is the yardstick to measure when health care personnel fail to recognize risks, lack interdisciplinary communication, or provide substandard care, thus resulting in complications during pregnancy, labor, or delivery.

Pregnancy-related death is defined by the International Classification of Diseases, 10th Revision (ICD-10) as the death of a woman while pregnant or within 42 days of termination of pregnancy, despite the cause of death. Although the risk for death from complications of pregnancy decreased dramatically during the 20th century in the United States, the Centers for Disease Control and Prevention (CDC) reports a fairly static maternal mortality ratio (MMR), of approximately 7.5 maternal deaths per 100,000 live births. In the year 2000, a collaborative effort involving World Health Organization (WHO), United Nations Children's Fund (UNICEF), and United Nations Population Fund (UNFPA) estimated 660 maternal deaths, thus averaging 11 maternal deaths per 100,000 live births, placing the MMR above the statistics reported by the CDC. These surveys on maternal mortality surveillances are limited in scope because the information is obtained from death certificates, and various states or academic institutions could be underreporting. Accurate statistics are lacking, thus resulting in only a snapshot of the actual maternal morbidity and mortality. The recent WHO estimate in the United States show that maternal mortality is approximately 17 in 100,000 pregnancies. This estimate is significantly higher than the goal set by the U.S. Department of Health and Human Services in *Healthy People 2010*, which sets the target for maternal mortality at less

---

* Corresponding author.
E-mail address: msuresh@bcm.tmc.edu (M.S. Suresh).

1932-2275/08/$ - see front matter © 2008 Elsevier Inc. All rights reserved.
doi:10.1016/j.anclin.2007.12.005   *anesthesiology.theclinics.com*

than 3.3 in 100,000 live births. Some regional reports document ratios as high as 22.8 per 100,000 live births, which is an unacceptably high rate.

In United States, the most common causes of maternal deaths, although they vary among states, include thromboembolism; amniotic fluid embolism; hemorrhage; complications of hypertension, including preeclampsia and eclampsia; and infection. Pulmonary disease, anesthesia-related deaths, and cardiomyopathy are also significant contributors to maternal morbidity and mortality.

In United Kingdom, the regularly conducted Confidential Enquiries into Maternal Deaths (CEMD) has the longest and most successful history of conducting and publishing findings triennially. The latest publication on "Why Mothers Die 2000–2002," was the first report of the new millennium and marks the 50th anniversary of the first triennial report [1]. In United Kingdom, maternal deaths are classified as direct (death caused by pregnancy occurring within 42 days of delivery), indirect (death from a preexisting condition aggravated by pregnancy), coincidental (death unrelated to pregnancy), and late (death occurring between 42 days and 1 year after delivery). In the triennium 2000 to 2002, 391 deaths were reported, of which 106 were classified as direct. The most common cause of direct death was thromboembolism, which remained unchanged since the previous triennium, 1997 to 1999. An increase in mortality rate from hemorrhage occurred, with it being the second leading cause of direct deaths and hypertensive disease as the fourth leading cause. Anesthesia ranked seventh among the top leading causes. Of the total deaths, 155 were classified as indirect. Cardiac disease remains a leading cause of indirect maternal deaths (Figs. 1 and 2).

The Confidential Enquiry into Maternal and Child Health (CEMACH) report (2000–2002) [1] is generally targeted toward health care professionals in the United Kingdom, and was originally criticized for its limited international scope. However, the lessons learned from the disciplined approach to rigorously collecting and analyzing data have had a far-reaching global impact, and the information is being disseminated in peer-reviewed journals in the United States [2]. Similarities are seen in the leading causes of maternal deaths in the United States and United Kingdom.

Thromboembolism

Maternal morbidity and mortality statistics

Thromboembolism remains the most common cause of direct pregnancy-related maternal death during live births in developed countries [3,4]. Because pregnancy is a hypercoagulable state, the risk for venous thromboembolism is 5 to 10 times higher in the pregnant population than the nonpregnant population [5,6]. The latest CDC data showed that thromboembolism accounted for 21.4% of pregnancy-related maternal mortality in

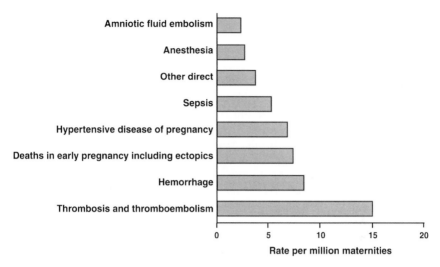

Fig. 1. Mortality rates per million maternities of leading causes of direct deaths as reported to the Confidential Enquiry into Maternal and Child Health in the United Kingdom, 2002–2002. (*From* Lewis G. Introduction and key findings 2002–2002. In: Confidential Enquiry into Maternal and Child Health. Why mothers die 2000–2002: the sixth report of the Confidential Enquiries into Maternal Death in the United Kingdom. London: RCOG Press; 2004. p. 32; with permission.)

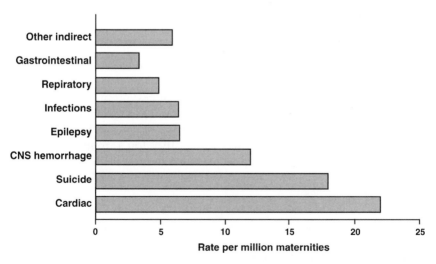

Fig. 2. Maternal mortality rate from leading causes of indirect deaths per million maternities as reported to the Confidential Enquiry into Maternal and Child Health in the United Kingdom, 2000–2002. (*From* Lewis G. Introduction and key findings 2002–2002. In: Confidential Enquiry into Maternal and Child Health. Why mothers die 2000–2002: the sixth report of the Confidential Enquiries into Maternal Death in the United Kingdom. London: RCOG Press; 2004. p. 32; with permission.)

the United States [3,4]. According to the CEMACH report (2000–2002), thromboembolism was the leading cause of direct maternal death in the United Kingdom, with two thirds occurring in the postpartum period. The overall incidence has continued to decline, probably because of improved thromboprophylaxis [7]. However, substandard practice from either failure to recognize risk factors and slow introduction or inadequate dosing of thromboprophylaxis and treatment was implicated in the report [7].

Deep vein thrombosis during pregnancy accounts for most pulmonary thromboembolism [8] occurring in the antepartum period [9]. If untreated, 13% to 24% parturients will have pulmonary embolism, with a high mortality rate of 12% to 15% [10]. Adequate treatment has helped reduce the incidence to 0.7% to 4.5% and the mortality to 0.7% [10].

Risk assessment

Risk factors for the increased incidence of thromboembolism during pregnancy include age older than 35 years, increased venous stasis, hypercoagulability, vascular injury from vaginal delivery or cesarean section, obstetric conditions (eg, preeclampsia, grand multiparity, multiple gestation) [11], and other comorbidities (eg, previous history of thromboembolism, smoking, obesity [BMI > 30 kg/m^2], gross varicose veins, antiphospholipid syndrome, protein C and S deficiency, antithrombin III deficiency, hyperhomocysteinemia, factor V Leiden mutation) [10].

Strategies to minimize risk and recommendations

Prepregnancy counseling should occur and include strategies designed to reduce thrombotic risk before, during, and after pregnancy. These strategies may include reduction of body weight [12] and cessation of smoking [13]. Use of elastic compression stockings (ECS) during pregnancy, intraoperative use of pneumatic stockings during cesarean section, and ECS use during puerperium have been shown to be effective for thromboprophylaxis [11,14,15]. Drugs commonly used to prevent and treat venous thromboembolism include heparin, low molecular weight heparin (LMWH), coumadin, and antiplatelet drugs.

Heparin is ideally suited for the parturient because it does not cross the placenta due to its large molecular size, strong polarity, and lipid insolubility [11]. Because of increased heparin requirements during pregnancy, dose adjustments must be made continuously to maintain the activated partial thromboplastin time (aPTT) ratio between 1.5 and 2.5 [16] or factor Xa level between 0.5 and 1.0 IU/mL [17]. However, large-dose heparin therapy has been associated with heparin-induced thrombocytopenia (HIT) [18] and osteoporosis [19]. Furthermore, the short half-life of intravenous heparin (60 minutes) requires administration by continuous infusion.

LMWH has a longer half-life, and doses are administered based on body weight. It has a lower risk for HIT [18] and osteoporosis [19] and is predominantly excreted by the kidney [11]. Because of the increased renal blood flow of pregnancy and associated increased renal clearance of LMWH in the parturient, it is administered as a twice-daily dose in contrast to the once-daily dose in the nonpregnant patient [11]. Factor Xa level monitoring is used in certain centers to adjust dosing, even though its efficacy is not well proven [20]. LMWH seems to be the preferred thromboprophylactic agent in pregnancy.

Warfarin has a low molecular weight, crosses the placenta, and is associated with teratogenicity, and is therefore contraindicated in pregnancy. Case reports exist of successful and safe use during pregnancy of antiplatelet drugs, such as aspirin [21], clopidogrel [22], and ticlopidine [23], as adjuvants to heparin or LMWH.

According to the American College of Chest Physicians Consensus Conference on Antithrombotic Therapy [24], no medication is necessary in women who have temporary risk factors, although they should remain under strict surveillance. However, thromboprophylaxis should be administered to women who have a previous history of venous thromboembolism if they are pregnant, using oral contraceptives, or have a thrombophilia.

Based on risk–benefit assessment, LMWH is the preferred treatment of venous thrombosis and established thromboembolism [11]. The typical dose for enoxaparin is 1 mg/kg twice daily; it has a predictable and adequate anticoagulant effect and [25] does not require anti–factor Xa monitoring [11]. Anticoagulated parturients are at special risk for developing neuraxial hematoma (epidural or spinal) during regional anesthesia. Individual risk evaluation based on The American Society for Regional Anesthesia Guidelines should be performed before neuraxial block placement [26].

Case reports exist of other successful treatment modalities, including thrombectomy [27] and use of inferior vena cava filters [28], in parturients who have a contraindication to anticoagulants.

Hemorrhage

Maternal morbidity and mortality statistics

Obstetric hemorrhage is one of the leading causes of maternal morbidity and mortality worldwide. In the United States, hemorrhage is the third most common cause of maternal mortality [4,29], with 17 % of maternal deaths attributed to obstetric hemorrhage [4]. Significant racial differences were seen in mortality rates between African American and Caucasian women in the United States [4,30].

The CEMACH (2000–2002) report from the United Kingdom showed that hemorrhage was the second most common cause of direct maternal death [1]. According to the CEMD, advanced maternal age older than

35 years seemed to increase the risk for maternal morbidity and mortality from obstetric hemorrhage in the United Kingdom from 1997–1999. Based on worldwide estimates, one woman dies of postpartum hemorrhage every 4 minutes, accounting for 140,000 deaths per year [31]. Maternal morbidity, from severe obstetric hemorrhage, was seen in 6.7 per 1000 deliveries in the United Kingdom [32].

WHO estimates show that postpartum hemorrhage alone has been incriminated in 25% of maternal mortality [33]. However, application of a temporal qualifier in obstetrics can be problematic, because exsanguinating hemorrhage in the late antepartum, intrapartum, and immediate postpartum periods is often related [34]. Patients at greatest risk for severe, life-threatening blood loss [35] include those who have abruptio placentae, placenta previa, placenta accreta, and uterine rupture.

Risk assessment

Risk factors for antepartum hemorrhage include placental abruption, trauma, uterine rupture, genetic, exposure to cocaine, methadone, and tobacco, hypertensive disorders of pregnancy, and presence of a uterine fibroid [34]. Risk factors for placenta previa include advanced maternal parity, advanced maternal age, prior placenta previa, and prior cesarean section [34].

The approximately 40% reduction in maternal mortality rates is attributed to improved prenatal care, improved blood banking techniques, better appreciation for the risks for hemorrhage, and improved anesthetic and obstetric management of excessive blood loss during pregnancy [34].

The most common causes of postpartum hemorrhage include uterine atony, genital trauma, retained placenta [36], placenta accreta (0%–5% in women who have an unscarred uterus [37], increasing to 67% in those who have a scarred uterus [38]), and uterine inversion (1/5000–1/10,000 pregnancies) [39].

Uterine atony leading to postpartum hemorrhage [39] is the most common indication for peripartum blood transfusion [40,41]. Risk factors for uterine atony include protracted labor requiring oxytocin augmentation, chorioamnionitis, obstructed labor, fetal macrosomia, polyhydramnios, placental abruption, placenta previa, grand multiparity, family history, uterine laceration, and prolonged tocolytic therapy [34].

Strategies to minimize risk and recommendations

In the antepartum period, vaginal delivery is pursued if no fetal or maternal compromise is present. Cesarean section is reserved for severe maternal hemorrhage or worsening coagulopathy. Blood product availability and continuous electronic fetal monitoring are essential for a successful and safe outcome.

Anesthetic management begins with careful preparation of patients. Preparation involves a multidisciplinary team effort. Open communication and frequent consultation should occur among anesthesiology, obstetric, blood banking, hematology, urology, neonatology, and nursing services. Preparation for adequate resuscitation requires placement of large-bore intravenous catheters. Monitoring and fluid management are managed with invasive arterial blood pressure, central venous pressure, and urine output catheter. A level-one rapid infuser is essential in severe hemorrhage requiring massive blood resuscitation. If time and hemodynamics permit, preoperative bilateral ureteric stents should be placed, particularly in patients who have placenta accreta/percreta, by the urology team to facilitate identification of ureters during intraoperative dissection by the obstetric team [34].

Patients presenting with severe ongoing obstetric hemorrhage, severe anticipated hemorrhage, or acute fetal compromise should receive general anesthesia for cesarean section. Regional anesthesia is contraindicated in hemorrhaging parturients with acute fetal distress, coagulopathy, or hypovolemia. Loss of compensatory mechanisms caused by the sympathectomy from regional anesthesia puts these patients at further risk. Hypotension is exacerbated by sympathectomy from regional anesthesia, ongoing hemorrhage, loss of compensatory mechanisms from sympathectomy, and use of magnesium for preeclampsia and preterm labor. If a patient is bleeding excessively under regional anesthesia, the airway should be secured electively. The anesthesia care team can then focus on massive volume resuscitation rather than dealing with airway management emergently during surgery. Massive volume resuscitation may result in airway edema, which can make tracheal intubation difficult if the surgery is performed under regional anesthesia, or may make tracheal extubation difficult at the end of surgery. Postoperatively, patients who have undergone massive volume resuscitation should be cared for in an intensive care unit.

Novel treatment options in severe hemorrhage

Uterine atony is a common cause of, or complication during, intractable obstetric hemorrhage. The uterine smooth muscle fails to contract after delivery of the fetus, resulting in hemorrhage from the dilated venous and arterial bleeders within the placenta. Pharmacologic treatment includes use of intravenous oxytocin, intramuscular methylergonovine, intramuscular 15-methyl prostaglandin $F_{2\alpha}$, and rectal misoprostol. If pharmacologic treatment fails, surgical therapy may be necessary, such as B-Lynch procedure, Bakri balloon placement, or hysterectomy.

The B-Lynch procedure involves suturing the uterus with a single, long, absorbable suture to avoid hysterectomy. The suture is run over the uterus to fold the uterus over itself, while compressing uterine blood vessels [42]. Bakri balloon, a fluid-filled balloon, inserted inside the uterine cavity to achieve hemostasis in cases of postpartum hemorrhage because of placenta previa/accreta, causes a tamponade effect and has been found useful in providing hemostasis [43]. Recently, the uterine sandwich technique, a combination of B-Lynch compression suture and Bakri balloon for patients who have uterine atony presenting with postpartum hemorrhage, has shown excellent results [44]. Hysterectomy may be the only option to control bleeding in uncontrolled hemorrhage.

Coagulation monitoring during massive obstetric hemorrhage is crucial to successful management. Thromboelastography has been used to detect coagulation defects associated with intraoperative blood loss in parturients and may help in monitoring coagulation parameters and reducing use of blood and blood components in hemorrhaging parturients [34,45].

Some blood conservation techniques that can be used rapidly and safely during intractable obstetric hemorrhage include acceptance of a lower hematocrit as a trigger for transfusion, erythrocyte salvage, rectal misoprostol, intravenous desmopressin, and intravenous recombinant factor VIIa. Additional techniques for hemorrhage prophylaxis, if time and hemodynamics allow, include use of preoperative subcutaneous recombinant erythropoietin [46,47], preoperative autologous blood donation [34,48], preoperative placement of bilateral hypogastric artery balloon catheters [49,50], and intraoperative autologous blood donation with acute normovolemic hemodilution [51].

Erythrocyte salvage has increased in obstetrics during the past few years. The main concern in obstetrics is amniotic fluid embolism [52–55]. Complete elimination of fetal squamous cells from filtered erythrocyte salvage suspension using a leukocyte reduction filter has been suggested [56].

Rectal administration of misoprostol has been recommended (1000 μg) as a means to control excessive blood loss during the third stage of labor [57]. Recommended doses of 400 to 600 μg (oral or per rectum) have had some success compared with placebo [58]. Intravenous desmopressin reduces intraoperative hemorrhage by increasing platelet aggregation [51,59]; the dosage is 0.15 to 0.3 μg/kg over 30 minutes.

Intravenous recombinant factor VIIa was recently reported to control intractable hemorrhage [60,61]. Its use in obstetrics is limited. It activates factor Xa production and increases the rate and amount of thrombin generation. The dosage is 60 μg/kg. It has a short half-life and redosing may be necessary.

Hypertension

Maternal morbidity and mortality statistics

Hypertensive disease affects roughly 6% to 8% of all pregnancies and is the second leading cause of maternal morbidity and mortality in the United States, whereas in the United Kingdom it ranks fourth. It accounts for almost 15% of pregnancy-related maternal deaths and is a major risk factor for fetal morbidity and mortality [62,63].

In the United Kingdom, although the trend has been toward a decline in maternal deaths from hypertension, 46% of patients showed clear evidence of substandard care in deaths that could have been avoidable. As the single largest cause of death, intracranial hemorrhage indicates failure of effective antihypertensive therapy. Late or failure to obtain consultation from an expert obstetrician was another factor in the mortality from hypertension.

Preeclampsia

Unique to humans, preeclampsia is a multiorgan disease of unknown origin. Symptoms present themselves in a normotensive woman after the 20th week of gestation. The risk for developing preeclampsia is greater in women who have preexisting conditions, such as chronic hypertension, diabetes, antiphospholipid syndrome, and collagen vascular disease.

Risk assessment

In risks associated with preeclampsia and eclampsia, the current CEM-ACH study (2000–2002) shows that among 14 accounted deaths from eclampsia and preeclampsia, 9 women died from intracranial hemorrhage, 1 from acute respiratory distress syndrome (ARDS), 2 from severe multiorgan failure, and 2 from disseminated intravascular coagulation [1]. Table 1 shows the causes of death compared with previous triennium reports. Risks from untreated hypertension, compounded by a low platelet count, place parturient women at increased risk for intracranial hemorrhage. Understanding the pathophysiology provides a basis for clinical and anesthetic management.

Table 1
Number of deaths by cause due to eclampsia and preeclampsia; United Kingdom 1988–2002

Cause of death	Triennium				
	1988–1990	1991–1993	1994–1996	1997–1999	2000–2002
Cerebral					
Intracranial hemorrhage	10	5	3	7	9
Subarachnoid	2	0	1	0	0
Infarct	2	0	0	0	0
Edema	0	0	3	0	0
Subtotal	14	5	7	7	9
Pulmonary					
ARDS	9	8	6	6	1
Edema	1	3	2	2	0
Subtotal	10	11	8	8	1
Hepatic					
Rupture	0	0	2	2	0
Failure/necrosis	1	0	1	1	0
Other	2	4	2	2	4
Subtotal	3	4	5	5	7
Total	27	20	20	20	14

From Neilson J. Pre-eclampsia and eclampsia. In: Confidential Enquiry into Maternal and Child Health. Why Mothers Die 2000–2002: the sixth report of the Confidential Enquiries into Maternal Death in the United Kingdom. London: RCOG Press; 2004. p. 79–84; with permission.

Complications from severe preeclampsia include pulmonary edema and the development of ARDS, resulting in maternal mortality. Pulmonary edema, both cardiogenic and noncardiogenic, is a serious complication of severe preeclampsia with an incidence of approximately 3% [64]. Cardiogenic pulmonary edema is caused by impaired left ventricular systolic or diastolic function and is more prevalent in patients who have severe chronic hypertension, valvular heart disease, or cardiomyopathy. Noncardiogenic pulmonary edema results from increased capillary permeability, iatrogenic fluid overload, an imbalance between colloid osmotic pressure and hydrostatic pressure, or a combination of these factors [65].

Strategies to minimize risk and prevent morbidity and mortality

Hospitalization and bed rest are effective treatment for women who have mild preeclampsia. The primary goals of minimizing the risks and goals of management include (1) prevention of convulsions, (2) control of hypertension, and (3) stabilization of cardiovascular status and optimization of intravascular volume.

Prevention of convulsions

Because of several positive effects, magnesium sulfate (Mg^{++}) remains the preferred prophylactic treatment for seizure in the United States and is gaining popularity in the United Kingdom [66]:

1. It depresses both central and peripheral nervous systems; its mechanism of action involves generalized central nervous system depression, which is mediated by N-methyl-D-aspartate receptors
2. It reduces hyperreflexia
3. It acts at the neuromuscular junction through decreasing the amount of acetylcholine liberated from the presynaptic junction, the sensitivity of the motor end plate to acetylcholine, and the excitability of muscle membrane
4. It produces mild to moderate vasodilation
5. It depresses uterine hyperactivity to improve uterine blood flow
6. It suppresses cortical neuronal burst firing and electroencephalographic spike generation
7. It opposes Ca^{++}-dependant arterial constriction and relieves vasospasm

Because Mg^{++} impairs peripheral neuromuscular transmission at the neuromuscular junction, the intensity of the neuromuscular block after muscle relaxants are administered during general anesthesia correlates with elevated serum magnesium and decreased serum calcium levels [67].

Control of hypertension

Another important goal is to control blood pressure to prevent exacerbation with the propensity for intracranial hemorrhage. Traditionally, the threshold for treating hypertension is a diastolic blood pressure of 105 to 110 mm Hg or a mean arterial pressure of 125 to 126 mm Hg. Diastolic blood pressure is a useful index of preeclampsia severity; current thinking is that the pressure during systole causes intracerebral hemorrhage. Recognition of this concept should be incorporated into guidelines to ensure effective reduction of systolic blood pressure. Therefore, the recommendation is for clinical protocols to identify a systolic blood pressure above which urgent and effective antihypertensive treatment is required [1].

Hydralazine. Hydralazine is no longer the preferred antihypertensive for acute blood pressure control during pregnancy. Recent studies have shown that it may decrease uterine blood flow by as much as 25% [68,69] and may be associated with neonatal thrombocytopenia [70]. Furthermore, the slow onset, delayed peak effect, and compensatory tachycardia make hydralazine a less than ideal agent for attenuating the hypertensive response to laryngoscopy and intubation during the administration of general anesthesia in women who have preeclampsia.

Labetalol. Labetalol a combined α- and β-adrenergic receptor antagonist (ratio 1:3 when given orally and 1:7 when given intravenously). Labetalol is found to be equally as, if not more, effective as hydralazine [71] in lowering the blood pressure. Labetalol decreases maternal systemic vascular resistance without increasing heart rate or decreasing cardiac index, uterine blood flow, or fetal heart rate [72]. The initial intravenous dose of labetalol is 10 to 20 mg, and this can be doubled every 10 minutes to a maximum dose of 300 mg. Labetalol crosses the placental barrier, but neonatal hypoglycemia and hypotension, initially believed to be a theoretic concern, are rarely seen [73]. Labetalol in doses of 1 mg/kg is effective in blunting the hypertensive response to tracheal intubation in patients who have preeclampsia undergoing general anesthesia [74].

Nicardipine, a calcium channel blocker, inhibits the influx of extracellular calcium into smooth muscle cells through the slow channels. The vascular effects predominate in arterial and arteriolar smooth muscle. Nicardipine has fewer negative inotropic effects and more selective action on peripheral vasculature than nifedipine, and effectively lowers blood pressure.

Optimization of intravascular volume

An important goal is to stabilize the patient's cardiovascular status and optimize the intravascular status, which includes (1) appropriate hemodynamic monitoring, (2) adequate volume resuscitation, and (3) adequate perfusion status. Evaluation of the patient's fluid balance must include a strict intake/output chart, placement of an indwelling urinary catheter, and (if possible) an assessment of the patient's current weight. The goal of fluid therapy is to provide an ideal intravascular volume, maintain a satisfactory urinary output, have immediate intravenous access for administration of therapeutic agents, and compensate for any reduction in preload and afterload during administration of epidural anesthesia.

A paucity of data exists regarding the ideal volume and type of intravenous fluid (crystalloid or colloid) for patients who have preeclampsia. Preeclampsia is associated with a complex set of hemodynamic changes, and predicting how patients will respond to fluid loading is difficult [75]. Excessive administration of crystalloid or colloid may result in pulmonary or cerebral edema. Little evidence shows that colloid preloading before regional anesthesia is more beneficial than crystalloid solutions. However, the use of certain colloids is debatable. A study comparing albumin use for plasma volume expansion versus no albumin in nonpregnant patients showed that albumin increased risk for death [76]. Similarly, increased mortality was associated with the use of colloid for resuscitation compared with crystalloid [77].

Invasive monitoring may become necessary in patients who have low urinary output whose preeclampsia does not respond to multiple fluid challenges, patients who have pulmonary edema, and those who have intractable hypertension [65].

Anesthetic management

Preanesthetic evaluation

It is important for the anesthesiologist, as part of the interdisciplinary team, to be involved early to help control hypertension, stabilize the hemodynamic status, and optimize intravascular resuscitation. It is also prudent to have a well-planned, yet flexible, anesthetic strategy, because the situation may change suddenly.

Maternal monitoring

For patients who have mild preeclampsia, close routine monitoring with pulse oximeter and automated blood pressure cuff are often sufficient. For those who have severe preeclampsia, a radial arterial catheter is recommended for accurate monitoring of arterial blood pressure and blood sampling (arterial blood gases, complete blood count with platelets, coagulation panel, renal and liver function tests, and appropriate drug levels).

Analgesia for labor and delivery

The appropriate anesthetic intervention, particularly with the well-timed placement of an epidural block, can minimize or negate the unnecessary hazards and risks for general anesthesia, including exacerbation of hypertension during induction, intubation, and emergence, and the problem of encountering difficult or failed intubation.

Other benefits of epidural labor analgesia include complete pain relief during labor; attenuation of any exaggerated hypertensive response to pain; reduction through sympathetic block of the circulating levels of catecholamines and stress-related hormones, which facilitates blood pressure control; vasodilation secondary to the sympathetic block, which improves intervillous blood flow; and stable cardiac output. Furthermore, the block can be extended to provide surgical anesthesia for instrumental or surgical delivery.

Maintenance of analgesia throughout labor can be accomplished with the use of a continuous infusion or patient-controlled epidural analgesia device. Currently, a mixture of a low concentration of bupivacaine (0.0625%) and a lipid-soluble narcotic such as fentanyl (2.0–2.5 µg/mL) has been shown to provide excellent sensory analgesia with minimal or no motor block [78]. Administration of 0.0625% or 0.125% bupivacaine with a lipid-soluble narcotic provides better analgesia than bupivacaine alone [79].

Anesthesia for cesarean section

General considerations

Patients who have preeclampsia scheduled for cesarean section have several important general considerations, including meticulous examination of the airway, administration of aspiration prophylaxis, availability of blood products, prevention of aortocaval compression, administration of increased FiO_2 (face mask), establishing a second peripheral intravenous line, immediate access to a difficult airway cart, application of standard American Society of Anesthesiologists (ASA) monitoring, invasive hemodynamic monitoring if required, and monitoring of the fetal heart rate pattern until the beginning of the surgery.

Regional anesthesia

Regional anesthesia (spinal or epidural) is the preferred method for cesarean deliveries because of the lower maternal morbidity compared to general anesthesia [80], it provides better hemodynamic control (to prevent exacerbation of blood pressure during induction and intubation), it blunts neuroendocrine stress response [81], patients are awake and able to interact with the infants, and it prevents transient neonatal depression associated with general anesthesia.

Epidural anesthesia is the regional anesthetic technique most commonly used for patients who have preeclampsia [82]. Investigators who have studied the systemic and pulmonary artery pressures in patients who have severe preeclampsia undergoing cesarean section have shown stable hemodynamic status with epidural anesthesia versus marked exacerbations in mean arterial pressure and pulmonary capillary wedge pressure during induction, intubation, and extubation with general anesthesia [82].

Ideally, in patients who have preeclampsia undergoing urgent cesarean section, a functioning epidural block should already be in place. The preexisting block can be augmented with either 3% 2-chloroprocaine or pH-adjusted 2% lidocaine to provide rapid surgical anesthesia. The fetal heart rate should be monitored in the operating room until immediately before preparation for and initiation of surgery. Several studies have shown the usefulness and safety of spinal anesthesia in patients who have severe preeclampsia undergoing cesarean section [83]. Furthermore, the hemodynamic effects of spinal anesthesia are also found to be stable [84–86]. The combined spinal and epidural technique has also been shown to be safe and effective in women who have severe preeclampsia undergoing cesarean section [87].

General anesthesia

General anesthesia is required in cases of nonreassuring fetal heart rate requiring emergency cesarean section (no preexisting epidural catheter), coagulopathy that precludes the use of regional anesthesia, and patient refusal of regional anesthesia. The risks for general anesthesia in women who have preeclampsia include difficult tracheal intubation, the potential for aspiration of gastric contents, exacerbated hypertensive response to endotracheal intubation, impairment of intervillous blood flow, and drug interaction between magnesium and muscle relaxants.

Airway evaluation in patients who have preeclampsia undergoing general anesthesia is critical because endotracheal intubation may be difficult. Two of four maternal deaths in 442 cases reviewed [88] resulted from cerebral hypoxia secondary to failed intubation. Therefore, airway evaluation is crucial and a predicted difficult airway requires appropriate airway management preparation. The authors recently reported the successful use of intubating laryngeal mask (ILMA) after a failed tracheal intubation in a patient who had eclampsia undergoing emergency cesarean section. Rapid intervention with the ILMA averted maternal and fetal catastrophes and resulted in a positive outcome for mother and baby [89].

General anesthesia used in patients who have preeclampsia with hypertension causes exacerbation of blood pressure from stimulation during laryngoscopy, tracheal intubation, and surgical incision. Any acute increase in blood pressure, particularly in the face of coagulopathy, places the patient at risk for intracranial hemorrhage. Other reasons to attenuate the hypertensive response include a maternal risk for increased myocardial oxygen consumption leading to myocardial infarction, cardiac arrhythmias, and pulmonary edema. The fetus is also at risk from maternal hypertensive surges secondary to a significant reduction in uterine blood flow [90].

Postoperative care/critical care

After labor and delivery, all patients who have preeclampsia should be monitored in the recovery room or obstetric intensive care unit for the next 24 hours or until adequate diuresis is established. Management of a subset of patients who have severe preeclampsia/eclampsia and HELLP syndrome who are critically ill requires involvement of a multidisciplinary team, including the obstetric, anesthetic, and critical care teams. Reassessment of this subgroup of critically ill patients in the immediate postpartum period is essential because of the high mortality rate. Patients who have multiorgan failure ARDS resulting from severe preeclampsia require postoperative mechanical ventilation [91] in the intensive care unit. Successful management of these patients who have high-risk severe preeclampsia/ eclampsia requires good communication among the obstetric, anesthesia, neonatology, nursing, and critical care teams.

Anesthesia-related maternal mortality

Anesthesia-related death is the seventh leading direct cause of maternal mortality in the United States and United Kingdom, and accounts for 1.6% of all pregnancy-related deaths in the United States [3,29]. Since the 1980s, a significant reduction has been seen in anesthesia-related maternal deaths, with the success being attributed to increased use of regional anesthesia, the widely adopted policy of limiting oral intake during labor, and the effective measure of providing aspiration prophylaxis before operative delivery. In the current CEMACH study [1], six direct deaths that were associated with general anesthesia, suggesting a risk of 1 death per 20,000 maternal general anesthetics administered, similar to the statistics reported in the 1982 to 1984 triennium [1]. Most anesthesia-related deaths in United States and United Kingdom are associated with general anesthesia for operative delivery and are related to difficult/failed intubation. Difficult pulmonary ventilation, resulting in failure to oxygenate, or pulmonary aspiration remain the primary factors responsible for anesthesia-related maternal mortality [29,92]. A maternal death is devastating to all involved; however, in obstetric patients (parturients), mortality is 200% (mother and baby) with significant medicolegal implications.

There were no direct deaths attributed to regional anesthesia in this triennium. However, as the use of general anesthesia in obstetrics continues to decline, the anesthesia trainees' experience in basic airway management in obstetrics also continues to decline. Given the fact that 80% of anesthesia-related fatalities occur during emergency cesarean sections, the incidence of failed intubation is higher during emergencies that occur during nights and weekends. The CEMACH report highlighted the lack of supervision of trainees during emergencies as an area of concern.

Protocols to manage difficult or failed tracheal intubation in obstetric anesthesia are absolutely essential. Every anesthesia practitioner must have a preformulated strategy before induction to deal with a difficult or failed intubation. The decision to abandon repeated attempts at tracheal intubation must be made promptly. The importance of prompt and competent decision making in these critical situations, having appropriate equipment immediately available in the labor and delivery suite operating room to deal with a difficult airway, and having advanced airway skills cannot be overemphasized.

Airway

Risk assessment

Pregnancy produces several anatomic and physiologic changes in the body, resulting in an increased risk for airway-related complications and pulmonary aspiration. Rocke and colleagues [93] suggested using the relative risk score to allow better prediction of difficult tracheal intubation in obstetric patients. This landmark study of obstetric patients showed that the relative risk for experiencing a difficult tracheal intubation compared with an uncomplicated class I airway assessment (risk ratio of 1.0) increased to 3.23 with class II; 7.58 with class III; 11.3 with class IV; 5.01 with a short neck indicating decreased mobility of neck; 8.0 with protruding maxillary incisors; and 9.71 with a receding mandible indicating decreased thyromental distance. Using the combination of risk factors showed that a combination of either Mallampati class III or IV airway plus protruding incisors, short neck, or receding mandible predicted a greater than 90% probability of encountering a difficult laryngoscopy. Other risk factors during pregnancy include, weight gain in pregnancy, increased breast size, and obesity. When these risk factors are encountered with a parturient who has a greater than 90% probability prediction of having a difficult airway, anesthesiologists should have a preformulated plan for dealing with a difficult airway or failed tracheal intubation.

In a recent review of maternal deaths in Michigan [94], anesthesia was the primary cause in eight of these deaths. However, no maternal deaths were associated with failed intubation during induction or with aspiration. Rather, all eight deaths occurred during emergence and recovery, which is becoming more frequent in surgical patients.

Strategies to minimize risk and prevent morbidity and mortality

Because most anesthesia-related deaths occur during operative delivery, strategies must be outlined to manage difficult or failed tracheal intubation. An emergency cesarean delivery is undertaken for either maternal or fetal indications, or both. Maternal hemorrhage or fetal distress dictates the need for an emergent or urgent delivery. Even in an emergency situation, a quick preanesthetic evaluation and determination of a difficult airway is possible, thus allowing for appropriate airway management [95].

The ASA Task force recently published a difficult airway algorithm (DAA) [96] for managing the difficult airway. The ASA Practice Guidelines for Obstetrical Anesthesia [97] recommend that labor and delivery units should have equipment (eg, basic airways, laryngeal mask airway [LMA], Combitube) and personnel readily available to manage airway emergencies, including during regional anesthesia. These resources can provide life-saving oxygenation and pulmonary ventilation, enable access for securing the airway to prevent pulmonary aspiration, and reduce the incidence of maternal complications [98].

Fundamental steps outlined in the ASA/DAA can be applied to special situations, such as obstetric anesthesia. Prioritizing the airway management strategies after a failed initial attempt at tracheal intubation can influence the final outcome for mother and baby. The priorities and management goals after a failed initial attempt should be (1) maternal oxygenation, and thereby fetal oxygenation, (2) airway protection, (3) prevention of pulmonary aspiration, and (4) expeditious delivery. The flow chart for an unanticipated, difficult, or failed tracheal intubation is shown in Fig. 3.

After failed tracheal intubation, the DAA recommends calling for help, returning to spontaneous ventilation, or awakening the patient. In all but the most urgent situations (eg, maternal hemorrhage or severe fetal distress), the mother is awakened after the failed first attempt and the fetus is reassessed (see Fig. 3). However, in an acute emergency (eg, umbilical cord prolapse and severe fetal distress) awakening the patient may not be possible. Therefore, balancing the priorities of oxygenation, prevention of pulmonary aspiration, and delivery of the fetus become critical (see Fig. 3).

Oxygenation becomes extremely critical. If pulmonary ventilation using conventional facemask is successful, a quick assessment for failed tracheal intubation should be performed to enhance the success rate of the second attempt. Failure to visualize the cords may be related to incorrect positioning, inadequate laryngoscopy, inadequate muscle relaxation, or failure to apply adequate external laryngeal pressure.

The recommendation is that the second attempt at laryngoscopy be considered the best attempt at intubation. To increase the success rate, it should be performed by a reasonably experienced anesthesiologist, the optimal sniff position used, and external laryngeal manipulation applied. Additionally, the laryngoscope blade type and handle may need to be changed.

If the best attempt at tracheal intubation is unsuccessful, a third attempt is really not an option in this emergent scenario; nonsurgical airway management techniques that allow ventilation and oxygenation must be implemented immediately. These approaches include the use of LMA for the nonemergency pathway (cannot intubate/can ventilate), and the Combitube, rigid scopes, and transtracheal jet ventilation for the emergency pathway (cannot intubate /cannot ventilate). After failed conventional facemask ventilation and tracheal intubation, the ASA/DAA recommends the use of the LMA [95].

Laryngeal mask airway
Classic laryngeal mask airway. The classic LMA has been widely used for difficult obstetric airways [99–104] without any episodes of gastric regurgitation or pulmonary aspiration. In parturients undergoing elective cesarean

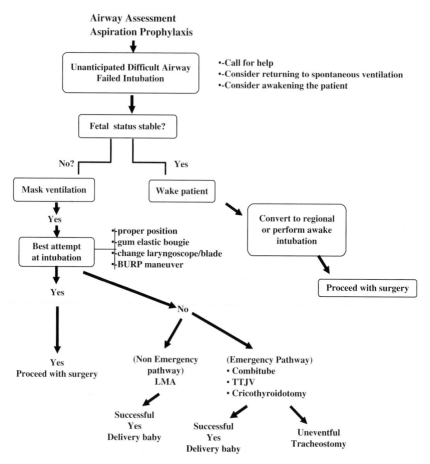

Fig. 3. Algorithm for an unanticipated difficult or failed intubation in a parturient undergoing an emergency cesarean section, with special emphasis on the goals of maintaining maternal oxygenation, airway protection, and delivery of the baby. BURP, backwards, upwards, rightwards pressure; LMA, laryngeal mask airway; TTJV, transtracheal jet ventilation.

delivery, Han and colleagues [105] reported the successful use of the classic LMA as a ventilatory device in 1060 of 1067 patients. No episodes of hypoxia, regurgitation, or aspiration occurred [105]. The successful use of the classic LMA after failed tracheal intubation in obstetrics has been reported in 17 instances.

Intubation through classic laryngeal mask airway. In patients requiring tracheal intubation, fiberoptic-guided tracheal intubation through the classic LMA is reliable [106]. However, a longer tracheal tube (eg, Endotrol, microlaryngeal, or nasal Ring-Adair-Elwyn) is needed. The Cook Aintree catheter

(Bloomington, Illinois) may also be used to facilitate intubation through the classic LMA.

Intubating laryngeal mask airway. The LMA Fastrach or Intubating LMA (ILMA) is designed to specifically overcome the problems associated with blind tracheal intubation through the classic LMA [107]. The ILMA is particularly useful during failed intubation in an emergency cesarean section because it provides oxygenation and a conduit for tracheal intubation, and prevents pulmonary aspiration. Several studies have shown the successful use of ILMA to help visually unassisted tracheal intubation in patients who have difficult airways [106–108]. The ILMA was used successfully after failed tracheal intubation during an emergency cesarean section in a patient who was morbidly obese and eclamptic [109]. The authors had a second case in which regional anesthesia had failed and was followed by general anesthesia, resulting in failed tracheal intubation. The ILMA again proved to be a life-saving device.

ProSeal laryngeal mask airway. The ProSeal LMA is a new, unique device that represents a substantial change in LMA design. The ProSeal LMA offers several advantages over the classic LMA for failed tracheal intubation in obstetrics: (1) the seal is 10 cm H_2O higher, giving it greater ventilatory capability [110]; (2) it enables correct positioning, isolating the glottis from the esophagus, and therefore may provide airway protection and protect against pulmonary aspiration [111,112]; (3) a gastric tube can be easily inserted to empty the stomach of fluid and air insufflated during difficult face mask ventilation. The ProSeal LMA has been used successfully in at least six case reports after failed intubation during emergency cesarean sections [111,113–117]. After failed tracheal intubation, and once the anesthesia practitioner is able to successfully achieve pulmonary ventilation and oxygenation, caution must be used in selecting a nonirritating inhalation anesthetic and an adequate depth of anesthesia. Recent studies show that sevoflurane provides rapid, smooth induction; adequate depth of anesthesia; and is the least irritating agent [118], and helps facilitate tracheal intubation through the LMA in patients who have a difficult airway [119].

Combitube. The Combitube should be considered in emergency airway situations, especially when patients are at risk for pulmonary aspiration and tracheal intubation has failed [120,121]. The DAA suggests using Combitube after failed pulmonary ventilation with conventional facemask and LMA [95]. The successful use of the Combitube has been described after failed tracheal intubation in an emergency cesarean section [120].

The DAA incorporated the use of Combitube in the emergency pathway (ie, the life-threatening "cannot ventilate, cannot intubate" situation. This situation is encountered in approximately 1 of 100,000 cases, and establishing ventilation and oxygenation is critical. Similarly, it may also be particularly

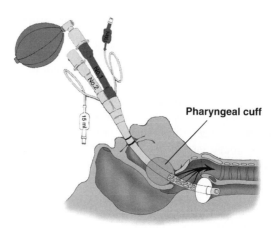

Fig. 4. Combitube in esophagus. The tube is advanced until the black rings are at the level of the teeth. The distal cuff is inflated with 10 mL of air to seal the esophagus, and the proximal cuff is inflated with 80 mL of air, securing the tube in position and occluding the nasal and oral passages. Ventilation is attempted through lumen.1. (*Courtesy of* Baylor College of Medicine, Houston, TX; with permission.)

useful for difficult or failed tracheal intubations in obstetric patients, who are especially at risk for gastric regurgitation and pulmonary aspiration. The Combitube may offer significant advantages over the LMA in the parturient. These advantages include isolation of the stomach from the glottic area and minimal preparation. Oxygenation and pulmonary ventilation can be achieved rapidly, especially because the parturient is prone to rapid arterial oxygen desaturation. The Combitube is shown to prevent pulmonary aspiration during cardiopulmonary resuscitation [122] and protect the airway from pulmonary aspiration of gastric contents during anesthesia [123]. Combitube

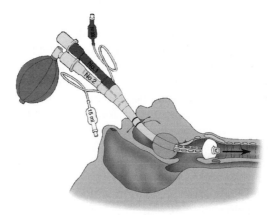

Fig. 5. Combitube placement in trachea. The Combitube is placed in trachea; the ventilation is shifted to lumen No. 2. (*Courtesy of* Baylor College of Medicine, Houston, TX; with permission.)

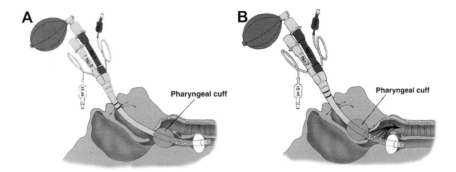

Fig. 6. (*A*) Improper placement of Combitube. Excessive insertion depth of the Combitube, causing obstruction of the glottic opening. Ventilation is not possible. (*B*) Correct position of the Combitube in the esophagus after readjustment. The Combitube is pulled back 2 cm (indicated by the two black rings) and ventilation from the side orifices into the trachea. (*Courtesy of* Baylor College of Medicine, Houston, TX; with permission.)

is a disposable double-lumen tube with two cuffs designed for blind insertion. Ventilation is initially attempted through lumen 1, which forces air into the trachea (Fig. 4).

Causes of failed ventilation with the Combitube include inadvertent tracheal placement (5%), deep insertion laryngospasm, and bronchospasm. The steps to troubleshoot are important to understand, especially when confronted with a critical airway. The Combitube is designed to enter the esophagus after blind insertion. If ventilation is difficult through the blue lumen 1, the Combitube could be in the trachea, which requires switching ventilation to the clear lumen 2, allowing air to enter the trachea directly through the open end (Fig. 5). Sometimes the Combitube is inserted too deep, in which case the pharyngeal balloon must be deflated, the Combitube pulled back 1 to 2 cm, and ventilation switched back to the blue lumen (Fig. 6A, B).

Other airway devices

Other airway devices include the LaryngealTube S (LTS) and the Airtraq. The LTS is a new supraglottic airway device. It has a second lumen for suctioning and gastric drainage. It may provide higher airway seal pressures than a classic LMA. In contrast to Combitube, it has only one adapter for ventilation. LTS may be useful in situations and patients who are at risk for aspiration. In a recent report, the LTS was used successfully to establish ventilation and oxygenation after failed intubation in an emergency cesarean section [124].

The Airtraq is a new disposable intubating laryngoscope. It is designed to provide a view of the glottis without alignment of oral, pharyngeal, and tracheal axes. Two cases of rapid tracheal intubation with Airtraq laryngoscope have been reported recently in morbidly obese parturients undergoing emergency cesarean delivery after failed tracheal intubation [125].

Cricothyroidotomy and transtracheal jet ventilation

When oxygenation and ventilation are not established with either the LMA or Combitube, this presents a grave life-threatening cannot ventilate, cannot intubate situation, and more invasive techniques such as cricothyroidotomy or transtracheal jet ventilation may become necessary [126].

Extubation

Having a strategy established for extubating the airway after difficult airway/failed tracheal intubation, including using an airway exchange catheter, is as crucial as the alternative plan for difficult tracheal intubation [95,127].

Local anesthetic toxicity

The problem of maternal deaths associated with local anesthetic toxicity has almost been eliminated in obstetrics.

Risk assessment

Almost 30 years ago, Albright [128] was the first to report several cases of fatal cardiac toxicity associated with use of the long-acting lipophilic local anesthetics, bupivacaine, and etidocaine in pregnant women. His editorial and a second one in 1984 [129], outlining scientific investigations and evidence of fatal cardiotoxicity, led to the eventual U.S. Food and Drug Administration withdrawal of 0.75% bupivacaine for epidural anesthesia in obstetrics. The common theme in those fatalities, who were otherwise healthy patients, was the apparent lack of response to standard resuscitative measures. Albright was prescient in his observation that both bupivacaine and etidocaine are lipophilic, a physical characteristic that has since been shown to correlate with particularly intransigent cardiac toxicity among local anesthetics [130].

Strategies to minimize risk and prevent morbidity and mortality

Albright's scientific observation led to implementation of practice standards that have reduced the incidence of cardiovascular catastrophes after local anesthetic use. These guidelines include implementing fractionated test doses, thus replacing the administration of concentrated local anesthetics as a bolus; an epinephrine-containing test dose to detect intravascular injection of local anesthetic through epidural catheter, and use of safe dose limits.

Clinical features of local anesthetic toxicity

The earliest clinical manifestations of local anesthetic toxicity include lightheadedness, altered mental status, agitation, slurred speech, and visual disturbance [131]. Early changes in vital signs include tachycardia and hypertension [131]. The clinical presentation of more severe toxicity is classically a combination of central nervous system excitation, cardiac arrhythmias, conduction blockade, and myocardial depression. Typically severe bupivacaine cardiac toxicity presents as hypotension with bradycardia leading quickly to malignant ventricular arrhythmias and cardiovascular collapse that is highly resistant to standard resuscitation [128,132]. Most recommended drugs are supportive: sympathomimetics for blood pressure and inotropic support, and amiodarone for arrhythmias [130]. Use of β-adrenoceptor antagonists, calcium channel agonists, and local anesthetics for treating rhythm disturbances from local anesthesia toxicity are contraindicated.

Mechanism of toxicity

The standard model, established by Clarkson and Hondeghem [133], holds that the pronounced inhibition of cardiac voltage–gated sodium ion channels accounts for the differential toxicity of bupivacaine. Furthermore, it is well established that hypoxia exacerbates bupivacaine toxicity [134], suggesting that respiration is a clinically important target of bupivacaine.

Lipid reversal resuscitation

Animal studies have shown successful resuscitation from local anesthetic toxicity with the administration of lipid solutions. These observations suggest that lipid infusion might be useful in treating local anesthetic toxicity, and a recent editorial [135] described lipid rescue as a possible "silver bullet" for bupivacaine overdose.

Mechanisms of lipid rescue

Lipid-treated hearts showed a more rapid decline in myocardial bupivacaine content than controls; mean time constants (95% CIs) were 37 [32,43] and 83 seconds [66,107] for lipid-treated and control hearts, respectively (n = 5 for both groups, $P < .0002$). Stehr and colleagues [136] recently found in isolated rat hearts that lipid emulsion reverses bupivacaine-induced contractile depression at concentrations that are too low to provide a lipid sink effect, thus proposing a metabolic explanation for this beneficial effect.

Recommendations based on evidence of clinical efficacy for lipid rescue resuscitation

Given the highly reproducible benefit in reversing animal models of bupivacaine-induced toxicity, some have suggested that lipid emulsion should be stocked at sites where regional anesthesia is performed [137]. Currently, 0.5% bupivacaine is used for patients undergoing cesarean section with epidural anesthesia. Therefore, educating anesthesiologists is the first step to achieving this goal. Secondly, stocking lipid solutions in all labor and delivery suites is recommended. Experts have proposed that lipid be stocked and kept with a recommended dosing regimen in operating rooms and locations where regional anesthesia is performed.

Lipid infusion is reserved for use in cardiac arrest caused by local anesthetic toxicity that resists standard resuscitative measures. If asystole, malignant arrhythmias, or severe hypotension persist, standard advanced cardiac life support (including ventilation with 100% oxygen and chest compressions) should be continued, and then 20% intralipid intravenously should be infused a bolus injection of 1.5 mL/kg, followed by continuous infusion 0.25 mL/kg per minute for 30 minutes. If no improvement is seen, the bolus should be repeated one to two times. For declining blood pressure, rate of infusion should be increased to 0.5 mL/kg per minute. Once sinus rhythm is restored, ventricular ectopy or other arrhythmias may persist, but additional bolus doses are probably not required. The infusion should continue for a full hour and may need to be restarted if blood pressure declines after it is stopped.

Propofol is formulated with 10% lipid and has been reported to improve bupivacaine toxicity, which has prompted some clinicians to consider, or perhaps confuse, using propofol as a lipid source during resuscitation from bupivacaine toxicity. However, propofol should not be used when there is any sign of cardiac compromise.

Infusing a lipid emulsion during resuscitation from local anesthetic toxicity reliably rescues animals from overwhelming and otherwise fatal bupivacaine overdose. Recent case reports of clinical efficacy of lipid rescue resuscitation [130] support the value of this technique in treating patients who have severe local anesthetic toxicity. To improve survival from this potentially catastrophic complication of regional anesthesia, general use of the regimen for treating local anesthetic cardiac toxicity should be incorporated into the standard approach for treating local anesthetic systemic toxicity.

Obesity

Maternal morbidity and mortality statistics

Obesity has increased worldwide, especially in developed countries, over the past decade. In the United States, one third of adult women were found to be obese based on the 1999–2002 National Health and Nutrition examination survey [138]. Additionally, women are delaying pregnancy until after 35 years of age, further compounding comorbidities [96,139]. Obese women also have a propensity to pregnancy-related complications, such as gestational diabetes, gestational hypertension, preeclampsia, fetal macrosomia, shoulder dystocia, failure to progress during labor [140–143], cesarean section [142], and spontaneous abortion after natural conception [144] or infertility treatment [145]. Intraoperative complications in obese parturients include prolonged operative time and excessive hemorrhage [146]. Postoperative complications include endometritis, obstructive sleep apnea [96,139], and wound infection [147]. Problems associated with regional and local anesthesia are increased in the obese parturient [148]. A maternal mortality review in Michigan from 1985 to 2003 showed eight anesthesia-related deaths; 75% of the patients were obese (body mass index >30) and 75% were African American [94], suggesting body weight and race are incriminating factors. Obesity increases the risk for death during pregnancy [149] and obstetric anesthesia [150].

Risk assessment

Prepregnancy education is vital for obese women to have a successful and safe outcome for mother and baby. Obstetricians must discuss the importance of weight reduction, dietary planning, exercise regime, and behavior modification with their obese patients before they become pregnant [151]. Obese parturients should also be counseled about possible obstetric complications and worsening of preexisting medical comorbidities in the peripartum period. Screening for gestational diabetes should be provided at the earliest possible stage and followed up later. Obstetricians must educate obese parturients about intrapartum difficulties, such as estimating fetal weight, external fetal heart rate monitoring and tocodynamometry, and fetal access during emergency cesarean section [151].

Strategies to minimize risk and recommendations

Pregnancy-related complications, such as gestational diabetes, gestational hypertension, and preeclampsia, are greater in the pregnant patients who are obese. The incidence of fetal complications, such as prematurity, stillbirths, and neural tube defects, is higher in maternal obesity [140,152]. Fetal macrosomia is a common finding in obese parturients [153]. Cesarean section is recommended for fetal macrosomia (fetal weight > 5000 g in the nondiabetic parturient [154] and fetal weight > 4500 g in the diabetic parturient) [155]. Obstetricians must obtain multidisciplinary consultation from anesthesiology [156], neonatology, and cardiology [157] services. An anesthesiology consultation, early in labor, allows adequate time to develop an anesthetic plan [151]. Anesthetic challenges include difficult intravenous and arterial access, difficult sizing of noninvasive blood pressure cuff, positioning issues for regional and general anesthesia, transportation problems, and finding an adequately sized Herculean operating table. Obese parturients should receive aspiration and thromboembolism prophylaxis [151]. Antibiotic prophylaxis is recommended for elective and emergency cesarean section because of the higher incidence of wound dehiscence and infections in obese parturients [147]. Additional blood products may need to be available, because incidence of intraoperative hemorrhage is higher [146].

Neuraxial analgesia for labor and delivery may be provided through continuous epidural analgesia or continuous spinal analgesia. Combined spinal epidural technique is not desirable because of an untested epidural catheter in the first few hours after the initial spinal injection. A continuous neuraxial (epidural or spinal) catheter technique in labor allows for extension to continuous neuraxial anesthesia for cesarean section. Obese parturients are at risk for an unplanned cesarean section, difficult neuraxial block placement, and difficult airway management [148]. Hence, a well-functioning neuraxial catheter is essential to proceed safely with an urgent or emergent cesarean section [158]. Neuraxial analgesia issues include difficulty identifying landmarks, which may require use of ultrasound guidance [159] with a 5.0 MHz curved array probe, and use of long neuraxial needles to identify the epidural space or obtain cerebrospinal fluid [148].

General anesthesia in the obese parturient has the compounded risk for pregnancy-related airway complications, obesity-related airway complications, and airway complications related to other comorbidities, such as pre-eclampsia and diabetes. Airway management strategies should include optimizing patient positioning, using a ramped pillow (straight line between sternal notch to external auditory meatus), an easily accessible difficult airway cart, and availability of experienced anesthesia personnel. The difficult airway cart should be stocked with 6- or 7-mm tracheal tubes, short-handle laryngoscope, Eschmann bougie, Levitan scope (fiberoptic stylet), videolaryngoscope, intubating laryngeal mask airway, Combitube, cricothyrotomy kit, and equipment for transtracheal jet ventilation [160,161].

Postoperatively, patients should be advised about the use of elastic compression stockings, adequate hydration, incentive spirometry, and early ambulation. Adequate analgesia must be provided, preferably neuraxially, to minimize postoperative pulmonary complications [162]. Dietetic education, exercise regimes, and weight reduction planning must be continued in the puerperium [151].

Summary

Maternal deaths in developed countries continue to decline and are rare. Maternal mortality statistics are essentially similar in the United States and United Kingdom. However, the situation is completely different in developing countries, where maternal mortality exceeds 0.5 million every year [163]. This article not only assesses morbidity risks in some of the leading causes of maternal death but also highlights strategies to minimize the risks and prevent maternal morbidity and mortality.

Venous thromboembolism is the leading cause of direct maternal mortality. Risk evaluation and reduction should begin before pregnancy and continue during and after pregnancy. LWMH is the preferred method for prophylaxis and treatment.

Obstetric hemorrhage can be life-threatening. Novel treatments, including nonsurgical and surgical options, should be attempted before cesarean hysterectomy, especially in young patients who desire future pregnancy. Excellent communication and teamwork among obstetric, anesthesia, nursing, and blood bank teams is critical for successful outcome.

Airway-related issues in obstetrics during induction and emergence continue to be problematic. Preoperative airway evaluation, risk assessment, having a preformulated strategy to deal with difficult or failed tracheal intubation, and acquisition of advanced airway skills are critical to avoid maternal morbidity and mortality from airway catastrophes.

Preeclampsia poses serious threats to mother and fetus. The dangers of high systolic blood pressure leading to intracranial hemorrhage require greater recognition and timely antihypertensive intervention. Magnesium sulfate is the preferred anticonvulsant. To avoid potentially serious consequences of fluid overload, careful monitoring of fluid input and output and invasive monitoring are essential. Regional anesthesia is the preferred technique, and offers several advantages over general anesthesia.

Finally, the virtual elimination of local anesthetic toxicity, particularly in obstetrics, is an anesthesia-related success story. Therefore, a heightened awareness of risks, proper communication among disciplines, and a multidisciplinary team approach toward the care of high-risk parturients helps physicians not only execute appropriate care and elevate standard care but also ensures safe outcomes for mothers and babies. Obesity, a growing epidemic, increases anesthesia-related maternal and fetal risks. Preoperative airway evaluation and functional neuraxial analgesia are critical in the safe management of mother and baby. Dietetic modification and behavioral therapy should be undertaken in the peripartum period.

References

[1] Confidential Enquiry into Maternal and Child Health. Why mothers die 2000–2002: the sixth report of the confidential enquiries into maternal death in the United Kingdom. London: RCOG Press; 2004.

[2] de Swiet M. Maternal mortality: confidential enquiries into maternal deaths in the United Kingdom. Am J Obstet Gynecol 2000;182(4):760–6.

[3] Berg CJ, Chang J, Callaghan WM, et al. Pregnancy-related mortality in the United States, 1991–1997. Obstet Gynecol 2003;101(2):289–96.

[4] Chang J, Elam-Evans LD, Berg CJ, et al. Pregnancy-related mortality surveillance—United States, 1991–1999. MMWR Surveill Summ 2003;52(2):1–8.

[5] Lindqvist P, Dahlback B, Marsal K. Thrombotic risk during pregnancy: a population study. Obstet Gynecol 1999;94(4):595–9.

[6] Simpson EL, Lawrenson RA, Nightingale AL, et al. Venous thromboembolism in pregnancy and the puerperium: incidence and additional risk factors from a London perinatal database. BJOG 2001;108(1):56–60.

[7] Clyburn PA. Early thoughts on 'Why Mothers Die 2000–2002'. Anaesthesia 2004;59(12): 1157–9.

[8] Weiner CP. Diagnosis and management of thromboembolic disease during pregnancy. Clin Obstet Gynecol 1985;28(1):107–18.

[9] Barbour LA, Pickard J. Controversies in thromboembolic disease during pregnancy: a critical review. Obstet Gynecol 1995;86(4 Pt 1):621–33.

[10] Malinow A. Embolic disorders. In: Chestnut DH, editor. Obstetric anesthesia principles and practice. Philadelphia: Elsevier Mosby; 2004. p. 683–94.

[11] Nelson SM, Greer IA. Thromboembolic events in pregnancy: pharmacological prophylaxis and treatment. Expert Opin Pharmacother 2007;8(17):2917–31.

[12] Darvall KA, Sam RC, Silverman SH, et al. Obesity and thrombosis. Eur J Vasc Endovasc Surg 2007;33(2):223–33.

[13] Larsen TB, Sorensen HT, Gislum M, et al. Maternal smoking, obesity, and risk of venous thromboembolism during pregnancy and the puerperium: a population-based nested case-control study. Thromb Res 2007;120(4):505–9.

[14] Casele H, Grobman WA. Cost-effectiveness of thromboprophylaxis with intermittent pneumatic compression at cesarean delivery. Obstet Gynecol 2006;108(3 Pt 1):535–40.

[15] Kakkos SK, Daskalopoulou SS, Daskalopoulos ME, et al. Review on the value of graduated elastic compression stockings after deep vein thrombosis. Thromb Haemost 2006; 96(4):441–5.

[16] Chunilal SD, Young E, Johnston MA, et al. The APTT response of pregnant plasma to unfractionated heparin. Thromb Haemost 2002;87(1):92–7.

[17] Rodie VA, Thomson AJ, Stewart FM, et al. Low molecular weight heparin for the treatment of venous thromboembolism in pregnancy: a case series. BJOG 2002;109(9):1020–4.

[18] Warkentin TE, Greinacher A. Heparin-induced thrombocytopenia: recognition, treatment, and prevention: the Seventh ACCP Conference on Antithrombotic and Thrombolytic Therapy. Chest 2004;126(Suppl 3):311S–37S.

[19] Murray WJ, Lindo VS, Kakkar VV, et al. Long-term administration of heparin and heparin fractions and osteoporosis in experimental animals. Blood Coagul Fibrinolysis 1995;6(2): 113–8.

[20] Greer I, Hunt BJ. Low molecular weight heparin in pregnancy: current issues. Br J Haematol 2005;128(5):593–601.

[21] Imperiale TF, Petrulis AS. A meta-analysis of low-dose aspirin for the prevention of pregnancy-induced hypertensive disease. J Am Med Assoc 1991;266(2):260–4.

[22] Klinzing P, Markert UR, Liesaus K, et al. Case report: successful pregnancy and delivery after myocardial infarction and essential thrombocythemia treated with clopidogrel. Clin Exp Obstet Gynecol 2001;28(4):215–6.

[23] Ueno M, Masuda H, Nakamura K, et al. Antiplatelet therapy for a pregnant woman with a mechanical aortic valve: report of a case. Surg Today 2001;31(11):1002–4.

[24] Bates SM, Greer IA, Hirsh J, et al. Use of antithrombotic agents during pregnancy: the Seventh ACCP Conference on Antithrombotic and Thrombolytic Therapy. Chest 2004; 126(Suppl 3):627S–44S.

[25] Greer IA, Nelson-Piercy C. Low-molecular-weight heparins for thromboprophylaxis and treatment of venous thromboembolism in pregnancy: a systematic review of safety and efficacy. Blood 2005;106(2):401–7.

[26] Horlocker TT, Wedel DJ, Benzon H, et al. Regional anesthesia in the anticoagulated patient: defining the risks (the second ASRA Consensus Conference on Neuraxial Anesthesia and Anticoagulation). Reg Anesth Pain Med 2003;28(3):172–97.

[27] Pillny M, Sandmann W, Luther B, et al. Deep venous thrombosis during pregnancy and after delivery: indications for and results of thrombectomy. J Vasc Surg 2003;37(3): 528–32.

[28] Jamjute P, Reed N, Hinwood D. Use of inferior vena cava filters in thromboembolic disease during labor: case report with a literature review. J Matern Fetal Neonatal Med 2006; 19(11):741–4.

[29] Hawkins JL. Anesthesia-related maternal mortality. Clin Obstet Gynecol 2003;46(3): 679–87.

[30] NCCDPHP, CDC. State-specific maternal mortality among black and white women— United States, 1987–1996. MMWR Morb Mortal Wkly Rep 1999;48:492–6.

[31] ACOG Practice Bulletin. Clinical management guidelines for obstetrician-gynecologists number 76, October 2006: postpartum hemorrhage. Obstet Gynecol 2006;108(4):1039–47.

[32] Waterstone M, Bewley S, Wolfe C. Incidence and predictors of severe obstetric morbidity: case-control study. BMJ 2001;322(7294):1089–93.

[33] Li XF, Fortney JA, Kotelchuck M, et al. The postpartum period: the key to maternal mortality. Int J Gynaecol Obstet 1996;54(1):1–10.

[34] Wali A, Suresh MS, Gregg AR. Antepartum Hemorrhage. In: Datta S, editor. Anesthetic and obstetric management of high-risk pregnancy; 2004. p. 87–111.

[35] American College of Obstetricians and Gynecologists. Hemorrhagic shock. ACOG Technical Bulletin No 82, Washington, DC. The College 1984;1:82.

[36] King PA, Duthie SJ, Dong ZG, et al. Secondary postpartum haemorrhage. Aust N Z J Obstet Gynaecol 1989;29(4):394–8.

[37] Chattopadhyay SK, Kharif H, Sherbeeni MM. Placenta praevia and accreta after previous caesarean section. Eur J Obstet Gynecol Reprod Biol 1993;52(3):151–6.

[38] Clark SL, Koonings PP, Phelan JP. Placenta previa/accreta and prior cesarean section. Obstet Gynecol 1985;66(1):89–92.

[39] Mayer D, Spielman FBE. Antepartum and postpartum hemmorrhage. In: Chestnut DH, editor. Obstetric anesthesia principles and practice. Philadelphia: Elsevier Mosby; 2004. p. 662–82.

[40] Clark SL, Yeh SY, Phelan JP, et al. Emergency hysterectomy for obstetric hemorrhage. Obstet Gynecol 1984;64(3):376–80.

[41] Kamani AA, McMorland GH, Wadsworth LD. Utilization of red blood cell transfusion in an obstetric setting. Am J Obstet Gynecol 1988;159(5):1177–81.

[42] Lynch C, Coker A, Lawal AH, et al. The B-Lynch surgical technique for the control of massive postpartum haemorrhage: an alternative to hysterectomy? Five cases reported. Br J Obstet Gynaecol 1997;104(3):372–5.

[43] Bakri YN, Amri A, Abdul JF. Tamponade-balloon for obstetrical bleeding. Int J Gynaecol Obstet 2001;74(2):139–42.

[44] Nelson WL, O'Brien JM. The uterine sandwich for persistent uterine atony: combining the B-Lynch compression suture and an intrauterine Bakri balloon. Am J Obstet Gynecol 2007; 196(5):e9–10.

[45] Sharma SK, Philip J, Wiley J. Thromboelastographic changes in healthy parturients and postpartum women. Anesth Analg 1997;85(1):94–8.

[46] Rutherford CJ, Schneider TJ, Dempsey H, et al. Efficacy of different dosing regimens for recombinant human erythropoietin in a simulated perisurgical setting: the importance of iron availability in optimizing response. Am J Med 1994;96(2):139–45.

[47] Sowade O, Warnke H, Scigalla P, et al. Avoidance of allogeneic blood transfusions by treatment with epoetin beta (recombinant human erythropoietin) in patients undergoing open-heart surgery. Blood 1997;89(2):411–8.

[48] Droste S, Keil K. Expectant management of placenta previa: cost-benefit analysis of outpatient treatment. Am J Obstet Gynecol 1994;170(5 Pt 1):1254–7.

[49] Kidney DD, Nguyen AM, Ahdoot D, et al. Prophylactic perioperative hypogastric artery balloon occlusion in abnormal placentation. AJR Am J Roentgenol 2001;176(6):1521–4.

[50] Dubois J, Garel L, Grignon A, et al. Placenta percreta: balloon occlusion and embolization of the internal iliac arteries to reduce intraoperative blood losses. Am J Obstet Gynecol 1997;176(3):723–6.

[51] Estella NM, Berry DL, Baker BW, et al. Normovolemic hemodilution before cesarean hysterectomy for placenta percreta. Obstet Gynecol 1997;90(4 Pt 2):669–70.

[52] Jackson SH, Lonser RE. Safety and effectiveness of intracesarean blood salvage. Transfusion 1993;33(2):181.

[53] Potter PS, Waters JH, Burger GA, et al. Application of cell-salvage during cesarean section. Anesthesiology 1999;90(2):619–21.

[54] Rainaldi MP, Tazzari PL, Scagliarini G, et al. Blood salvage during caesarean section. Br J Anaesth 1998;80(2):195–8.

[55] Rebarber A, Lonser R, Jackson S, et al. The safety of intraoperative autologous blood collection and autotransfusion during cesarean section. Am J Obstet Gynecol 1998; 179(3 Pt 1):715–20.

[56] Waters JH, Biscotti C, Potter PS, et al. Amniotic fluid removal during cell salvage in the cesarean section patient. Anesthesiology 2000;92(6):1531–6.

[57] Goldberg AB, Greenberg MB, Darney PD. Misoprostol and pregnancy. N Engl J Med 2001;344(1):38–47.

[58] Surbek DV, Fehr PM, Hosli I, et al. Oral misoprostol for third stage of labor: a randomized placebo-controlled trial. Obstet Gynecol 1999;94(2):255–8.

[59] Lighthall GK, Morgan C, Cohen SE. Correction of intraoperative coagulopathy in a patient with neurofibromatosis type I with intravenous desmopressin (DDAVP). Int J Obstet Anesth 2004;13(3):174–7.

[60] Alfirevic Z, Elbourne D, Pavord S, et al. use of recombinant activated factor VII in primary postpartum hemorrhage: the Northern European Registry 2000–2004. Obstet Gynecol 2007;110(6):1270–8.

[61] Franchini M, Lippi G, Franchi M. The use of recombinant activated factor VII in obstetric and gynaecological haemorrhage. BJOG 2007;114(1):8–15.

[62] Longo SA, Dola CP, Pridjian G. Preeclampsia and eclampsia revisited. South Med J 2003; 96(9):891–9.

[63] Berg CJ, Atrash HK, Koonin LM, et al. Pregnancy-related mortality in the United States, 1987–1990. Obstet Gynecol 1996;88(2):161–7.

[64] Mabie WC, Ratts TE, Ramanathan KB, et al. Circulatory congestion in obese hypertensive women: a subset of pulmonary edema in pregnancy. Obstet Gynecol 1988;72(4):553–8.

[65] Young P, Johanson R. Haemodynamic, invasive and echocardiographic monitoring in the hypertensive parturient. Best Pract Res Clin Obstet Gynaecol 2001;15(4):605–22.

[66] Sibai B. The case for magnesium sulfate in preeclampsia-eclampsia. Int J Obstet Anesth 1992;1:167–71.

[67] Ramanathan J, Sibai BM, Pillai R, et al. Neuromuscular transmission studies in preeclamptic women receiving magnesium sulfate. Am J Obstet Gynecol 1988;158(1):40–6.

[68] Lipshitz J, Ahokas RA, Reynolds SL. The effect of hydralazine on placental perfusion in the spontaneously hypertensive rat. Am J Obstet Gynecol 1987;156(2):356–9.

[69] Lunell NO, Lewander R, Nylund L, et al. Acute effect of dihydralazine on uteroplacental blood flow in hypertension during pregnancy. Gynecol Obstet Invest 1983;16(5):274–82.

[70] Vink GJ, Moodley J. The effect of low-dose dihydralazine on the fetus in the emergency treatment of hypertension in pregnancy. S Afr Med J 1982;62(14):475–7.

[71] Mabie WC, Gonzalez AR, Sibai BM, et al. A comparative trial of labetalol and hydralazine in the acute management of severe hypertension complicating pregnancy. Obstet Gynecol 1987;70(3 Pt 1):328–33.

[72] Morgan MA, Silavin SL, Dormer KJ, et al. Effects of labetalol on uterine blood flow and cardiovascular hemodynamics in the hypertensive gravid baboon. Am J Obstet Gynecol 1993;168(5):1574–9.

[73] Rogers RC, Sibai BM, Whybrew WD. Labetalol pharmacokinetics in pregnancy-induced hypertension. Am J Obstet Gynecol 1990;162(2):362–6.

[74] Ramanathan J, Sibai BM, Mabie WC, et al. The use of labetalol for attenuation of the hypertensive response to endotracheal intubation in preeclampsia. Am J Obstet Gynecol 1988;159(3):650–4.

[75] Young PF, Leighton NA, Jones PW, et al. Fluid management in severe preeclampsia (VESPA): survey of members of ISSHP. Hypertens Pregnancy 2000;19(3):249–59.

[76] Cochrane injuries group Albumin Reviewers. Human albumin administration in critically patients: systemic review of randomized trials. Br J Anaesth 1998;317:235–40.

[77] Alderson P, Schierhout G, Roberts I. Fluid resuscitation with colloid or crystalloid solutions in critically ill patients: a systematic review of randomised trials. BMJ 1998;316:961–4.

[78] Ferrante FM, Rosinia FA, Gordon C, et al. The role of continuous background infusions in patient-controlled epidural analgesia for labor and delivery. Anesth Analg 1994;79(1):80–4.

[79] Russell R, Reynolds F. Epidural infusion of low-dose bupivacaine and opioid in labour. Does reducing motor block increase the spontaneous delivery rate? Anaesthesia 1996; 51(3):266–73.

[80] Hawkins JL, Koonin LM, Palmer SK, et al. Anesthesia-related deaths during obstetric delivery in the United States, 1979–1990. Anesthesiology 1997;86(2):277–84.

[81] Ramanathan J, Coleman P, Sibai B. Anesthetic modification of hemodynamic and neuroendocrine stress responses to cesarean delivery in women with severe preeclampsia. Anesth Analg 1991;73(6):772–9.

[82] Hodgkinson R, Husain FJ, Hayashi RH. Systemic and pulmonary blood pressure during caesarean section in parturients with gestational hypertension. Can Anaesth Soc J 1980; 27(4):389–94.

[83] Hood DD, Curry R. Spinal versus epidural anesthesia for cesarean section in severely preeclamptic patients: a retrospective survey. Anesthesiology 1999;90(5):1276–82.

[84] Wallace DH, Leveno KJ, Cunningham FG, et al. Randomized comparison of general and regional anesthesia for cesarean delivery in pregnancies complicated by severe preeclampsia. Obstet Gynecol 1995;86(2):193–9.

[85] Karinen J, Rasanen J, Alahuhta S, et al. Maternal and uteroplacental haemodynamic state in pre-eclamptic patients during spinal anaesthesia for Caesarean section. Br J Anaesth 1996;76(5):616–20.

[86] Aya AG, Mangin R, Vialles N, et al. Patients with severe preeclampsia experience less hypotension during spinal anesthesia for elective cesarean delivery than healthy parturients: a prospective cohort comparison. Anesth Analg 2003;97(3):867–72.

[87] Ramanathan J, Vaddadi AK, Arheart KL. Combined spinal and epidural anesthesia with low doses of intrathecal bupivacaine in women with severe preeclampsia: a preliminary report. Reg Anesth Pain Med 2001;26(1):46–51.

[88] Sibai BM, Ramadan MK, Usta I, et al. Maternal morbidity and mortality in 442 pregnancies with hemolysis, elevated liver enzymes, and low platelets (HELLP syndrome). Am J Obstet Gynecol 1993;169(4):1000–6.

[89] Suresh M, Wali A, Felton E. Survey questionnaire: difficult airway management during emergent cesarean section and availability of difficult airway equipment in the labor and delivery quite: a comparison between academic and private practice hospitals [abstract]. Society of Airway Management 2004.

[90] Jouppila P, Kuikka J, Jouppila R, et al. Effect of induction of general anesthesia for cesarean section on intervillous blood flow. Acta Obstet Gynecol Scand 1979;58(3):249–53.

[91] Catanzarite V, Willms D, Wong D, et al. Acute respiratory distress syndrome in pregnancy and the puerperium: causes, courses, and outcomes. Obstet Gynecol 2001;97(5 Pt 1):760–4.

[92] Ross BK. ASA closed claims in obstetrics: lessons learned. Anesthesiol Clin North America 2003;21(1):183–97.

[93] Rocke DA, Murray WB, Rout CC, et al. Relative risk analysis of factors associated with difficult intubation in obstetric anesthesia. Anesthesiology 1992;77(1):67–73.

[94] Mhyre JM, Riesner MN, Polley LS, et al. A series of anesthesia-related maternal deaths in Michigan, 1985–2003. Anesthesiology 2007;106(6):1096–104.

[95] An updated report by the American Society of Anesthesiologists Task Force on Management of the Difficult Airway. Practice guidelines for management of the difficult airway. Anesthesiology 2003;98:1269–77.

[96] Gross JB, Bachenberg KL, Benumof JL, et al. Practice guidelines for the perioperative management of patients with obstructive sleep apnea: a report by the American Society of Anesthesiologists Task Force on Perioperative Management of patients with obstructive sleep apnea. Anesthesiology 2006;104(5):1081–93.

[97] American Society of Anesthesiologists Task Force on Obstetrical Anesthesia. Practice guidelines for obstetrical anesthesia: a report by the American Society of Anesthesiologists Task Force on Obstetrical Anesthesia. Anesthesiology 1999;90:600–11.

[98] American Society of Anesthesiologists. Equipment for management of airway emergencies. Practice Guidelines for Obstetrical Anesthesia. Park Ridge (IL): Task Force on Obstetrical Anesthesia. ASA; 1998. p. 18.

[99] Hawthorne L, Wilson R, Lyons G, et al. Failed intubation revisited: 17-yr experience in a teaching maternity unit. Br J Anaesth 1996;76(5):680–4.

[100] Godley M, Reddy AR. Use of LMA for awake intubation for caesarean section. Can J Anaesth 1996;43(3):299–302.

[101] Brimacombe J. Emergency airway management in rural practice: use of the laryngeal mask airway. Aust J Rural Health 1995;3:10–1.

[102] Chadwick IS, Vohra A. Anaesthesia for emergency caesarean section using the brain laryngeal airway. Anaesthesia 1989;44(3):261–2.

[103] Gataure PS, Hughes JA. The laryngeal mask airway in obstetrical anaesthesia. Can J Anaesth 1995;42(2):130–3.

[104] Vanner RG. The laryngeal mask in the failed intubation drill. Int J Obstet Anesth 1995;4: 191–2.

[105] Han TH, Brimacombe J, Lee EJ, et al. The laryngeal mask airway is effective (and probably safe) in selected healthy parturients for elective Cesarean section: a prospective study of 1067 cases. Can J Anaesth 2001;48(11):1117–21.

[106] Parr MJ, Gregory M, Baskett PJ. The intubating laryngeal mask. Use in failed and difficult intubation. Anaesthesia 1998;53(4):343–8.

[107] Lim CL, Hawthorne L, Ip-Yam PC. The intubating laryngeal mask airway (ILMA) in failed and difficult intubation. Anaesthesia 1998;53(9):929–30.

[108] Brain AI, Verghese C, Addy EV, et al. The intubating laryngeal mask. II: a preliminary clinical report of a new means of intubating the trachea. Br J Anaesth 1997;79(6): 704–9.

[109] Suresh M, Gardner M, Key E. Intubating laryngeal mask airway (ILMA): a life saving rescue device following failed tracheal intubation during cesarean section (CS) [abstract]. Anesthesiology Submitted to Society for Obstetric Anesthesia and Perinatology (SOAP) [100] 2004;A135:1–30.

[110] Brimacombe J, Keller C, Fullekrug B, et al. A multicenter study comparing the ProSeal and Classic laryngeal mask airway in anesthetized, nonparalyzed patients. Anesthesiology 2002;96(2):289–95.

[111] Keller C, Brimacombe J, Lirk P, et al. Failed obstetric tracheal intubation and postoperative respiratory support with the ProSeal laryngeal mask airway. Anesth Analg 2004;98(5): 1467–70, table.

[112] Miller DM, Light D. Laboratory and clinical comparisons of the Streamlined Liner of the Pharynx Airway (SLIPA) with the laryngeal mask airway. Anaesthesia 2003;58(2): 136–42.

[113] Awan R, Nolan JP, Cook TM. Use of a ProSeal laryngeal mask airway for airway maintenance during emergency Caesarean section after failed tracheal intubation. Br J Anaesth 2004;92(1):144–6.

[114] Bailey SG, Kitching AJ. The Laryngeal mask airway in failed obstetric tracheal intubation. Int J Obstet Anesth 2005;14(3):270–1.

[115] Bullingham A. Use of the ProSeal laryngeal mask airway for airway maintenance during emergency Caesarean section after failed intubation. Br J Anaesth 2004;92(6):903–4.

[116] Sharma B, Sahai C, Sood J, et al. The ProSeal laryngeal mask airway in two failed obstetric tracheal intubation scenarios. Int J Obstet Anesth 2006;15(4):338–9.

[117] Vaida SJ, Gaitini LA. Another case of use of the ProSeal laryngeal mask airway in a difficult obstetric airway. Br J Anaesth 2004;92(6):905.

[118] Doi M, Ikeda K. Airway irritation produced by volatile anaesthetics during brief inhalation: comparison of halothane, enflurane, isoflurane and sevoflurane. Can J Anaesth 1993;40(2):122–6.

[119] MacIntyre PA, Ansari KA. Sevoflurane for predicted difficult tracheal intubation. Eur J Anaesthesiol 1998;15(4):462–6.

[120] Baraka A, Salem R. The Combitube oesophageal-tracheal double lumen airway for difficult intubation. Can J Anaesth 1993;40(12):1222–3.

[121] Eichinger S, Schreiber W, Heinz T, et al. Airway management in a case of neck impalement: use of the oesophageal tracheal Combitube airway. Br J Anaesth 1992;68(5):534–5.

[122] Frass M, Frenzer R, Rauscha F, et al. Evaluation of esophageal tracheal Combitube in cardiopulmonary resuscitation. Crit Care Med 1987;15(6):609–11.

[123] Urtubia RM, Aguila CM, Cumsille MA. Combitube: a study for proper use. Anesth Analg 2000;90(4):958–62.

[124] Zand F, Amini A. Use of the laryngeal tube-S for airway management and prevention of aspiration after a failed tracheal intubation in a parturient. Anesthesiology 2005;102(2): 481–3.

[125] Dhonneur G, Ndoko S, Amathieu R, et al. Tracheal intubation using the Airtraq in morbid obese patients undergoing emergency cesarean delivery. Anesthesiology 2007;106(3): 629–30.

[126] Munnur U, de Boisblanc B, Suresh MS. Airway problems in pregnancy. Crit Care Med 2005;33(Suppl 10):S259–68.

[127] Daley MD, Norman PH, Coveler LA. Tracheal extubation of adult surgical patients while deeply anesthetized: a survey of United States anesthesiologists. J Clin Anesth 1999;11(6): 445–52.

[128] Albright GA. Cardiac arrest following regional anesthesia with etidocaine or bupivacaine. Anesthesiology 1979;51(4):285–7.

[129] Marx GF, Berman JA. Anesthesia-related maternal mortality. Bull N Y Acad Med 1985; 61(4):323–30.

[130] Weinberg GL. Current concepts in resuscitation of patients with local anesthetic cardiac toxicity. Reg Anesth Pain Med 2002;27(6):568–75.

[131] Scott DB. Evaluation of clinical tolerance of local anaesthetic agents. Br J Anaesth 1975; 47(Suppl):328–31.

[132] Groban L, Deal DD, Vernon JC, et al. Cardiac resuscitation after incremental overdosage with lidocaine, bupivacaine, levobupivacaine, and ropivacaine in anesthetized dogs. Anesth Analg 2001;92(1):37–43.

[133] Clarkson CW, Hondeghem LM. Mechanism for bupivacaine depression of cardiac conduction: fast block of sodium channels during the action potential with slow recovery from block during diastole. Anesthesiology 1985;62(4):396–405.

[134] Rosen MA, Thigpen JW, Shnider SM, et al. Bupivacaine-induced cardiotoxicity in hypoxic and acidotic sheep. Anesth Analg 1985;64(11):1089–96.

[135] Groban L, Butterworth J. Lipid reversal of bupivacaine toxicity: has the silver bullet been identified? Reg Anesth Pain Med 2003;28(3):167–9.

[136] Stehr SN, Ziegler J, Pexa A, et al. Lipid effects on myocardial function in L-bupivacaine induced toxicity in the isolated rat heart [abstract]. Reg Anesth Pain Med 2005;30:5.

[137] Picard J, Meek T. A response to 'lipid emulsion to treat bupivacaine toxicity'. Anaesthesia 2005;60(11):1158.

[138] Hedley AA, Ogden CL, Johnson CL, et al. Prevalence of overweight and obesity among US children, adolescents, and adults, 1999–2002. J Am Med Assoc 2004;291(23):2847–50.

[139] D'Angelo R. Anesthesia-related maternal mortality: a pat on the back or a call to arms? Anesthesiology 2007;106(6):1082–4.

[140] Baeten JM, Bukusi EA, Lambe M. Pregnancy complications and outcomes among overweight and obese nulliparous women. Am J Public Health 2001;91(3):436–40.

[141] Cedergren MI. Maternal morbid obesity and the risk of adverse pregnancy outcome. Obstet Gynecol 2004;103(2):219–24.

[142] Weiss JL, Malone FD, Emig D, et al. Obesity, obstetric complications and cesarean delivery rate–a population-based screening study. Am J Obstet Gynecol 2004;190(4):1091–7.

[143] Robinson HE, O'Connell CM, Joseph KS, et al. Maternal outcomes in pregnancies complicated by obesity. Obstet Gynecol 2005;106(6):1357–64.

[144] Lashen H, Fear K, Sturdee DW. Obesity is associated with increased risk of first trimester and recurrent miscarriage: matched case-control study. Hum Reprod 2004;19(7):1644–6.

[145] Bellver J, Rossal LP, Bosch E, et al. Obesity and the risk of spontaneous abortion after oocyte donation. Fertil Steril 2003;79(5):1136–40.

[146] Kabiru W, Raynor BD. Obstetric outcomes associated with increase in BMI category during pregnancy. Am J Obstet Gynecol 2004;191(3):928–32.

[147] Myles TD, Gooch J, Santolaya J. Obesity as an independent risk factor for infectious morbidity in patients who undergo cesarean delivery. Obstet Gynecol 2002;100(5 Pt 1):959–64.

[148] Mhyre JM. Anesthetic management for the morbidly obese pregnant woman. Int Anesthesiol Clin 2007;45(1):51–70.

[149] Kaunitz AM, Hughes JM, Grimes DA, et al. Causes of maternal mortality in the United States. Obstet Gynecol 1985;65(5):605–12.

[150] Endler GC, Mariona FG, Sokol RJ, et al. Anesthesia-related maternal mortality in Michigan, 1972 to 1984. Am J Obstet Gynecol 1988;159(1):187–93.

[151] ACOG. ACOG Committee Opinion number 315, September 2005. Obesity in pregnancy. Obstet Gynecol 2005;106(3):671–5.

[152] Cnattingius S, Bergstrom R, Lipworth L, et al. Prepregnancy weight and the risk of adverse pregnancy outcomes. N Engl J Med 1998;338(3):147–52.

[153] Stephansson O, Dickman PW, Johansson A, et al. Maternal weight, pregnancy weight gain, and the risk of antepartum stillbirth. Am J Obstet Gynecol 2001;184(3):463–9.

[154] Spellacy WN, Miller S, Winegar A, et al. Macrosomia–maternal characteristics and infant complications. Obstet Gynecol 1985;66(2):158–61.

[155] Lipscomb KR, Gregory K, Shaw K. The outcome of macrosomic infants weighing at least 4500 grams: Los Angeles County + University of Southern California experience. Obstet Gynecol 1995;85(4):558–64.

[156] Rode L, Nilas L, Wojdemann K, et al. Obesity-related complications in Danish single cephalic term pregnancies. Obstet Gynecol 2005;105(3):537–42.

[157] Tomoda S, Tamura T, Sudo Y, et al. Effects of obesity on pregnant women: maternal hemodynamic change. Am J Perinatol 1996;13(2):73–8.

[158] D'Angelo R, Dewan DD. Obesity. In: Chestnut DH, editor. Obstetric anesthesia. principles and practice. Philadelphia: Elsevier Mosby; 2004. p. 892–903.

[159] Wallace DH, Currie JM, Gilstrap LC, et al. Indirect sonographic guidance for epidural anesthesia in obese pregnant patients. Reg Anesth 1992;17(4):233–6.

[160] Felton E. Survey Questionnaire: difficult airway management during emergent cesarean section and availability of difficult airway equipment in the labor and delivery suite: a comparison between academic and private practice hospitals. Abstract Poster presentation at American Society of Anesthesiologist Annual Convention, Atlanta, GA [abstract poster # A583]. Anesthesiology 2005 [abstract].

[161] Suresh MS, Wali A. Failed intubation in obstetrics: airway management strategies. Anesthesiol Clin North America 1998;16(2):477–98.

[162] Wheatley RG, Schug SA, Watson D. Safety and efficacy of postoperative epidural analgesia. Br J Anaesth 2001;87(1):47–61.

[163] Liljestrand J. Reducing perinatal and maternal mortality in the world: the major challenges. Br J Obstet Gynaecol 1999;106(9):877–80.

ELSEVIER
SAUNDERS

Anesthesiology Clin
26 (2008) 231–240

ANESTHESIOLOGY
CLINICS

Index

Note: Page numbers of article titles are in **boldface** type.

A

Abruptio placentae, antepartum hemorrhage due to, 54

Acquired thrombophilias, in pregnancy, neuraxial blocks and, 4–5

Activated protein C resistance, in pregnant women, 3

Airtraq, maternal morbidity and mortality with, 217

Airway management, in obstetric anesthesia, **109–125**
  practices, 116–120
    management, 117–119
    prevention, 116–117
    rescue devices and alternative airways, 119–120
  principles, 109–116
    airway changes in pregnancy, 115–116
    difficulty of intubation in pregnant patients, 113–115
    epidemiology and maternal mortality data, 109–111
    nonphysiologic factors, 112
    physiologic factors, 111–112
  maternal morbidity and mortality related to, 212–218

Amniotic fluid embolism, antepartum hemorrhage due to, 56

Analgesia, remifentanil for, during labor, 169–175
  concomitant use of Entonox, 174
  efficacy of analgesia, 170–171
  fetal and neonatal effects, 174
  maternal effects, 173–174
  optimal dosing regimen, 171–173
  practical experience, 175
  suitability as labor analgesic, 169–170

Anesthesia, for pregnant patients outside the labor and delivery unit, **89–108**
  approach to the pregnant patient, 90–92
  maternal management challenges, 92–103
    fear of litigation, 97–98
    fear of medication, 98–100
    fear of radiation, 100–103
    inaction and undertreatment of pregnant patients, 97
    pregnant patients in nonobstetric areas, 92–97
  solutions, 103–105
    consideration of pregnant patients in policies hospital-wide, 104
    multidisciplinary education, 104–105
    pharmacology research, 103–104
  obstetric. *See* Obstetric anesthesia.

Angiotensin II, 79

Antibiotics, in prevention of neuraxial infections in obstetric patients, 46–47

Anticardiolipin antibodies, acquired thrombophilias in pregnant women related to, 5

Anticoagulants, commonly used in pregnancy, neuraxial blocks and, 10–17
  aspirin, 12
  intravenous and subcutaneous unfractionated heparin, 15–16
  low-molecular-weight heparin, 16–17
  warfarin, 12–15

Anticoagulation, in pregnancy, neuraxial blocks and, **1–22**
  commonly used anticoagulants in, 10–17

Anticoagulation (*continued*)
      aspirin, 12
      intravenous and
            subcutaneous
            unfractionated
            heparin, 15–16
      low-molecular-weight
            heparin, 16–17
      warfarin, 12–15
      in women with prosthetic heart
            valves, 7–9
      indications for thrombophylaxis,
            5–7
      spinal hematoma, 9–10
            diagnosis and treatment of,
            17–20
      thrombophilias, 2–5
            acquired, 4–5
            inherited, 3–4
      thrombosis, incidence and timing
            of, 1–2

Antiphospholipid syndrome, in pregnant
      women, 4

Antiretroviral medications, and anesthesia
      for pregnant HIV patients, 130–134
            complications in children, 132
            drug interactions with, 133–134
            effects on pregnancy outcome,
            134
            maternal complications, 132–133
            teratogenicity, 131–132

Antithrombin III deficiency, in pregnant
      women, 3–4

Apgar, Virginia, in history of obstetric
      anesthesia, 73

Arterial embolization, uterine, for obstetric
      hemorrhage, 60

Aspirin, use as anticoagulant in pregnant
      women, 12
            neuraxial anesthesia and, 12

Asthma, β_2-adrenergic receptor and
      polymorphisms in obstetric anesthesia,
      186–187

Atopy, uterine, postpartum hemorrhage due
      to, 57–58

B

B-Lynch suture, for obstetric hemorrhage,
      61

Balloon tamponade, uterine, for obstetric
      hemorrhage, 60

Beta$_1$-adrenergic receptor, clinically relevant
      polymorphisms and pharmacogenetics
      in obstetric anesthesia, 185–186

Beta$_2$-adrenergic receptor, clinically relevant
      polymorphisms and pharmacogenetics
      in obstetric anesthesia, 186–188
            asthma, 186–187
            hemodynamic regulation and
                  cardiovascular conditions,
                  187–188
            preterm labor and delivery, 187

C

Cardiovascular conditions, β_2-adrenergic
      receptor and polymorphisms in
      obstetric anesthesia, 187–188

Cardiovascular system, assessment of, in
      pregnant HIV-infected patients, 136

Catechol-*O*-methyltransferase gene,
      clinically relevant polymorphisms and
      pharmacogenetics in obstetric
      anesthesia, 190–191

Catheterization, avoidance of prolonged,
      in prevention of neuraxial infections
      in obstetric patients, 46–47

Cell salvage, intraoperative, for major
      obstetric hemorrhage, 63

Central nervous system, assessment of,
      in pregnant HIV-infected patients,
      136–137

Cervical lacerations, postpartum
      hemorrhage due to, 58

Cesarean section, complications in
      HIV-infected patients, 135
            general anesthesia with remifentanil
                  for, 176–177
            maternal morbidity, mortality, and
                  risk assessment, 209–211
            general anesthesia, 210
            postoperative care/critical care,
                  210–211
            regional anesthesia,
                  209–210

Chlorhexidine, in prevention of neuraxial
      infections in obstetric patients, 44–46

Coagulation disorders, postpartum
      hemorrhage due to, 58

Combitube, maternal morbidity and
      mortality with, 215–216

Cricothyroidotomy, and transtracheal jet
      ventilation, maternal morbidity and
      mortality with, 218

Cytochrome P450, clinically relevant
      polymorphisms and pharmacogenetics
      in obstetric anesthesia, 190–191

D

Deaths, maternal. *See* Mortality.

Disinfection, chlorhexidine in prevention of neuraxial infections in obstetric patients, 44–46

Dressings, for catheter entry points, in prevention of neuraxial infections in obstetric patients, 44–46

Drug interactions, antiretroviral medications in pregnant patients with HIV, 133–134, 139

Drug targets, pharmacology and polymorphisms in obstetric anesthesia, 184

E

Education, multidisciplinary, to improve nonobstetric hospital care of pregnant patients, 104–105

Embolism, amniotic fluid, antepartum hemorrhage due to, 56

Embolization, uterine arterial, for obstetric hemorrhage, 60

Entonox, concomitant use with remifentanil during labor, 174

Enzymes, drug-metabolizing, pharmacology and polymorphisms in obstetric anesthesia, 184

Ephedrine, for maternal hypotension, 77–78
side effects, 81

Epidural abscess, in obstetric patients, 33–42
causative organisms, 37–40
clinical features and management, 33–42
infection related to, 37
possible risk factors, 40–42
potential routes of infection, 40

Epidural analgesia/anesthesia, obstetric, history of, 71–72
remifentanil supplementation of, 175–176
ultrasound-facilitated, in obstetrics, **145–158**

Epidural blood patch, use in pregnant HIV-infected patients, 139

Errors, medical, in labor and delivery, reduction of with medical simulation and team training, **159–168**

Ether, rectal, in history of obstetric anesthesia, 70–71

F

Factor V Leiden, in pregnant women, 3

Fetal effects, of remifentanil analgesia during labor, 174

Fingernails, false, removal of, in prevention of neuraxial infections in obstetric patients, 43

G

Gastrointestinal system, assessment of, in pregnant HIV-infected patients, 137

General anesthesia, maternal morbidity, mortality, and risk assessment for cesarean section, 210
with remifentanil for cesarean section, 176–177

Gloves, sterile, in prevention of neuraxial infections in obstetric patients, 44

H

Hand washing, in prevention of neuraxial infections in obstetric patients, 44

Hats, in prevention of neuraxial infections in obstetric patients, 43

Heart valves, prosthetic, anticoagulation in pregnant women with, 7–8

Hematologic abnormalities, assessment of, in pregnant HIV-infected patients, 137

Hematoma, spinal, in obstetric patients, 9–10
diagnosis and treatment, 17–20

Hemodynamic regulation, [beta]$_2$-adrenergic receptor and polymorphisms in obstetric anesthesia, 187–188

Hemorrhage, major obstetric, **53–66**
antepartum, 53–56
abruptio placentae, 54
amniotic fluid embolism, 56
placenta accreta/increta/ percreta, 54–55
placenta previa, 54
uterine rupture, 55
vasa previa, 56
intraoperative cell salvage, 63
invasive therapy, 59–62
B-Lynch suture, 61
hysterectomy, 61–62
surgical iliac (or uterine) artery ligation, 61
uterine arterial embolization, 60

Hemorrhage (*continued*)
   planning for, 58–59
   postpartum, 56–58
      cervical vaginal lacerations, 58
      coagulation disorders, 58
      retained placenta, 56–57
      uterine atony, 57–58
      uterine inversion, 58
      recombinant factor VIIA, 63–64
      transfusion therapy and resuscitation, 62
      vasopressors, 83–84
   maternal morbidity, mortality, and risk assessment, 201–204

Heparin, low-molecular-weight, use as anticoagulant in pregnant women, 16–17
      neuraxial anesthesia and, 17
   unfractionated, use as anticoagulant in pregnant women, 15–16
      neuraxial anesthesia and, 15–16

History, of obstetric anesthesia, **67–74**
   discovery, 68–69
   epidural analgesia and anesthesia, 71–72
   professionalism, 69–70
   rectal ether, 70–71
   Virginia Apgar, 73

HIV. *See* Human immunodeficiency virus (HIV).

Human immunodeficiency virus (HIV), anesthesia for pregnant HIV patients, **127–143**
   anesthetic considerations, 135–140
      assessment of, 135–136
      choice of anesthetic technique, 137–139
      drug interactions, 139
      epidural blood patch, 139
      universal precautions and occupational exposure to HIV, 139–140
   antenatal HIV testing, 130
   antiretroviral medications, 130–134
      complications in children, 132
      drug interactions with, 133–134
      effects on pregnancy outcome, 134
      maternal complications, 132–133
      teratogenicity, 131–132

complications of cesarean section in, 135
   effect of pregnancy on HIV progression, 128–129
   management of delivery, 134–135
   mother to child transmission, 129–130
   pathophysiology of HIV, 127–128
      seroconversion and diagnosis, 128
      transmission, 128

Hypertension, maternal morbidity, mortality, and risk assessment, 204–208

Hypotension, maternal, vasopressors for, **75–88**
   administration of, 79–81
      combination therapy, 81
      prophylaxis, 79–81
   history, 76–77
   other situations, maternal hemorrhage, 83–84
      preeclampsia, 82–83
   side effects of, 81–82
      ephedrine, 81
      other situations, 82–84
      phenylephrine, 81–82
   treatment, 77–79
      ephedrine, 77–78
      other vasoconstrictors, 78–79
      phenylephrine, 78

Hysterectomy, for obstetric hemorrhage, 61–62

I

Iliac artery ligation, for obstetric hemorrhage, 61

Imaging, fear of radiation, in nonobstetric care of pregnant patients, 100–103

Infections, neurological, after neuraxial anesthesia in pregnant women, **23–52**
   epidural abscess and related infection, 33–42
   incidence, 24–26
   measures to prevent, 42–47
   meningitis, 26–33

Inherited thrombophilias, in pregnancy, neuraxial blocks and, 3–4
   activated protein C resistance (Factor V Leiden), 3
   antithrombin III deficiency, 3–4
   protein C and S deficiency, 4
   prothrombin gene mutation G2010A, 4

Intraoperative cell salvage, for major obstetric hemorrhage, 63

Intubating laryngeal mask airway, maternal morbidity and mortality with, 215

Intubation, in pregnant patients, difficulty of, 113–115

Inversion, uterine, cervical/vaginal, postpartum hemorrhage due to, 58

J

Jewelry, removal of, in prevention of neuraxial infections in obstetric patients, 43

L

Labor, preterm, β₂-adrenergic receptor and polymorphisms in obstetric anesthesia, 187
    remifentanil for analgesia during, 169–175
        concomitant use of Entonox, 174
        efficacy of analgesia, 170–171
        fetal and neonatal effects, 174
        maternal effects, 173–174
        optimal dosing regimen, 171–173
        practical experience, 175
        suitability, 169–170

Lacerations, cervical/vaginal, postpartum hemorrhage due to, 58

Laryngeal mask airway, for failed intubation in pregnant patients, 119–120
    maternal morbidity and mortality and, 213–217

LaryngealTube S, maternal morbidity and mortality with, 217

Lipid reversal resuscitation, for local anesthetic toxicity during obstetric anesthesia, 219–220

Litigation, fear of, in nonobstetric anesthesia for pregnant patients, 97–98

Local anesthetics, toxicity of, maternal morbidity and mortality related to, 218–220

Low-molecular-weight heparin, use as anticoagulant in pregnant women, 16–17
    neuraxial anesthesia and, 17

Lupus anticoagulant, acquired thrombophilias in pregnant women related to, 5

M

Masks, in prevention of neuraxial infections in obstetric patients, 43

Maternal effects, of remifentanil analgesia during labor, 173–174

Maternal morbidity and mortality, risk assessment and, **197–230**
    anesthetic management and, 208–209
    for cesarean section, 209–211
    local anesthetic toxicity, 218–220
    maternal mortality related to, 211–218
    hemorrhage, 201–204
    hypertension, 204–208
    obesity and, 220–222
    thromboembolism, 198–201

Medical simulation, team training and, to reduce errors in labor and delivery, **159–168**

Medications, fear of, in nonobstetric anesthesia for pregnant patients, 98–100

Meningitis, in pregnant women after neuraxial anesthesia, 26–33
    causative organisms, 32
    clinical features and management, 27–32
    risk factors, 32–33

Metaraminol, 78

Methoxamine, 78–79

Morbidity, maternal, risk assessment and, **197–230**
    anesthetic management and, 208–209
    for cesarean section, 209–211
    local anesthetic toxicity, 218–220
    maternal mortality related to, 211–218
    hemorrhage, 201–204
    hypertension, 204–208
    obesity and, 220–222
    thromboembolism, 198–201

Mortality, maternal, anesthesia-related, 211–219
    airway, 211–218
    local anesthetic toxicity, 218–220
    obesity and, 220–222

Mu-opioid receptor, clinically relevant
    polymorphisms and pharmacogenetics
    in obstetric anesthesia, 190–191

Multidisciplinary education, to improve
    nonobstetric hospital care of pregnant
    patients, 104–105

N

Neonatal effects, of remifentanil analgesia
    during labor, 174

Neuraxial blocks, anticoagulation in
    pregnancy and, **1–22**
        commonly used anticoagulants
            in, 10–17
        aspirin, 12
        intravenous and
            subcutaneous
            unfractionated
            heparin, 15–16
        low-molecular-weight
            heparin, 16–17
        warfarin, 12–15
    in women with prosthetic heart
        valves, 7–9
    indications for thrombophylaxis,
        5–7
    spinal hematoma, 9–10
        diagnosis and treatment of,
            17–20
    thrombophilias, 2–5
        acquired, 4–5
        inherited, 3–4
    thrombosis, incidence and timing
        of, 1–2
    neurological infections after, in
        pregnant women, **23–52**
        epidural abscess and related
            infection, 33–42
        incidence, 24–26
        measures to prevent, 42–47
        meningitis, 26–33

Neurological infections, after neuraxial
    anesthesia in pregnant women, **23–52**
        epidural abscess and related
            infection, 33–42
        incidence, 24–26
        measures to prevent, 42–47
        meningitis, 26–33

NovoSeven. See Recombinant Factor VIIA.

O

Obesity, maternal morbidity and mortality
    related to, 220–222

Obstetric anesthesia, 1–230

airway management, **109–125**
    practices, 116–120
    principles, 109–116
anticoagulation in pregnancy and
    neuraxial blocks, **1–22**
        commonly used anticoagulants
            in, 10–17
        aspirin, 12
        intravenous and
            subcutaneous
            unfractionated
            heparin, 15–16
        low-molecular-weight
            heparin, 16–17
        warfarin, 12–15
    in women with prosthetic heart
        valves, 7–9
    indications for thrombophylaxis,
        5–7
    spinal hematoma, 9–10
        diagnosis and treatment of,
            17–20
    thrombophilias, 2–5
        acquired, 4–5
        inherited, 3–4
    thrombosis, incidence and timing
        of, 1–2
for pregnant HIV patients, **127–143**
    anesthetic considerations,
        135–140
        assessment of, 135–136
        choice of anesthetic
            technique, 137–139
        drug interactions, 139
        epidural blood patch, 139
        universal precautions and
            occupational exposure
            to HIV, 139–140
    antenatal HIV testing, 130
    antiretroviral medications,
        130–134
        complications in children,
            132
        drug interactions with,
            133–134
        effects on pregnancy
            outcome, 134
        maternal complications,
            132–133
        teratogenicity, 131–132
    complications of cesarean section
        in, 135
    effect of pregnancy on HIV
        progression, 128–129
    management of delivery, 134–135
    mother to child transmission,
        129–130
    pathophysiology of HIV,
        127–128

historical narrative, **67–74**
  discovery, 68–69
  epidural analgesia and
    anesthesia, 71–72
  professionalism, 69–70
  rectal ether, 70–71
  Virginia Apgar, 73
major obstetric hemorrhage, **53–66**
  antepartum, 53–56
  intraoperative cell salvage, 63
  invasive therapy, 59–62
  planning for, 58–59
  postpartum, 56–58
  recombinant factor VIIA,
    63–64
  transfusion therapy and
    resuscitation, 62
maternal morbidity, mortality, and
  risk assessment, **197–230**
  anesthetic management and,
    208–209
    for cesarean section,
      209–211
    local anesthetic toxicity,
      218–220
    maternal mortality related
      to, 211–218
  hemorrhage, 201–204
  hypertension, 204–208
  obesity and, 220–222
  thromboembolism, 198–201
medical simulation and team training
  in, **159–168**
neurological infections after neuraxial
  anesthesia, **23–52**
  epidural abscess and related
    infection, 33–42
  incidence, 24–26
  measures to prevent, 42–47
  meningitis, 26–33
outside the labor and delivery unit,
  89–108
  approach to the pregnant patient,
    90–92
  maternal management
    challenges, 92–103
    fear of litigation, 97–98
    fear of medication, 98–100
    fear of radiation, 100–103
    inaction and
      undertreatment of
      pregnant patients, 97
    pregnant patients in
      nonobstetric areas,
      92–97
  solutions, 103–105
    consideration of pregnant
      patients in policies
      hospital-wide, 104

    multidisciplinary education,
      104–105
    pharmacology research,
      103–104
pharmacogenetics and, **183–195**
  clinically relevant
    polymorphisms, 184–191
  pharmacology and
    polymorphisms, 184
remifentanil use in, **169–182**
  concomitant use of Entonox, 174
  efficacy of analgesia, 170–171
  fetal and neonatal effects, 174
  for anesthesia interventions, 175
  for sedation in critically ill
    patients, 177–179
  general anesthesia with, for
    cesarean sections, 176–177
  maternal effects, 173–174
  off-label use, 179
  optimal dosing regimen, 171–173
  practical experience, 175
  suitability as labor analgesic,
    169–170
  supervision and monitoring, 175
  supplementation of epidural
    anesthesia, 175–176
ultrasound-facilitated epidurals and
  spinals, **145–158**
vasopressors for maternal
  hypotension, **75–88**
  administration of, 79–81
    combination therapy, 81
    prophylaxis, 79–81
  history, 76–77
  other situations, maternal
    hemorrhage, 83–84
    preeclampsia, 82–83
  side effects of, 81–82
    ephedrine, 81
    other situations, 82–84
    phenylephrine, 81–82
  treatment, 77–79
    ephedrine, 77–78
    other vasoconstrictors,
      78–79
    phenylephrine, 78

Occupational exposure, to pregnant patients
  with HIV, 139–140

Off-label use, of remifentanil in obstetric
  patients, 179

P

Pain-related candidate genes, clinically
  relevant polymorphisms and
  pharmacogenetics in obstetric
  anesthesia and, 189–191

Pain-related (*continued*)
μ-opioid receptor, 190–191
catechol-*O*-methyltransferase
gene, 190
cytochrome P450, 189–190

Pharmacogenetics, obstetric anesthesia and,
183–195
clinically relevant polymorphisms,
184–191
β₁-adrenergic receptor, 185–186
β₂-adrenergic receptor, 186–188
asthma, 186–187
hemodynamic regulation
and cardiovascular
conditions, 187–188
preterm labor and delivery,
187
analgesia and pain-related
candidate genes, 189–191
μ-opioid receptor, 190–191
catechol-*O*-methyltransferase
gene, 190
cytochrome P450, 189–190
pharmacology and polymorphisms,
184
drug targets, 184
drug-metabolizing enzymes, 184
drug-transporting proteins, 184

Phenylephrine, for maternal hypotension,
78
side effects, 81–82

Placenta accreta vera, antepartum
hemorrhage due to, 54–55

Placenta increta, antepartum hemorrhage
due to, 54–55

Placenta perceta, antepartum hemorrhage
due to, 54–55

Placenta previa, antepartum hemorrhage
due to, 54

Placenta, retained, postpartum hemorrhage
due to, 56–57

Polymorphisms, and pharmacogenetics in
obstetric anesthesia, **183–195**
clinically relevant, 184–191
β₁-adrenergic receptor, 185–186
β₂-adrenergic receptor, 186–188
asthma, 186–187
hemodynamic regulation
and cardiovascular
conditions, 187–188
preterm labor and delivery,
187
analgesia and pain-related
candidate genes, 189–191

μ-opioid receptor, 190–191
catechol-*O*-methyltransferase
gene, 190
cytochrome P450,
189–190
pharmacology and, 184
drug targets, 184
drug-metabolizing enzymes, 184
drug-transporting proteins, 184

Precautions, universal, with pregnant
patients with HIV, 139–140

Preeclampsia, vasopressors and spinal
anesthesia in women with, 82–83

Pregnancy. *See* Obstetric anesthesia.

Pregnant patients, requiring anesthesia
outside the labor and delivery unit,
89–108
approach to the pregnant patient,
90–92
maternal management
challenges, 92–103
fear of litigation, 97–98
fear of medication, 98–100
fear of radiation, 100–103
inaction and
undertreatment of
pregnant patients, 97
pregnant patients in
nonobstetric areas,
92–97
solutions, 103–105
consideration of pregnant
patients in policies
hospital-wide, 104
multidisciplinary education,
104–105
pharmacology research,
103–104

Preterm labor and delivery,
[beta]₂-adrenergic receptor and
polymorphisms in obstetric anesthesia,
187

Professionalism, in history of obstetric
anesthesia, 69–70

Prophylaxis, vasopressor, in obstetric
anesthesia, 79–81

ProSeal laryngeal mask airway, maternal
morbidity and mortality with, 215

Prosthetic heart valves, anticoagulation in
pregnant women with, 7–8

Protein C deficiency, in pregnant women, 4

Protein S deficiency, in pregnant women, 4

Proteins, drug-transporting, pharmacology and polymorphisms in obstetric anesthesia, 184

Prothrombin gene mutation G2010A, in pregnant women, 4

R

Radiation, fear of, in nonobstetric anesthesia for pregnant patients, 100–103

Recombinant Factor VIIA, for major obstetric hemorrhage, 63–64

Rectal ether, in history of obstetric anesthesia, 70–71

Remifentanil, use in obstetrics, **169–182**
        concomitant use of Entonox, 174
        efficacy of analgesia, 170–171
        fetal and neonatal effects, 174
        for anesthesia interventions, 175
        for sedation in critically ill patients, 177–179
        general anesthesia with, for cesarean sections, 176–177
        maternal effects, 173–174
        off-label use, 179
        optimal dosing regimen, 171–173
        practical experience, 175
        suitability as labor analgesic, 169–170
        supervision and monitoring, 175
        supplementation of epidural anesthesia, 175–176

Renal abnormalities, assessment of, in pregnant HIV-infected patients, 137

Rescue devices, for failed intubation in pregnant patients, 119–120

Research, pharmacology, on effects on fetus, 103–104

Respiratory system, assessment of, in pregnant HIV-infected patients, 136

Retained placenta, postpartum hemorrhage due to, 56–57

Rupture, uterine, antepartum hemorrhage due to, 55

S

Salvage, cell, intraoperative, for major obstetric hemorrhage, 63

Sedation, remifentanil for, in critically ill obstetric patients, 177–178

Simulation, medical, team training and, to reduce errors in labor and delivery, **159–168**

Spinal anesthesia, ultrasound-facilitated, in obstetrics, **145–158**

Spinal hematoma, in obstetric patients, 9–10
        diagnosis and treatment, 17–20

T

Tamponade, balloon, uterine, for obstetric hemorrhage, 60

Targets, drug, pharmacology and polymorphisms in obstetric anesthesia, 184

Team training, medical simulation and, to reduce errors in labor and delivery, **159–168**

Teratogenicity, of antiretroviral medications in pregnant patients with HIV, 131–132

Thromboembolism, maternal morbidity, mortality, and risk assessment, 198–201

Thrombophilias, in pregnancy, neuraxial blocks and, 2–5
        acquired, 4–5
        inherited, 3–4
                activated protein C resistance (Factor V Leiden), 3
                antithrombin III deficiency, 3–4
                protein C and S deficiency, 4
                prothrombin gene mutation G2010A, 4

Thromboprophylaxis, indications for, during pregnancy, delivery, and postpartum, 5–7

Thrombosis, in pregnancy, incidence and timing of, 1–2

Training, team, medical simulation and, to reduce errors in labor and delivery, **159–168**

Transfusion therapy, for major obstetric hemorrhage, 62

U

Ultrasound, to facilitate epidurals and spinals in obstetrics, **145–158**

Unfractionated heparin, use as anticoagulant in pregnant women, 15–16
  neuraxial anesthesia and, 15–16

Universal precautions, with pregnant patients with HIV, 139–140

Uterine arterial embolization, for obstetric hemorrhage, 60

Uterine artery ligation, for obstetric hemorrhage, 61

Uterine atopy, postpartum hemorrhage due to, 57–58

Uterine balloon tamponade, for obstetric hemorrhage, 60

Uterine inversion, cervical/vaginal, postpartum hemorrhage due to, 58

Uterine rupture, antepartum hemorrhage due to, 55

V

Vaginal lacerations, postpartum hemorrhage due to, 58

Valves, prosthetic heart, anticoagulation in pregnant women with, 7–8

Vasa previa, antepartum hemorrhage due to, 56

Vasoconstrictors, for maternal hypotension, 78–79
  See also Vasopressors.

Vasopressors, for maternal hypotension, **75–88**
  administration of, 79–81
    combination therapy, 81
    prophylaxis, 79–81
  history, 76–77
  other situations, maternal hemorrhage, 83–84
    preeclampsia, 82–83
  side effects of, 81–82
    ephedrine, 81
    other situations, 82–84
    phenylephrine, 81–82
  treatment, 77–79
    ephedrine, 77–78
    other vasoconstrictors, 78–79
    phenylephrine, 78

W

Warfarin, use as anticoagulant in pregnant women, 12–15
  neuraxial anesthesia and, 15